THE PEDIATRIC ANESTHESIA HANDBOOK

Department of Anesthesiology
Yale University School of Medicine

EDITORS

Charlotte Bell, M.D.
Cindy W. Hughes, M.D.
Tae Hee Oh, M.D.

with fifty-two illustrations

Mosby Year Book

St. Louis Baltimore Boston Chicago London Philadelphia Sydney Toronto

Mosby Year Book
Dedicated to Publishing Excellence

Editor: Susan M. Gay
Assistant Editor: Janet R. Livingston
Project Manager: Linda J. Daly
Designer: Laura Steube

Great care has been used in compiling and checking the information in this book to ensure its accuracy. However, because of changing technology, recent discoveries, research, and individualization of prescriptions according to patient needs, the uses, effects, and dosages of drugs may vary from those given here. Neither the publisher nor the authors shall be responsible for such variations or other inaccuracies. We urge that before you administer any drug you check the manufacturer's dosage recommendations as given in the package insert provided with each product.

Printed in the United States of America

Mosby–Year Book, Inc.
11830 Westline Industrial Drive
St. Louis MO 63146

Library of Congress Cataloging-in-Publication Data

The Pediatric anesthesia handbook / Department of Anesthesiology, Yale University School of Medicine; editors, Charlotte Bell, Cindy W. Hughes, Tae Hee Oh.
p. cm.
Includes bibliographical references and index.
ISBN 0-8016-0230-0
1. Pediatric anesthesia—Handbooks, manuals, etc. I. Bell, Charlotte. II. Hughes, Cindy W. III. Oh, Tae Hee. IV. Yale University. Dept. of Anesthesiology.
[DNLM: 1. Anesthesia—in infancy & childhood—handbooks. WO 231 P371]
RD139.P423 1991
617.9′6798—dc20
DNLM/DLC
for Library of Congress
90-13698
CIP

GW/DC/DC 9 8 7 6 5 4 3 2 1

CONTRIBUTORS

Department of Anesthesiology
Yale University School of Medicine

Professor
Tae Hee Oh, M.D.

Associate Professor
Roberta H. Hines, M.D.
Kathryn E. McGoldrick, M.D.

Associate Clinical Professor
Boonsri Kosarussavadi, M.D.

Assistant Professor
Charlotte Bell, M.D.
Stephen A. Eige, M.D.
Jonathan D. Halevy, M.D.
Francis X. McGowan, M.D.
A. Pamela Reichheld, M.D.
Stephen Rimar, M.D.
Christine S. Rinder, M.D.
Harvey Stern, M.D.
Michael K. Urban, M.D.
Howard A. Zucker, M.D.

Assistant Clinical Professor
Cindy W. Hughes, M.D.

Instructor
William H. Rosenblatt, M.D.

Resident Contributors
Susan M. Chlebowski, M.D.
Richard A. DuBose, M.D.
Michael D. Ho, M.D.
Frederick C. Jacobson, M.D.
Karen M. Kabat, M.D.
Kevin S. Morrison, M.D.
Gail E. Rasmussen, M.D.
Anne M. Savarese, M.D.
Jody Lynn Shapiro, M.D.
Mary M. Stenger, M.D.
Edward Weingarden, M.D.

To

Paul G. Barash, M.D.

whose role as a physician and educator
has served as the model for our practice of Pediatric Anesthesia,
and whose inspiration, encouragement, and support
made this book possible.

FOREWORD

Pediatric anesthesiology is now established as one of the essential core subspecialties of Anesthesiology. Previously, the pediatric patient was cared for clinically by two types of practitioners. The first group consisted primarily of physicians with training in pediatrics, followed by training in anesthesiology and specialty training in pediatric anesthesia. The second and larger group consisted of practicing anesthesiologists who became interested in the subspecialty of pediatrics by the frequent contact with children in their daily practice. It has only been recently that specific training is provided for pediatric anesthesiologists.

Historically, the teaching of anesthesiology and the availability of didactic materials for its instruction were limited for a number of reasons. The classic textbook by Dr. Robert Smith serves as a foundation for all pediatric anesthesia texts in the field. With the formal introduction of pediatric anesthesia into residency training programs, there arose a need to supplement this reference text with a handbook that would guide the resident (and practitioner who infrequently cares for children) through the intricate minutiae of managing the pediatric patient.

Drs. Charlotte Bell, Cindy Hughes and Tae Oh, pediatric anesthesiologists at Yale-New Haven Hospital, developed a teaching program extraordinarily popular with our trainees as well as practitioners in the community. Instruction was based on a series of outlines by which the novice was guided through the various disciplines of pediatric anesthesia. The format for these was adapted from the *Harriet Lane Pediatric Handbook,* a widely used and well known pediatric text. A number of us will fondly recall those occasions when, attempting to treat critically ill infants in the middle of the night, this succinct yet definitive manual provided the only written documentation of treatment modalities and drug dosages. THE PEDIATRIC ANESTHESIA HANDBOOK can be considered a logical extension of the classic Harriet Lane text. It features an efficient graphic style consisting of numerous tables, outlines and illustrations, in which information can be easily located. Duplication of data is minimal. Additionally, the text is used for the advancement of certain conceptual ideas, as well as emphasizing different approaches to managing complex clinical problems. In this regard, the authors have tried to avoid the "this is how I do it" approach. Rather, treatment alternatives are provided with various formulas and equations included which form the scientific foundation for clinical action.

As such, THE PEDIATRIC ANESTHESIA HANDBOOK serves as an excellent starting point for the inexperienced trainee who wishes to assimilate quickly a considerable amount of information in this area. It facilitates acquisition of data for the experienced practitioner who manages pediatric patients only occasionally, and finally serves as a comprehensive yet concise source of reference for drug infusions, eponyms and rare syndromes for the pediatric anesthesiologist.

In summary, Charlotte Bell, Cindy Hughes, and Tae Oh have crafted a superb handbook which is a natural extension of two of the standards in pediatrics and anesthesia, *Smith's Anesthesia for Infants and Children* and the *Harriet Lane Pediatric Handbook*.

Paul G. Barash, M.D.

PREFACE

This book was originally conceived as a means to assist residents and nonpediatric anesthesiologists overwhelmed by the endless amount of detail relevant to the administration of anesthetics to pediatric patients. To make matters worse, the volume of information seemed to be exceeded only by the immense task of locating it quickly. This handbook was designed to simplify minutiae, organize detail, and present more complete lists of eponyms and drug pharmacology in a single easily accessible, cross-referenced volume.

In the course of completing this book, residents and practicing anesthesiologists (both pediatric and nonpediatric) provided us with several other goals which we have tried to achieve. Different approaches to the same problem have been included, whether the task be as simple as selecting endotracheal tube sizes or as complex as acute pain management techniques. The need was also expressed for tabular advice and protocols on rarely encountered but potentially life-threatening emergencies, such as acute electrolyte imbalance, malignant hyperthermia, neonatal resuscitation and transport, etc.

The same monitoring standards that apply to adults also apply to infants and children despite the difficulties of application and interpretation as monitoring becomes increasingly sophisticated. Consequently, we have tried to include sufficient information about pediatric physiology in order that data obtained from current monitoring may be appropriately interpreted. Some methods for technical modifications to improve accuracy in pediatric monitoring have also been described.

Finally, we have tried to incorporate timely information on complicated new procedures such as heart, lung and liver transplant, and the management of these patients for future anesthetics.

Concerning style, a general bibliographic format was selected to support material found in each chapter. Specific references are cited for factual information and drug dosaging. Whenever possible, a tabular format is used instead of text for the rapid extraction of information when necessary in urgent clinical situations.

We have taken the liberty of using poetry and nursery rhymes to introduce each chapter as a reminder that this book is fundamentally about the care of children. Some of these provide levity and humor, lest we become too overwhelmed by the tragedy of illness in children and our own limitations to intervene in their behalf. Other poems were quoted from works by Marguerite R. Lerner, M.D., Professor of Dermatology at Yale University School of Medicine, educator, and author of countless medical books for children before her death in 1987 from Alzheimer's disease. We are particularly grateful to Rivian Bell and Caitlin Loeffler (in the special roles of editorial sister and daughter) whose eleventh-hour poetry helped to capture the essence of this book.

We would like to express our gratitude to several people for their help and assistance. We are deeply indebted to Kristina Knobelsdorff whose dual titles of Editorial Assistant and Artist only begin to reflect the many essential roles she fulfilled during completion of the manuscript. Special thanks go to Jill Fuggi and Marion Mangino who repeatedly typed the numerous chapters and tables without complaint. We are very grateful to Doris Barclay for her photographic contributions and to Peter Rosenblatt, M.D. for his classic medical illustrations. We would also like to thank Stephen Sullman, R.Ph., Director of Drug Information Services at Yale-New Haven Hospital for his careful review of the Drug Appendix.

Finally, we would like to thank our spouses, John Loeffler, M.D., Stephen Hughes, M.D., and Vivian Oh for their understanding, support, encouragement and patience throughout this project which seemed to be endless. And a special hug for our children for their tolerance, understanding and sense of humor about the many late dinners and missed carpools.

Charlotte Bell
Cindy W. Hughes
Tae Hee Oh
October 1990

CONTENTS

1

NEWBORN PHYSIOLOGY AND DEVELOPMENT

Stephen Rimar
Michael K. Urban

My brother Jack Jimbo was just born today.
He cries, eats and sleeps in a very strange way.
He has a round face and a small button nose,
and the teeniest, tiniest, littlest toes.
I thought he was cute, so I picked him right up,
and all of a sudden (Oh, yuck!), he threw up!
CAITLIN LOEFFLER, AGE 10

NEWBORN PHYSIOLOGY

The newborn period includes the first 30 days of extrauterine life. At birth the parasitic fetus becomes an autonomous organism by securing oxygen and delivering it to tissue, metabolizing food, eliminating waste, and synthesizing macromolecules for growth and development.

See Table 1-1 for neonatal physiology.

Cardiac Function

Fetal Circulation (Fig. 1-1)

1. Unsaturated blood is carried by the two umbilical arteries to the placenta for oxygenation and then returned to the fetus via the single umbilical vein (PO_2 = 30 to 35 mm Hg).
2. Umbilical vein blood primarily enters the inferior vena cava (IVC) from the ductus venosus and mixes with desaturated blood from the lower extremities. A small amount of umbilical vein blood enters the liver.
3. Blood enters the right atrium from the IVC and superior vena cava (SVC) and is shunted across the patent foramen ovale into the left atrium. Blood from the right atrium entering the pulmonary artery is shunted across the ductus arteriosus to the aorta.

TABLE 1-1. Normal physiologic characteristics of the newborn

System	Characteristics
Cardiovascular	Closure of PDA Closure of foramen ovale Decrease in PVR Cardiac output is heart-rate dependent because of fixed stroke volume
Respiratory	Increased work of breathing because of: Compliant chest wall Noncompliant lung Fewer Type I diaphragmatic muscle fibers Prone to hypoxia because of: High O_2 consumption High closing capacity/FRC ratio Periodic breathing
Metabolic	Physiologic jaundice
Renal	Decreased GFR Poor ability to concentrate or dilute urine Obligate sodium loss
Temperature	Nonshivering thermogenesis
Neurologic	Immature autonomic nervous system with parasympathetic predominance and poor sympathetic tone Immature CNS Incomplete myelination

4. Blood is shunted away from the nonfunctioning lungs by high pulmonary vascular resistance (PVR) caused by:
   a. the relatively hypoxic environment;
   b. compression of vessels by fluid-filled alveoli.
5. Oxygenated blood goes from the left atrium (LA) into the left ventricle (LV) and out the ascending aorta to the coronary, carotid, and subclavian arteries. Carotid artery blood has a PO_2 of 23 to 25 mm Hg.
6. About half the desaturated blood in the descending aorta (PO_2 = 18 to 19 mm Hg) perfuses the abdomen and lower extremities, and the rest is returned to the placenta.

Fig. 1-1. Fetal circulation. The unbroken line demonstrates the pathway of oxygenated blood from the placenta. Desaturated blood returns to the placenta through the umbilical arteries via the broken line. (Legend: *PL* = placenta; *UV* = umbilical vein; *DV* = ductus venosus; *LB* = lower body; *IVC* = inferior vena cava; *SVC* = superior vena cava; *RA* = right atrium; *FO* = foramen ovale; *RV* = right ventricle; *PA* = pulmonary artery; *DA* = ductus arteriosus; *LA* = left atrium; *LV* = left ventricle; *AO* = aorta; *UA* = umbilical artery; *L* = liver.)

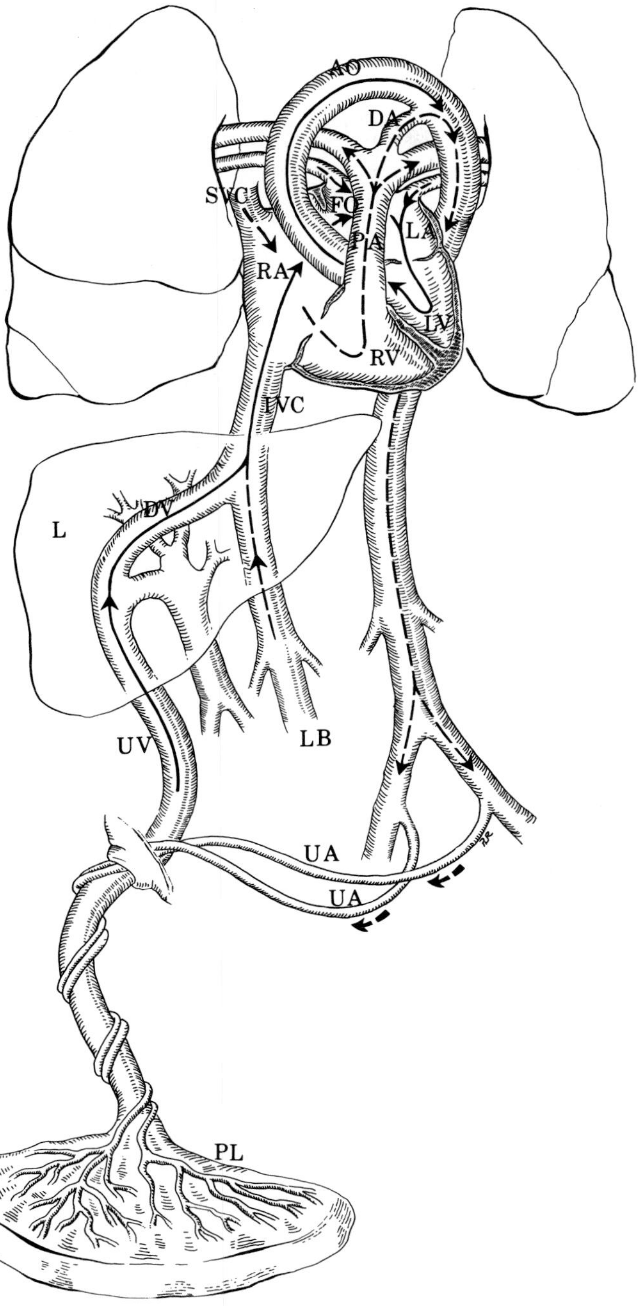
AO
DA
SVC
FO
LA
PA
RA
LV
RV
IVC
DV
L
LB
UV
UA
UA
PL

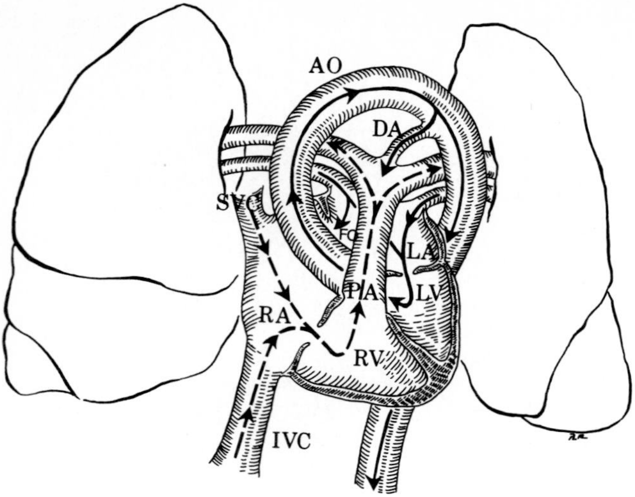

Fig. 1-2. Circulatory changes at birth. Decreased pulmonary vascular resistance at birth results in increased pulmonary blood flow and subsequent flow to the left atrium and ventricle. Increased PO_2 and left-sided pressures typically result in closure of the ductus arteriosus and foramen ovale. A left to right shunt will be present if patency persists in either structure. (Legend: *IVC* = inferior vena cava; *SVC* = superior vena cava; *RA* = right atrium; *RV* = right ventricle; *PA* = pulmonary artery; *FO* = foramen ovale; *DA* = ductus arteriosus; *LA* = left atrium; *LV* = left ventricle; *AO* = aorta.)

Circulatory Changes at Birth (Fig. 1-2)

1. Expansion of the lungs and increased PO_2 to 60 mm Hg leads to an 80% decrease in the PVR. As a result, pulmonary circulation and oxygenation increase. A further decrease in PVR occurs over the next 8 weeks.
2. The ductus arteriosus is composed of tissue that is uniquely sensitive to oxygen, prostaglandins, and pH. The ductus will close over the first week of life as PO_2 increases, pH becomes less acidic, and the placental contribution of prostaglandins is stopped. Permanent closure may take 2 to 3 weeks.
3. The increase in pulmonary blood flow will result in increased blood volume in the left atrium and subsequent closure of the flap of the foramen ovale as left atrial pressures rise above right atrial pressures. A small left-to-right shunt may persist for several weeks because of incomplete closure, and probe patency persists in approximately 20% of the adult population.

Neonatal Myocardial Function

The resting neonate's cardiac output is very close to maximal because of a relatively fixed stroke volume (SV), low systemic vascular resistance (SVR), and immature sympathetic innervation.

1. The neonatal heart has fewer contractile elements per gram of tissue than the adult heart.
2. It is richer in mitochondria and endoplasmic reticulum that are needed for future growth and protein synthesis, but make the neonate's heart stiffer and less contractile than the adult's.
3. The Frank-Starling mechanism is limited by poor contractility resulting in a relatively fixed stroke volume. Increases in cardiac output (CO) are accomplished by increases in heart rate (HR):

$$CO = SV \times HR$$

4. The neonate has a relatively low systemic vascular resistance because of pristine vessels and other immature systems that modulate blood pressure. The mean arterial pressure is 35 to 40 mm Hg.
5. The parasympathetic supply to the heart is developed completely at birth and the sympathetic supply is not. The neonate therefore is predisposed to bradycardia with minimal chronotropic and inotropic counterbalance.

Respiratory Function

Conversion to Aerobic Life

At birth the lungs undergo the transition from a fluid-filled organ to an air-filled organ for gaseous exchange. Most of the fluid is expelled from the lungs by compression of the fetal chest during vaginal delivery with the remainder removed by the lymphatic system over the next 24 hours. In order to overcome surface active forces and fully expand the lungs the neonate must generate negative intrathoracic pressures of 40 to 60 cm of water, the same pressure needed for the first few breaths during newborn resuscitation.

Compliance and Work of Breathing

1. The increased compliance of the chest wall (because of pliable and cartilaginous ribs) and the decreased compliance of the lungs require *increased work of breathing* for the infant to maintain a fixed functional residual capacity (FRC).
2. Respiratory movement is generated mostly by diaphragmatic and abdominal muscles. The diaphragmatic and intercostal muscles of a newborn have a smaller proportion of Type I fibers, the high oxidative fibers used for repetitive movement.
3. During periods of partial airway obstruction or increased respiratory demands (sepsis, pneumonia) the neonate is more susceptible to respiratory failure from fatigue.

Pulmonary Volumes

Tidal volume (V_T) is the same for neonates and adults (7 to 10 ml/kg). However, because neonatal oxygen consumption ($\dot{V}O_2$) is two to three times that of the adult, alveolar ventilation must be increased proportionally.

1. FRC is normal after the first 10 to 20 minutes.
2. The high minute ventilation/FRC ratio produces rapid desaturation

in the neonate during apnea or airway obstruction and a more rapid induction of inhalation anesthetics.

3. Neonatal closing volumes are higher than in the adult. The high closing capacity/FRC ratio increases pulmonary shunt and therefore desaturation, especially when tidal volumes are inadequate.

Ventilatory Drive

Hypoxia initially stimulates ventilation, which is followed by a decrease in ventilation.

1. Chemoreceptors are functional in the full-term infant so that an increase in CO_2 will stimulate ventilation.
2. Periodic breathing with intermittent apneic spells of less than 10 seconds is common in neonates. Anesthesia, hypoxia, and sepsis may accentuate periodic breathing or apnea in the newborn.

Neonatal Hematology

1. Blood volume in the newborn is about 90 ml/kg.
2. Hemoglobin content is about 19 g/100 ml.
3. About 80% of hemoglobin at birth is fetal hemoglobin (Hgb F), which has a higher affinity for oxygen, causing a shift to the left of the oxyhemoglobin dissociation curve.
4. This shift to the left is compensated for by an increased hematocrit (45% to 55%).
5. The level of Hgb F will fall as it is replaced by adult hemoglobin (Hgb A; see Chapter 12).
6. Fetal hematopoiesis occurs in the liver and shifts completely to the bone marrow by the sixth week of life.

Hepatic Metabolism and Physiologic Jaundice

Phase I reactions (degradative) include oxidation, reduction, and hydrolysis. These reactions appear to be fully functional at birth. Phase II reactions (synthetic) are found in the cytochrome p450 microsomal enzyme fraction and are not fully developed in the neonate.

1. A reduced amount of UDP-glucuronyl transferase results in deficient glucuronide conjugation, which does not reach normal levels until age 3. This enzyme is necessary for bilirubin (partially metabolized heme) to be rendered water soluble for excretion in the bile or by renal filtration.
2. The normal newborn produces bilirubin at twice the rate of an adult, 75% of which is from red blood cell destruction.
3. Much larger quantities of unconjugated bilirubin are reabsorbed by the enterohepatic circulation in the neonate than the adult.
4. Ninety percent of term newborns have a serum unconjugated bilirubin level of 2 mg/dl or greater, which produces a jaundiced appearance.
5. In normal newborns 48 hours after birth, the median bilirubin concentration is 6 mg/dl with a range from 1 to 12 mg/dl. If the bilirubin concentration exceeds 12 mg/dl in a full-term infant and 15 mg/dl

in a premature infant, then other causes of jaundice are considered (ABO incompatibility, infection, spherocytosis, etc).

6. Phototherapy usually is instituted at bilirubin levels of 8 mg/dl in infants between 1500 and 2000 g and at levels greater than 12 mg/dl in normal-weight neonates. Exchange transfusions may be necessary when the bilirubin approaches 20 mg/dl.

Renal Function

The newborn's limited renal function contributes to the problems the infant has with fluid and electrolyte homeostasis.

Glomerular Filtration (GFR)

1. Because fetal waste is removed by the placenta, the fetal kidney produces a minimal amount of urine, which is excreted into the amniotic sac.
2. At birth, renal vascular resistance decreases and both renal blood flow and GFR increase.
3. The term newborn has the same number of nephrons as an adult, but they are smaller so that the GFR is considerably lower.
4. The GFR at birth is 30% of an adult's, with a rapid increase in function over the next 2 weeks.
5. GFR approaches adult levels by the end of the first year.
6. The newborn has a low normal plasma creatinine level (0.4 mg/dl) resulting from a small muscle-mass/body-weight ratio and a high anabolic rate.

Concentrating Ability

1. Because renal tubular development and function will not reach adult capacity for 2 to 3 years, the newborn kidney has a limited ability to concentrate and dilute urine.
2. The maximal urine concentration of a premature infant is 600 mOsm/L, for a full-term infant it is 700 mOsm/L, and for an adult it is 1200 mOsm/L.

Sodium Homeostasis and Acid/Base

1. The newborn kidney is an obligate sodium loser and will continue to excrete sodium even during a severe sodium deficit.
2. Antidiuretic hormone (ADH) synthesis and secretion appears to be intact in the neonate as does the production of renin, angiotensin, and aldosterone. However, there may be an inability of immature tubular cells to respond to aldosterone.
3. The renal threshold for bicarbonate is low, about 20 mmol/L, which makes the normal plasma pH for the neonate about 7.34.

Temperature Regulation

1. The newborn has several disadvantages with regard to its ability to regulate temperature: large surface area, poor insulation, a small mass from which heat is generated, and an inability to shiver.

TABLE 1-2. Neutral thermal temperature

Age	Neutral temp*	Critical temp**
Preterm	34° C	28° C
Full term	32° C	23° C
Adult	28° C	1° C

*Neutral temperature is the ambient room temperature that results in minimal oxygen consumption.
**Critical temperature is the temperature below which an unclothed unanesthetized person cannot maintain a normal core temperature.
From Krishna G and others: The pediatric patient. In Stoelting RK and Dierdorf SF, editors: Anesthesia and co-existing disease, ed 1, New York, 1983, Churchill-Livingston. Used by permission.

2. Catecholamine-stimulated nonshivering thermogenesis by brown fat is the major source of heat production in the cold-stressed neonate. Complications of increased catecholamine release include elevated pulmonary and systemic vascular resistance and higher O_2 consumption with resultant stress on the newborn heart.
3. The newborn infant should be maintained in a "neutral thermal environment" (Table 1-2). The term refers to the ambient temperature at which an infant can maintain core body temperature with minimal metabolic activity. The use of radiant heat lamps, warming blankets, hats, wrapping limbs, the delivery of warmed and humidified gases, and the infusion of warmed intravenous fluids in the operating room will help to maintain a neutral thermal environment.

Central Nervous System (CNS)

1. The CNS of a newborn infant is very immature and will undergo major growth and myelination in the first 3 to 4 years of life.
2. The presence of primitive reflexes at birth such as the rooting reflex, Moro response, and grasp reflex are indicative of normal fetal CNS development.
3. The appearance of developmental milestones at the appropriate ages is indicative of normal CNS maturation (Table 1-3).

TABLE 1-3. Neurologic signs

Response	Age of appearance	Age of disappearance
Moro reflex	Birth	1-3 months
Babinski response	Birth	Variable
Horizontal following vision	4-6 weeks	—
Rooting response—awake	Birth	3-4 months
Handedness	2-3 years	—

NORMAL PATTERNS OF GROWTH AND DEVELOPMENT

The infant or child's failure to achieve developmental landmarks is indicative of underlying pathology and can help guide the anesthesiologist in selecting anesthetic plans and assigning risk.

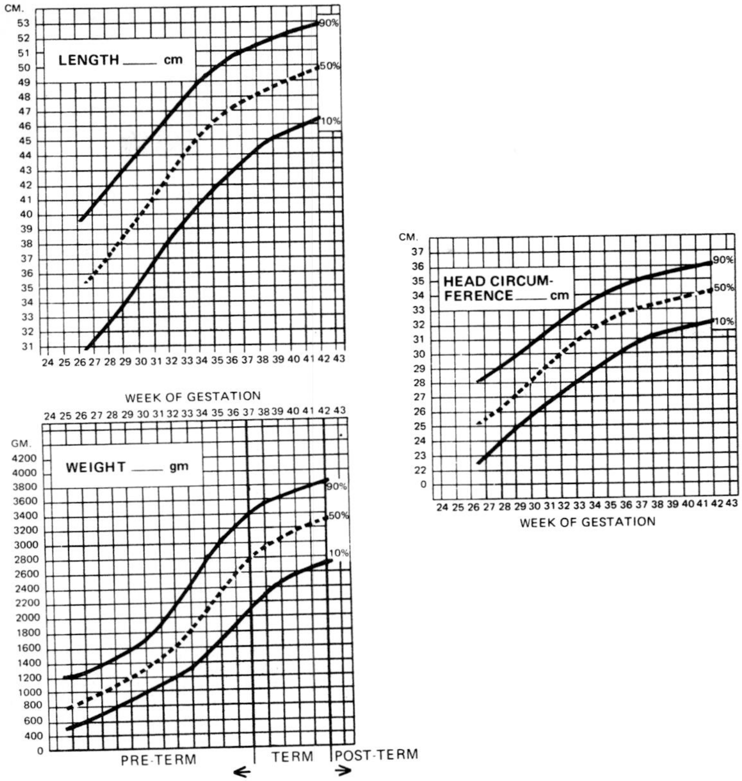

Fig. 1-3. Classification of newborns based on maturity and intrauterine growth. (Adapted from Lubchenco LC, Hansman C, and Boyd E: Pediatrics 37:403, 1966; Battaglia FC and Lubchenco LC: Pediatrics 71:159, 1967. Reproduced by permission of Pediatrics.)

Gestational Age

Importance of Post Conceptual Age (PCA) Determination

Multisystem immaturity in the preterm infant necessitates different anesthetic considerations than those for a full-term infant. Postconceptual age has been used widely by many investigators as the most important factor for determining increased anesthetic risk in preterm infants. However, the age at which increased postoperative apnea and respiratory complications are noted varies from 44 weeks to 60 weeks PCA depending on the study cited. Recently other preoperative factors such as presence of respiratory distress syndrome (RDS) or patent ductus arteriosus (PDA) in the medical history have been noted to be important predictors of postoperative complications.

Determinations of Gestational Age

Maternal dates are often misleading when estimating the gestational age. More accurate indicators of maturity include external physical criteria and neuromuscular maturity (Table 1-4). A less accurate method is to estimate gestational age based upon weight and size (Fig. 1-3 and Table 1-5).

TABLE 1-4. Estimation of gestational age by neurologic and physical criteria

Exam	Preterm (<38 wks)	Full term (38-41 wks)	Post term (>42 wks)
Skin	Thin, visible veins	Thick	Leathery, wrinkled
Lanugo	Present	Thinning or absent	Absent
Ear	Pliable, no recoil	Formed, firm recoil	Stiff, thick cartilage
Sole of foot	Creases anteriorly only	Creases cover sole	As full term
Breast tissue	Flat areola 1-mm bud	Full areola 3- to 4-mm bud	Full areola 5-10 mm bud
Genitalia			
male	Empty scrotum	Testes descended, scrotum rugated	As full term
female	Prominent clitoris, labia minoria; gaping labia majora	Clitoris and labia minora covered by majora	As full term
Limbs	Hypotonic	Tonic	Possibly hypertonic (hip flexion >90°)
Grasp reflex	Weak	Strong	As full term
Sucking reflex	Weak	Strong	As full term
Rooting reflex	Weak	Strong	As full term

Adapted from Todres ID: Growth and development. In Ryan JF, Todres ID, Cote CJ, and Gondsonzian NG, editors: A practice of anesthesia for infants and children, Orlando, Fla, 1986, Grune & Stratton, Inc.

TABLE 1-5. Relationship of gestational age to birth weight

Age	Weight
28 wks	1.0 kg
32 wks	1.7 kg
36 wks	2.5 kg
40 wks	3.4 kg

From Todres ID: Growth and development. In Ryan JF, Todres ID, Cote CJ, Gondsonzian NG, editors: A practice of anesthesia for infants and children, Orlando, Fla, 1986, Grune & Stratton, Inc. Used by permission.

Birth Weight/Size

- The *low birth weight (LBW)* infant (less than 2500 g) has a much higher risk of a complicated postnatal course requiring respiratory and nutritional support. Low birth weights are usually the result of poor prenatal care, smoking, drugs, alcohol, maternal malnutrition, toxemia, and placental insufficiency. A *very low birth weight (VLBW)* infant weighs less than 1500 g.
- The infant with weight below the 10th percentile is *small for gestational age (SGA),* and must be suspected of having an intrauterine infection (CMV, rubella), congenital malformations, or chromosomal abnormalities. Many SGA infants are also the result of toxemia or placental insufficiency.
- The *large for gestational age (LGA)* infant has weight above the 90th percentile, a condition which is commonly associated with maternal diabetes. Such an infant should be observed for hypoglycemia.
- An *appropriate for gestational age (AGA)* infant's weight is between the 10th and 90th percentiles.

Patterns of Growth

Height, weight, and head circumference are followed routinely and plotted on a percentile chart (Fig. 1-4 on pp. 14 and 15); a deviation from the normal percentiles given may indicate significant pathology. It is anticipated that the full-term infant (3 to 4 kg birth weight) will double the birth weight at 6 months and triple it at 1 year. Most preterm infants catch up to their full-term counterparts by the end of the first year.

Development

Maturation of the central nervous system can be followed by noting the appearance of developmental landmarks. Familiarity with these milestones will aid the anesthesiologist in making an accurate assessment of the child and formulating an appropriate anesthetic plan (Table 1-6).

The areas of development that have been identified are as follows:

1. Gross motor skills: head, trunk, and limbs
2. Fine motor skills: small muscle control, coordination
3. Language skills: cognitive function
4. Social skills: environment influences

TABLE 1-6. Developmental landmarks

Age	Gross motor skills	Fine motor skills	Language skills	Social skills
Newborn	Complete head lag	—	—	—
3 mos	Supports head	Grasps rattle, reaches objects	Coos	Smiles
6 mos	Sits alone	Transfers objects from hand to hand	Recognizes voices (mom/dad)	Feeds self cookies
9 mos	Crawls, cruises	Bangs together two cubes held in hands	Imitates sounds (mama/dada)	Holds bottle
12 mos	Walks	Pincer grip, scribbles spontaneously	Comes when called	Uses cup
18 mos	Runs	Stacks blocks	Vocabulary (mama/dada + three other words), uses two words together	Feeds self with spoon
24 mos	Walks up and down stairs	Draws a straight line	Composes short sentences	Plays interactive games

COMMON PROBLEMS OF PREMATURITY

Pulmonary Problems

Respiratory Distress Syndrome

Description: Absence or deficiency of surfactant characterized by respiratory distress, cyanosis, and "ground glass" appearance with air bronchograms on chest x-ray.

Treatment: Endobronchial surfactant, oxygen therapy, often with some form of positive pressure ventilation (CPAP, PEEP) and supportive care.

Meconium Aspiration Syndrome

Description: Perinatal aspiration of meconium characterized by respiratory distress, pneumonia, and asphyxia.

Treatment: Oxygen, positive pressure ventilation, and supportive care.

Apnea

Description: Absence of breathing for 15 to 30 seconds, often accompanied by bradycardia and cyanosis.

Differential Diagnosis: Hypoxemia, respiratory depression from metabolic disorders (hypoglycemia, hypocalcemia, electrolyte disorders, sepsis), intracranial bleed, airway obstruction and hyperthermia or hypothermia.

Treatment: Theophylline, mechanical ventilation, and supportive care.

Bronchopulmonary Dysplasia (BPD)

Description: Chronic obstructive lung disease of neonates characterized by persistent respiratory difficulty and radiographic progression resulting in cystic lung changes.

Treatment: Oxygen, bronchodilators, diuretics, and mechanical ventilation.

Cardiac Problems

Patent Ductus Arteriosus

Description: Left-to-right shunt from the aorta to the pulmonary artery resulting in congestive heart failure.

Treatment: Surgical ligation of the ductus, indomethacin therapy.

A

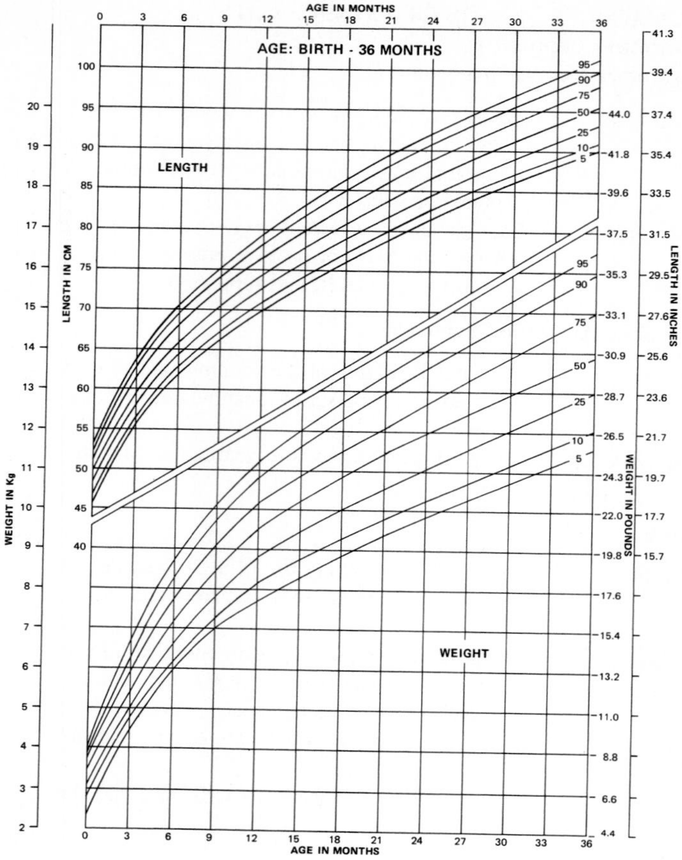

Fig. 1-4. **A,** Infant growth chart for girls. (From National Center for Health Statistics.)

Continued.

Congenital Heart Disease

Description: Characterized by congestive heart failure or cyanosis unresponsive to oxygen therapy.

Treatment: Pulmonary artery banding, palliative shunt, complete repair.

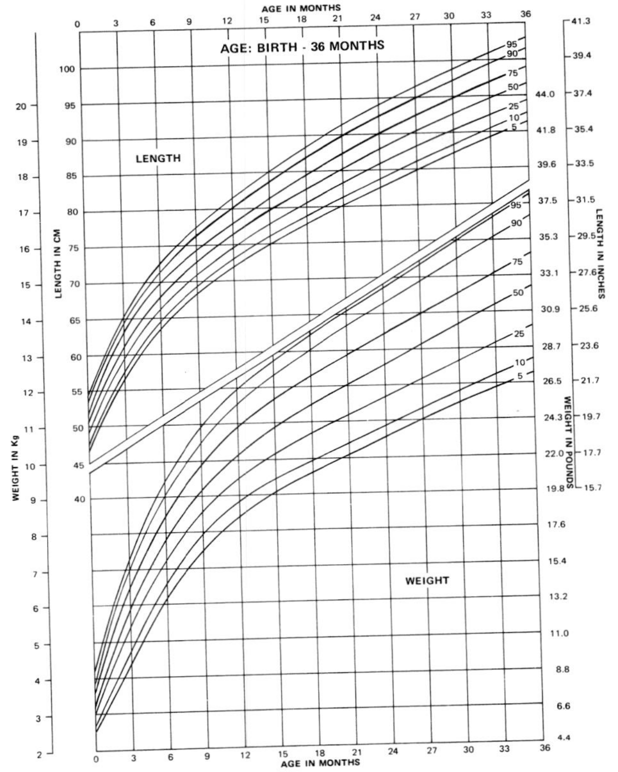

B

Fig. 1-4, cont'd. **B,** Infant growth chart for boys. (From National Center for Health Statistics.)

GI Problems

Necrotizing Enterocolitis (NEC)

Description: Disorder of intestinal mucosa causing abdominal distention, bloody diarrhea, acidosis, apnea, and septic shock.

Treatment: IV hydration, antibiotics, discontinuation of feeds, surgical exploration and resection of damaged intestine.

Hematologic Problems

Jaundice

Description: Hyperbilirubinemia secondary to increased bilirubin load and poor hepatic conjugation (unconjugated, physiologic) or abnormalities of bilirubin production, metabolism, or excretion (nonphysiologic).

Treatment: Phototherapy, exchange transfusion, and treatment of underlying medical disorder.

Anemia

Description: Low hematocrit caused by decreased erythropoiesis (physiologic), blood loss, and hemolysis.

Treatment: Elimination of causes, transfusion.

Metabolic Disorders

Hypoglycemia

Description: Blood sugar less than 40 mg/100 ml; characterized by lethargy, limpness, tremors, apnea, and seizures.

Treatment: PO or IV glucose.

Hypocalcemia

Description: Total serum calcium concentration less than 7 mg/100 ml or ionized calcium less than 3.0 to 3.5 mg/dl. Characterized by irritability, jitteriness, hypotonia, and seizures.

Treatment: Administration of IV or PO calcium.

Infections

Congenital Infections

Description: Characteristic syndromes caused by TORCH (toxoplasmosis, rubella, CMV, herpes, syphilis).

Treatment: Supportive care.

Group B Streptococcal Infection

Description: Characterized by pneumonia, sepsis, and meningitis syndromes.

Treatment: Antibiosis and supportive care.

Problems of the Central Nervous System

Intraventricular Hemorrhage (IVH)

Description: Periventricular-intraventricular hemorrhage associated with immaturity and hypoxemia. Characterized by bradycardia, respiratory irregularity, apnea, seizures, and hypotonia.

Treatment: Supportive.

Neonatal Seizures

Description: Convulsion with infectious, metabolic, or traumatic (IVH) etiology.

Treatment: Anticonvulsants and supportive care.

BIBLIOGRAPHY

Avery GB, editor: Neonatology, pathophysiology and management of the newborn, New York, 1987, JB Lippincott Co.

Berry FA, editor: Anesthetic management of difficult and routine pediatric patients, New York, 1986, Churchill Livingston.

Carlo WA and Chatburn RL, editors: Neonatal respiratory care, Chicago, 1988, Year Book Medical Publishers.

Dubose R and others: Predictors of postoperative respiratory failure in the preterm infant after inguinal hernia repair, Anesth Analg 68:S73, 1989.

Graef JW and Cone TE: Manual of pediatric therapeutics, Boston, 1985, Little Brown & Co.

Katz J and Steward DJ, editors: Anesthesia and uncommon pediatric diseases, Philadelphia, 1987, WB Saunders Co.

Klaus MH and Fanaroff AA: Care of the high-risk neonate, Philadelphia, 1987, WB Saunders Co.

Kurth CD and others: Postoperative apnea in preterm infants, Anesthesiology 66:483-488, 1987.

Welborn LB and others: Postanesthetic apnea and periodic breathing in infants, Anesthesiology 65:658-661, 1986.

2

NEWBORN RESUSCITATION

William H. Rosenblatt

Where did you come from, baby dear?
Out of the everywhere into here.
GEORGE MACDONALD
AT THE BACK OF THE NORTH WIND

FETAL MONITORING

Knowledge of fetal monitoring techniques allows the physician to anticipate resuscitation and helps to predict treatment and outcome.

Monitors for Uterine Activity

Noninvasive

Tocodynamometry is a technique that uses a pressure-sensitive device to give a qualitative tracing of uterine contraction.

Invasive

A catheter is inserted transvaginally to measure uterine pressure during labor.

1. The transducer should be at the level of parturient's xiphoid process.
2. Normal baseline pressure:
   - Latent phase <5 mm Hg
   - Active phase 10-12 mm Hg
3. Normal peak pressure:
   - Early stage 1 20-30 mm Hg above baseline
   - Early stage 2 up to 100 mm Hg

Fetal Heart Rate Monitors (Table 2-1 and the box on p. 20)

Noninvasive

An external transabdominal Doppler probe monitors fetal heart rate.

1. A poor trace may be present in the obese parturient.
2. The signal is easily lost during maternal or fetal motion.
3. False beat-to-beat variability may be seen, and this technique can be unreliable in a parturient with multiple gestations.
4. The parturient's discomfort is an additional disadvantage.

TABLE 2-1. Abnormal fetal heart rate tracings[1]

Type	Description	Etiology
Early decelerations	10-30 beats/min decrease from baseline U-shaped curve Deceleration ends at or before end of contraction	Compression of fetal head causing increased vagal tone
Baseline bradycardia	Rate <120; variability indicates a well-compensated fetus	Common in infants of >42 weeks gestation Potential etiologies: β-blockers, hypothermia, decreased uterine blood flow, atrioventricular block, congenital cytomegalovirus infection
Baseline tachycardia	>160 beats/min	Maternal causes: sepsis, thyrotoxicosis, use of atropine, ritodrine, sympathomimetic Fetal causes: early hypoxia, congestive heart failure, supraventricular tachycardia
Variable decelerations	Alternate rise and fall in fetal heart rate; fetal HR <70 beats/min for more than 60 sec is considered severe	Umbilical cord compression: umbilical vein compression decreases preload and transiently increases heart rate; hypertension and baroreceptor mediated bradycardia is caused by loss of low resistance placental bed
OMINOUS TRACINGS: Loss of baseline variability (only reliably assessed by internal monitors)	No beat-to-beat or cyclic changes in rate	Prolonged hypoxia and myocardial depression; CNS depressant drugs
Late decelerations	Begin 15 sec or more after contraction has peaked	Vagal responses to peripheral chemoreceptor hypoxia; associated with uteroplacental insufficiency
Prolonged deceleration	Decrease of more than 30 beats/min for more than 2 min	Hypoxia, uterine tetany (oxytocin), cord prolapse, local anesthetic toxicity, vasa previa

Invasive

More precise measurement of rate and beat-to-beat variability is obtained with a fetal scalp electrode.

Scalp pH

Scalp pH should be obtained in the presence of a worrisome fetal heart tracing to document the degree of fetal distress. Levels of pH are classified as follows:

Normal	7.25 to 7.35
Preacidotic	7.20 to 7.25
Acidotic	<7.20

A pH value of less than 7.20 usually indicates the need for immediate delivery (cesarean section) if not improved within 15 minutes.

Treatment of Fetal Compromise

1. O_2 to mother
2. Left uterine displacement
3. Maternal volume expansion (without dextrose)
4. Discontinuation of oxytocin

NORMAL FETAL HEART RATE[1]

Rate
120-150 beats per minute

Pattern
Short-term (± 10 beats per minute) rate changes from beat-to-beat
Long-term cyclic changes (two to five times each minute)

1. Increased systemic vascular resistance (SVR) by loss of placental bed
2. Increased left atrial pressure as a result of increased SVR
3. Decreased flow via foramen ovale
4. Decreased pulmonary vascular resistance (PVR) as lungs expand and receive right ventricular cardiac output

↓

1. Increased PaO_2
2. Increased pH

↓ ↑

1. Decreased PVR below SVR to halt R to L shunt via ductus arteriosus
2. Increased PaO_2 above 60 mm Hg resulting in ductus closure

Fig. 2-1. Normal changes at birth.

GOALS OF NEWBORN RESUSCITATION

Normal physiologic changes (Fig. 2-1) at birth are directed toward converting the newborn from dependence on the placenta and fetal circulation to self-sufficient gas exchange.

The *goals of resuscitation* are directed at aiding the infant in completing the above transition to independent life by:

A. Assuring airway patency
B. Maintaining ventilation/oxygenation
C. Maintaining cardiac output
D. Reducing metabolic requirements

A. Airway

The airway may be obstructed by secretions, flaccid musculature, or dysmorphic anatomy. As a result of a relatively low functional residual capacity and high closing capacity, the PO_2 of a newborn can fall 40 mm Hg in 15 seconds during acute airway obstruction. Successful resuscitation depends on rapid assessment and treatment of the problem.

Light Suction

This technique recognizes neonatal susceptibility to reflex bradycardia.

1. Thumb control is necessary to prevent applying prolonged, uncontrolled suction to the airway.
2. Intermittent suction allows a period for ventilation (5 seconds may cause hypoxia). Suction bulbs cause fewer bradyarrhythmias but are less efficient.
3. A trap should be present in the suction circuit for examining aspirated material (e.g., blood, meconium).
4. Traumatic suction to bronchi, trachea, or carina may cause bleeding or edema and worsen airway patency.

Positioning

1. When the neonate is supine, the retropharynx and glossopalatine channel can become sealed by soft tissue.
2. Hyperextension of the neck may worsen obstruction and actually cause tracheal collapse. Chin lifts and mandibular extension are more useful for opening the airway.
3. The neonate's shoulders can be elevated if occipital edema is present.

Airway Patency

1. Congenital anomalies such as choanal atresia, paralyzed vocal cords, laryngeal webs, or the ptotic tongue of Pierre Robin syndrome may obstruct the airway. Often a nasal trumpet can bypass oral lesions. However, because neonates are obligate nose breathers, an oral airway may precipitate bradycardia or laryngospasm and may not improve ventilation.
2. The ultimate assurance of airway patency is the oral endotracheal tube (ETT). The ETT should be advanced under direct vision only 1 to 1.5 cm past the cords to prevent endobronchial intubation.
3. Complications of intubation in vigorous infants include stridor, hoarse cry (which may persist up to 6 months of age), and an increased incidence of meconium aspiration syndrome.

B. Ventilation/Oxygenation

After 3 to 4 minutes of apnea, acidosis will cause a drop in cardiac output. PaO_2 is too low to measure by 5 minutes of total asphyxia. Treatment of neonatal asphyxia includes basic resuscitative techniques (Table 2-4 on pp. 26 and 27).

C. Cardiac Output

The cardiac output of the neonate is rate dependent. The normal heart rate is greater than 120 beats per minute and is best palpated at the umbilicus where it can be appreciated as a brief forceful (often bounding) pulse.

1. A heart rate of 100 beats per minute may be tolerated in the presence of adequate oxygenation and ventilation.
2. A heart rate of 80 to 100 beats per minute demands assisted ventilation with 100% oxygen.
3. A heart rate of less than 60 beats per minute demands immediate chest compressions.
4. A heart rate between 60 and 80 beats per minute may be acceptable for the first 30 seconds, but chest compressions should begin if there is no improvement with adequate oxygenation.
5. Chest compressions should continue until the heart rate is greater than 100 beats per minute.
6. A newborn who requires chest compressions should be intubated. If the cardiac output does not improve with oxygenation and volume expansion, resuscitative drugs may be indicated (Table 2-2).
7. Inadequate cardiac output (low perfusion) with an adequate heart rate may indicate hypovolemia; if volume loss is suspected (as in placental/uterine catastrophe and delayed cord clamping), 10 ml/kg of normal saline or Ringer's lactate can be pushed repeatedly as necessary.
8. Other causes of electromechanical dissociation should be considered: hypoxia, hypercapnia, acidosis, pneumothorax, or pneumomediastinum.

D. Metabolism (Heat Production)

Heat is produced in the newborn by metabolism of brown fat (nonshivering thermogenesis). Oxygen consumption ($\dot{V}O_2$) in neonates is normally 2 to 3 times that of the adult. $\dot{V}O_2$ doubles at a skin-to-air temperature gradient of 10° C and triples at 15° C.

Hypothermia causes hypoxia, hypercapnia, acidosis, and hypoglycemia. These factors increase pulmonary vascular resistance and right-to-left shunting. Normally, 10% of cardiac output goes to brown fat. During hypothermia, 75% of cardiac output is diverted to brown fat. Treatment and prevention are aimed at reducing all forms of heat loss (Table 2-3).

BASIC RESUSCITATION IN THE DELIVERY ROOM

APGAR scores (Tables 2-4 and 2-5) are useful in defining the level of neonatal depression. The resuscitator, however, should not stop to calculate the score if therapy will be delayed. A gross impression of neonatal status (vigorous, mildly depressed, depressed, morbid) can be made after delivery to a prewarmed resuscitation area, quick drying with a warm towel, and suctioning of the mouth and nose. Generally the signs appear in the following order: color, respiration, tone, reflex irritability, and heart rate. Regression of signs (i.e., improvement) is generally in the reverse order. It is also unnecessary to delay definitive action in order to count out the heart rate; an impression of normal (>120 beats per minute), slow (80 to 100 beats per minute), or morbid (<80 beats per minute) heart rate is sufficient to initiate therapy. Documentation of the 1, 5, and 10 minute APGAR score is important and can be done by a second observer, or calculated after resuscitation is completed.

Text continued on p. 28.

TABLE 2-2. Drugs used in neonatal resuscitation[3,4]

Drug	Standard concentration	Dose (per/kg)	Dose (ml/kg)	Endotracheal route
Epinephrine	0.1 mg/ml	0.01 mg	0.1 ml	yes
Atropine	0.1 mg/ml	0.01-0.03 mg	0.1-0.3	yes
Bicarbonate	8.4% = 1 mEq/ml	1 mEq*	1 ml	no
Calcium chloride	100 mg/ml	20 mg	0.2 ml	no
Glucose	$D_{10}W$ (100 mg/ml)	200 mg	2 ml	no
Naloxone (neonatal)	0.02 mg	0.01 mg	0.5 ml	yes
PGE_1†	0.05 μg/kg/min continuous infusion × 30 min, then titrate according to PaO_2			

*Should be diluted 1:1 with normal saline or Ringer's lactate.

†Side effects of PGE infusion include: apnea, systemic hypotension, CNS irritability (hyperthermia, seizure-like activity), and cardiac arrhythmias.

TABLE 2-3. Mechanism and treatment of heat loss in the delivery room[1]

Method	Mechanism in neonate	Treatment
Evaporation: vaporization of liquids from surface requires energy	Via: Amniotic fluid from skin Respiratory tract fluids Wet delivery table or blankets Ventilation with dry gases	Dry infant Replace wet blankets Humidify gases for resuscitation
Conduction: transfer of heat from skin to air or to solid objects in contact with skin	Wrapping infant in cold blankets Cold ambient temperature in delivery suite	Warm blankets Increase air temperature Radiant warmers
Convection: heat loss via air currents moving past body surfaces	Greater with wet infant because of water/air gradients	Dry infant Cover body parts with dry, warm blankets
Radiation: infrared heat loss by flow of heat from warmer to cooler surface	Larger body surface area	Radiant lamps Keep covered

TABLE 2-4. Resuscitation of neonates by APGAR scores

Score	Physical condition	Resuscitation
8-10 vigorous*	Heart rate >100 Slow—good respiratory effort Good motion Grimace or cough Pink or acrocyanotic	1. Suction 2. Dry blankets/radiant warmer 3. Stimulate to cry (rub back, flick feet) 4. Light percussion with mask on back to clear fluid
5-7 mildly depressed	Heart rate >100 Poor respiratory effort and weak cry Decreased tone No grimace to suction Pale or acrocyanosis	1. Vigorous drying and stimulation/radiant warmer 2. "Blow-by" O_2 3. Bag mask ventilation if heart rate <80 4. Naloxone 0.01 mg/kg if appropriate history 5. Observe in intensive care nursery (ICN) if continued depression or naloxone responsive
3-4 depressed	Heart rate > or < 100 Apneic or gasping Floppy No response to tactile stimulation Blue or pale	1. Immediate bag mask ventilation (rate 30-40/min, 100% O_2, PIP <30) 2. Simultaneous vigorous drying and stimulating 3. Intubate if no improvement at one minute 4. If heart rate <80 after 1 min of positive pressure ventilation, begin cardiac compression and treat as morbid

0-2 morbid	Heart rate <100 beats/min Rare gasp or apneic Limp No response to stimulation Pale, blue or "black" color	1. Brief bag mask ventilation while drying 2. Immediate intubation if no improvement (within 30 sec) 3. Cardiac compressions immediately if HR <60 beats/min or any time HR <80 beats/min after adequate ventilation established 4. If depressed HR + CO, epinephrine 0.1 cc/kg of 1:10,000 (1 mg epi in 10 cc diluent) via ETT or IV (10 μg/kg) 5. Treat acidosis 2-3 mEq bicarbonate via umbilical vein 6. Volume: 10 ml/kg normal saline or Ringer's lactate 7. Dextrose 2 ml/kg $D_{10}W$ or 200 mg/kg 8. Naloxone 0.01 mg/kg 9. Transport to ICN with 100% O_2, cardiac compressions if needed, warm blankets and warmer

*If premature or suspicion of intrauterine asphyxia, respiratory distress can occur 5 min to 12 hours after successful resuscitation. Any sign of nasal flaring, retractions, or grunting on reassessment dictates intensive care nursery observation. Prolonged acrocyanosis is normal.

TABLE 2-5. APGAR scores[5]

Score	0	1	2
Heart rate (beats/min)	Absent	<100	>100
Respiratory effort	Absent	Slow, regular	Good crying
Muscle tone	Limp	Some flexion of extremities	Active motion
Reflex irritability (nasal catheter)	No response	Grimace	Cough or sneeze
Color	Blue/pale	Extremities blue	Completely pink

MANAGEMENT OF COMMON MATERNAL-NEONATAL DISORDERS

Maternal Problems

This category can include drug abuse, previous history of fetal and neonatal problems, analgesic administration, maternal sepsis, preeclampsia, hypotension and hypertension, magnesium therapy, anemia, and the elderly primipara. Infants born to mothers with these disorders often require only general support; specific treatment may be found in Table 2-7.

Diabetes

Infants born to diabetic mothers should have their blood glucose checked at 1/2, 1, 4, and 8 hours after birth. Neonates have a blood glucose of 80% of the maternal value at delivery. Infants of diabetic mothers may have a drop in glucose within the first hour caused by infant production of insulin. The glucose level may reach 20 to 30 mg/dl by 2 to 4 hours of age even though the child may remain asymptomatic.

Difficult Delivery

Use of forceps, vacuum extraction, an abnormal presentation, cord prolapse, presence of a nuchal cord, cephalopelvic disproportion, or early cord clamping may be responsible for an infant with lowered APGAR scores. Resuscitation should reflect the level of depression, and consists primarily of general supportive measures.

Cesarean Section

When participating in the emergency cesarean section, pertinent information about factors potentially compromising the fetus usually can be obtained from the obstetric team. In utero the lungs contain an ultrafiltrate of plasma (30 ml/kg), two-thirds of which is expelled during vaginal delivery. Infants born by cesarean section require oropharyngeal suction and often chest percussion to clear rales.

Placental Catastrophe/Hypovolemia

Abruption, previa, hemorrhage, umbilical vein compression by the fetal head, severe maternal hypotension, or being held above the introitus before cord clamping may all produce a depressed infant. Besides general supportive care, a bolus of 10 ml/kg of normal saline or Ringer's lactate should be considered for the infant with poor cardiac output.

Anesthetic Agents (Table 2-6)

All anesthetic agents cross the placenta and therefore pose a theoretical risk to the neonate that is rarely significant clinically.

Neonatal Problems

Meconium Aspiration/Staining

The presence of meconium may herald the birth of a vigorous or morbidly depressed infant.

1. The oropharynx is suctioned on the perineum before delivery of the thorax to clear the airway before negative inspiratory pressure draws the meconium into the trachea and lungs.
2. The infant is carried to the resuscitation table in the Trendelenburg lateral decubitus position, with the hands about the thorax applying gentle circumferential pressure to impede inspiration.
3. If particulate meconium is present in the amniotic fluid or aspirate, immediate laryngoscopy and intubation is indicated with "one-pass" suction (3 to 5 seconds) via a catheter passed through the endotracheal tube or by withdrawing the endotracheal tube while suction is being applied, and immediate reintubation. Stimulating the infant is avoided during this period, but the umbilical pulse is palpated continuously and the infant is warmed with a radiant warmer and blankets.
4. Intubation should not be performed in a vigorous child when lightly stained fluid is present. Increased morbidity is associated with intubation in infants with APGAR scores of greater than 8.
5. Either spontaneous (preferred) or gentle positive pressure ventilation should occur for 15 to 30 seconds between repeat one-pass suction.
6. Suction through the endotracheal tube should continue until the aspirate is nearly clear. Rotating the head from side to side may facilitate endobronchial suction.
7. The stomach should be emptied before transportation and/or extubation.
8. Immediate bag-mask or bag-tube ventilation should proceed if the heart rate is less than 60 beats per minute. If the heart rate is less than 100 beats per minute, prolonged attempts at intubation should be abandoned in favor of bag-mask ventilation (i.e., basic resuscitation takes priority over treatment of meconium aspiration syndrome).

Neonatal Emergencies (Table 2-7)

Surgical Emergencies. If surgical anomalies are diagnosed in utero the neonate should be delivered at a hospital with an intensive care nursery and facilities for immediate repair. If the condition is not recognized in utero, the infant often requires resuscitation and stabilization before transport.

Nonsurgical Neonatal Emergencies. These conditions may occur immediately upon delivery or within the first few hours of life. They usually necessitate immediate treatment and transfer to a facility with an intensive care nursery.

Text continued on p. 38.

TABLE 2-6. Fetal effects of maternally administered anesthetics[6-8]

Drug	Placental transfer	Effect on neonate
Thiopental	Rapidly crosses placenta Most removed by fetal liver Diluted in fetal IVC	Little depression seen in doses <4 mg/kg
Succinylcholine	Limited transfer due to highly ionized molecule	Motor weakness only seen in neonate homozygous for pseudocholinesterase deficiency
Nondepolarizing muscle relaxants	Limited transfer due to large, bulky, rigid molecule with steroid nucleus and high ionization	Minimal effect
Nitrous oxide	Rapidly transferred	Exposure should be limited to less than 20 min for minimal neonatal depression
Halogenated agents	Transfer relative to uptake and distribution of agent	Can depress cardiovascular system if fetus is acidotic—effects rarely seen at levels of halothane 0.5%, enflurane 1%, isoflurane 0.75%
Narcotics	Easily transferred	May cause depression reversed by naloxone
Local anesthetics	Transfer dependent on degree of protein binding; fetal acidosis increases accumulation in fetus	
• Chloroprocaine	• Eliminated by cholinesterases and does not cross placenta	• No effect
• Bupivacaine	• Limited transfer due to high protein binding	• Little effect
• Lidocaine	• Moderate transfer due to less protein binding	• May see transient neurobehavioral changes

TABLE 2-7. Delivery room stabilization of neonatal emergencies*[1,9,10]

Pathology	Signs/symptoms	Treatment
Respiratory surgical emergencies		
Congenital diaphragmatic hernia (CDH)	Respiratory distress CXR shows bowel in thorax, usually on left Bowel sounds present over thorax Hypoplastic lungs Prone to pneumothorax on nonherniated side with immediate and profound decompensation	Nasogastric tube Intubation and support with small tidal volumes and PIP <30 cm H_2O Insertion of 20 g IV catheter if pneumothorax occurs At high risk for Group-B streptococcus pneumonia
Tracheoesophageal fistula	85% have blind esophageal pouch and a tracheal-to-lower esophagus fistula Polyhydramnios Excessive salivation Cyanotic spells, especially with feeding Gastric distention with ventilation Unable to pass NG (see in pouch on x-ray)	Prone to aspiration Placement of esophageal pouch suction tube If immediate intubation is necessary, see technique outlined in Chapter 18
Cystic hygroma	Neck mass with extrinsic airway obstruction	Awake intubation if needed while maintaining spontaneous ventilation
Vascular ring Double aortic arch Right arch with ligamentum arteriosum Pulmonary artery sling Anomalous innominate, subclavian or carotid	Stridor may be present at birth, but usually develops over first day to weeks	Awake intubation if airway obstruction occurs

*In these emergencies a neonatologist and/or intensive care nursery should be alerted immediately.

Continued.

TABLE 2-7. Delivery room stabilization of neonatal emergencies—cont'd

Pathology	Signs/symptoms	Treatment
Laryngeal/bronchial cysts	Stridor	Intubation and ventilatory support as needed Needle aspiration of cyst if its size prevents passage of ETT
Congenital adenomatoid cystic malformation of lung	Respiratory distress CXR reveals multiple cysts (may resemble CDH)	Respiratory support as needed
Congenital lobar emphysema	Respiratory distress CXR shows hyperlucent lung field	Respiratory support as needed
Choanal atresia	Cyanosis with feeding Improvement with crying Unable to pass nasal catheter Otoscope visualization of atresia	Oral airway Suspect associated anomalies
Laryngeal web (at level of true vocal cords)	Stridor if incomplete Visualization with laryngoscope	Intubation with forcible rupture of web if possible Needle cricothyrotomy
Tracheomalacia	Inspiratory stridor due to pliable airway tissues	Respiratory support as needed
Congenital subglottic stenosis	Stridor	Respiratory support or intubation as needed

Cyanotic congenital heart disease[1] (see also Fig. 2-2)		
Transposition of great vessels Tetralogy of Fallot Pulmonary stenosis or atresia Tricuspid atresia Truncus arteriosus Single or hypoplastic ventricle Total anomalous pulmonary venous return	Tachypnea Tachycardia Cyanosis Deterioration or worsened cyanosis with crying or ductus closure Often accompanied by septal defects	Intubation if needed Increased F_IO_2 to decrease pulmonary vascular resistance PGE_1 to keep ductus patent Correction of acidosis Inotropic support, emergent septostomy, valvotomy or shunt if not improving
Gastrointestinal surgical emergencies		
Omphalocele	Failure of midgut to return to abdominal cavity by 10th week of gestation Midline Umbilical location Bowel is covered with membrane	NG tube for decompression Cover intestines with saline-soaked gauze, plastic wrap Beware of coexisting malformations, Beckwith syndrome, congenital heart disease
Gastroschisis	Occurs frequently in premature infants Bowel is uncovered	Treat as above Not associated with other malformations
Neurological surgical emergencies		
Myelomeningocele	Posterior midline defect	Cover with saline-soaked gauze Keep infant in prone or lateral position

Continued.

TABLE 2-7. Delivery room stabilization of neonatal emergencies—cont'd

Pathology	Signs/symptoms	Treatment
Nonsurgical neonatal emergencies* **Early (first minutes)**		
Asphyxia	Low APGAR score	Resuscitation as needed (see Table 2-4)
Meconium aspiration	Meconium staining Respiratory distress May have low APGAR score	Clear mouth/pharynx before delivery of shoulders and body Laryngoscopy/intubation Suction via ETT, extubate when aspirate clear and stomach emptied May develop persistent fetal circulation
Maternal drugs: Narcotics; magnesium; anesthetic agents	History of recent drug administration Low APGAR score Failure to improve	Respiratory support as needed Naloxone 0.01 mg/kg/dose IM, IV, ETT Calcium gluconate (for hyper-Mg^+) 100 mg/kg/dose IV
Late (>30 min postpartum) (sepsis may be etiology for any of these conditions)		
Apnea	>20 seconds (more severe if associated with bradycardia)	Intubation and support if persistent Potential etiologies: narcotics, acidosis, hypoxia, hypoglycemia, anemia, sepsis, CNS trauma, pulmonary disease, maternal Mg^+ Apnea of prematurity (not seen until 2-5 days of age)
Respiratory distress syndrome (RDS)	Respiratory distress developing in first hours with grunting, nasal flaring, retractions Hx of maternal diabetes <36 weeks gestation Low APGAR score	Respiratory support as needed (may only require O_2) Peak airway pressures 20-25 cm H_2O PEEP 4-5 cm H_2O, I:E at 1:1-1:3 Maintain PaO_2 50-80, pH 7.25-7.45 Consider muscle relaxants to improve ventilation Culture and treat for sepsis

Meconium aspiration syndrome ([MAS] plugging of small airways with meconium, chemical pneumonitis)	History Respiratory distress as above Prone to pneumothorax	Respiratory support as above Frequent ABG Ventilate with I:E of 1:3 or greater in order to reduce air trapping Maintain PaO_2 50-80, pH 7.25-7.45 Consider muscle relaxant Culture and treat for sepsis
Bacterial pneumonia Group B β-hemolytic *streptococcus* *S. aureus*	Respiratory distress as above Signs of sepsis	Respiratory support as above Consider muscle relaxant Culture and treat as for sepsis (see below)
Transient tachypnea of the newborn	Respiratory distress as above, usually less severe	Respiratory support as above Self limited Check serial ABG Consider sepsis
Pneumothorax (may be due to resuscitation or associated with RDS, MAS, pneumonia)	Acute unexplained deterioration Decreased breath sounds	If life-threatening, may perform needle aspiration based on asymmetric transillumination If stable, CXR is obtained prior to treatment Chest tube

*In nonsurgical emergencies a pediatrician, neonatologist and/or level III nursery should be consulted.

Continued.

TABLE 2-7. Delivery room stabilization of neonatal emergencies—cont'd

Pathology	Signs/symptoms	Treatment
Persistent fetal circulation Hx of asphyxia in near term Post term infant Associated with MAS, CDH	Cyanosis in first 12 hr of life ECG: right ventricular hypertrophy	Hyperventilation to achieve hypocarbia (PCO_2 of 20-30 mm Hg) and alkalosis Consider muscle relaxation Inotropic support Vasodilatory support (e.g., tolazoline) after consultation
Seizures (multiple causes)	May present as eye fluttering, sucking, drooling, tonic posturing or apnea	Consider immediately treatable etiologies: sepsis, hypoxia, acidosis, hypoglycemia, hypokalemia, maternal drug addiction (withdrawal) Phenobarbital 10 mg/kg q 30 min up to 40 mg/kg to stop seizure Maintenance: 5 mg/kg/24 hr divided q 12 hr Diphenyl hydantoin 10 mg/kg/dose × 2 doses q 12 hr Maintenance: 5 mg/kg/24 hr divided q 12 hr
Sepsis (In newborn *E. coli*, *S. aureus*, Group B β-hemolytic *streptococcus*, Listeria)	History (maternal illness, rupture of fetal membranes >24 hr) Nonspecific symptoms Irritable, lethargic poor suck, hypothermia, respiratory distress, apnea, mottling of skin, jaundice, abdominal distention Neutropenia or neutrophilia Increased band forms Thrombocytopenia	Culture CSF, blood, urine, tracheal aspirate IV ampicillin 100 mg/kg per 24 hr divided q 12 hr IV gentamycin 5 mg/kg per 24 hr divided q 12 hr

Hypoglycemia (IUGR, IDDM, postdates, asphyxia premature)	History (IDDM), asphyxia May be asymptomatic Nonspecific symptoms including seizures, apnea, jitteriness, poor feeding	Stable: PO $D_{10}W$ Unstable or <34 weeks: IV $D_{10}W$ 100 ml/kg/24 hr PO If emergent: 2 ml/kg $D_{10}W$ bolus, repeat prn
Narcotic withdrawal	History Nonspecific symptoms including seizures, apnea, irritability, poor feeding	Phenobarbital 5 mg/kg/24 hr q 8-12 IV/IM Taper as tolerated over 3 weeks

TRANSPORTATION OF THE CRITICALLY ILL NEWBORN

The problem of stabilization and transportation of the critically ill child and newborn may be encountered by the anesthesiologist working in a hospital without pediatric or neonatal intensive care capability. The general practitioner, pediatrician, or obstetrician who rarely encounters a critically ill child may consult an anesthesiologist regarding airway management, intravenous access, pharmacotherapy, or general stabilization before transporting the infant to a tertiary care center.

The Receiving Team

Transportation of a critical child generally is performed by a specialized team from the accepting facility. The transport team usually is activated by telephone contact with the on-duty transport coordinator, usually a staff physician from the accepting intensive care unit, who also may advise on management. The coordinator also chooses the mode of transportation. In general, medicolegal responsibility is transferred to the accepting hospital when the transport team arrives at the bedside, and not with acceptance of transportation by telephone. In cases of interstate transportation, most states allow the transport team to function under the "Good Samaritan Act." Conversely, until the transport team arrives at the bed side, medicolegal responsibility falls on the referring physician, who may decide not to institute therapies recommended by telephone.

Conveyance Information

Information needed by the accepting tertiary care hospital when arranging transportation of a sick neonate is given in the following outline:

1. Parental involvement and understanding regarding the need for and specific details of the transfer
2. Full medical history of the neonate (maternal, prenatal, birth history)
   a. Weight, height, age
   b. History of resuscitation
   c. Current clinical status
   d. Current medical therapies that will need to be continued during transport
   e. Progression of symptoms and likelihood of the need for escalated therapy
   f. Results of laboratory tests, x-rays, particularly current CBC and arterial blood gases
3. Information that will help guide the accepting hospital's transport coordinator in selecting the mode of transportation
   a. Severity of illness and need for rapid transportation
   b. Distance, geography, and weather
   c. Suspected air in closed spaces such as mediastinum, peritoneum, and pericardium or ileus or pneumothorax, which can expand at increased altitudes if transportation by helicopter or plane is considered

Pretransport Therapies

In addition to therapies instituted at the referring hospital the transport coordinator at the accepting hospital may suggest therapies to be instituted before the arrival of the transporting vehicle. Many therapies/procedures are difficult to initiate in a moving vehicle and are better applied before transportation, even if only prophylactically.

1. Maternal and newborn blood clot is obtained along with signed consent for transport.
2. Children with an unstable airway, or whose (presumptive) diagnosis may later threaten the airway, may need elective endotracheal intubation and muscle relaxation.
3. Hyperventilation may be necessary in the child suspected of having increased intracranial pressure ($PaCO_2$ of 25 to 30 mm Hg).
4. Chest tubes may be needed when even a small pneumothorax is diagnosed.
5. Ideally, two sites of IV access should be available either via umbilical (see the box on pp. 44 and 45) or peripheral vessels.
6. A nasogastric tube usually is inserted for bowel obstruction or in patients at risk for aspiration (e.g., tracheoesophageal fistula).
7. All patients should be NPO as long as possible before transportation.
8. Omphalocele, gastroschesis, meningiomyelocele, bladder extrophy are covered with saline-soaked sterile gauze and plastic wrap.
9. If the child is to be transported by air, transfusion may be necessary to raise the hematocrit.
10. Blood, urine, and CSF should be cultured before beginning antibiotic administration, which usually is started before transfer.
11. Checking stools for occult blood helps in diagnosing necrotizing enterocolitis in the newborn.
12. A continuous infusion of PGE_1 is a reasonable therapeutic maneuver for most patients with cyanotic congenital heart disease to maintain a patent ductus arteriosus (see Table 2-2).
13. Dopamine may be used for renal perfusion or inotropic support.
14. Sodium nitroprusside is a peripheral and pulmonary vasodilator that can be useful for the treatment of persistent fetal circulation.
15. With the use of anticonvulsants, equipment for controlling the airway (i.e., endotracheal intubation) must be available.
16. Patients with a history of hypoglycemia should be transported with a continuous infusion of $D_{10}W$.

TABLE 2-8. Predelivery preparation and room set up[1,2]

The neonatal resuscitation set up should mimic the "SCOMLADI" mneumonic as outlined for the operating room in Chapter 5. Additionally, special attention must be paid to maintaining the neonate's temperature.

	Equipment	Comments
S—Suction	6, 8, 10 French catheters Suction bulb Negative pressure (− 20) to (− 30) mm Hg Thumb control and trap	Use largest possible suction to remove particulate matter from pharynx
C—Circuit	O_2 supply with connected, tested bag mask circuit Variety of clear, padded one-piece masks Manometer to measure peak inspiratory pressure	The ambu bag prevents delivering high pressure because of the pop off valve, but is unwieldy and does not easily yield information on compliance Several valve styles on ambu bags deliver varied concentrations of oxygen, especially during spontaneous ventilation
O—Oxygen	3-8 L/min flow Back-up tanks for transport or system failure	Humidifiers or nebulizers help to prevent hypothermia
M—Monitors	Neonatal stethoscope Hand on the base of the umbilical cord for heart rate and cardiac output Observation of color, tone, movement Pulse oximeter	An oximeter is useful for anesthesiologists who are more experienced with oximetry than umbilical cord monitoring. It is easy to apply, gives heart rate, SaO_2, and plethysmography and leaves two hands free when the resuscitator is working alone ECG leads often do not stay attached to a wet infant and may distract the resuscitator

L—Laryngoscope	Pediaric handle Miller 0, 1 blades	An oxygen port on the blade may be useful
A—Airway	Oral airway: 000, 00, 0, 1 Nasal airways Endotracheal tubes	ETT size by gestational age: less than 34 weeks 2.5, greater than 34 weeks 3.0, term 3.0, 3.5
D—Drugs	Atropine Epinephrine Bicarbonate Calcium Chloride Naloxone (neonatal) Glucose Prostaglandin E_1	See Table 2-2
I—Intravenous	Umbilical vein catheterization tray (see box on pp. 44 and 45)	ETT should serve as initial drug route IVs are placed in morbid infants when intensive care transport is not imminent
T—Temperature	Warmed blankets Radiant warmer	Blankets should be changed as they get wet

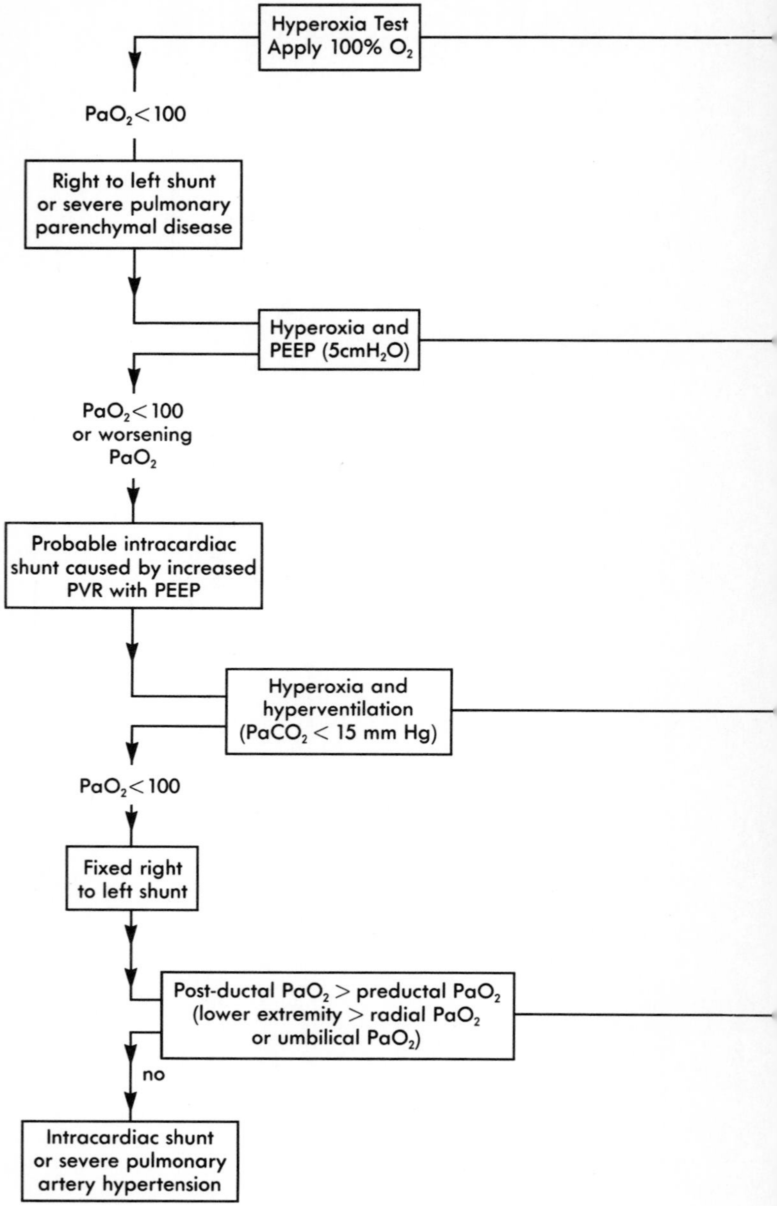

Fig. 2-2. Evaluation of the cyanotic newborn.[11] The tests shown can aid in the diagnosis and early treatment of a newborn with cyanosis. Pure oxygen and hyperventilation are used for diagnostic purposes and are potentially harmful if sustained for long periods.

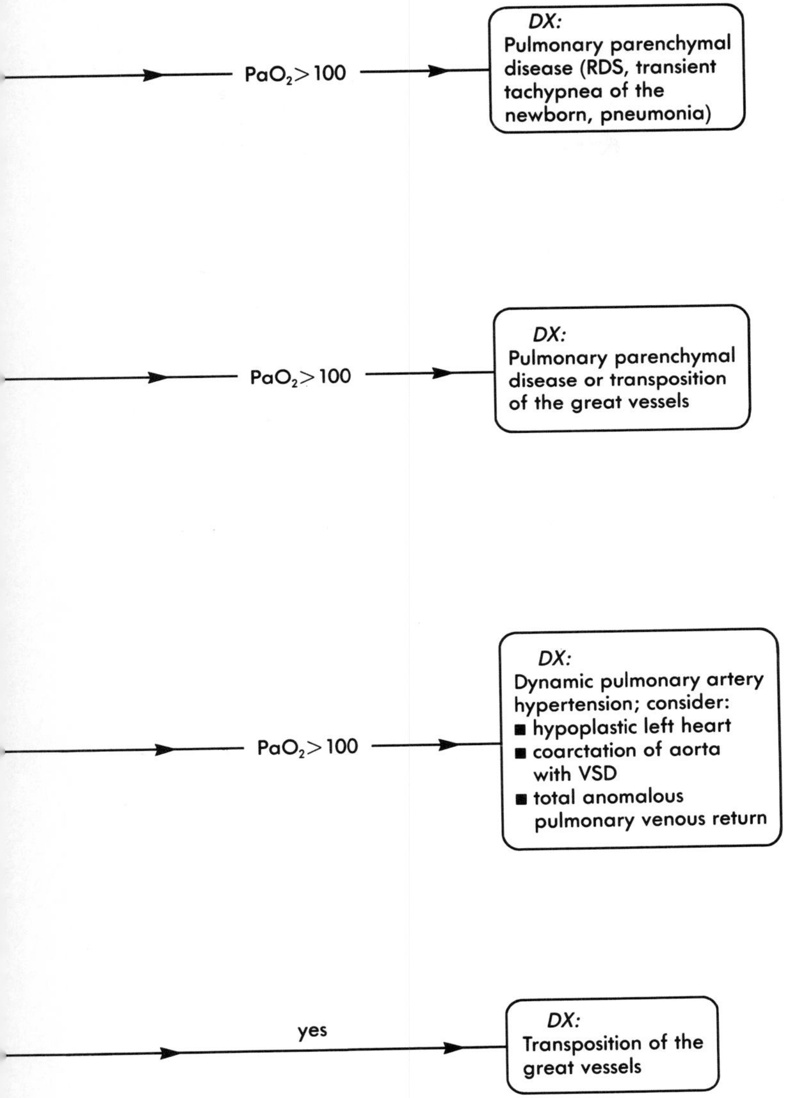
PaO₂>100
DX:
Pulmonary parenchymal disease (RDS, transient tachypnea of the newborn, pneumonia)
PaO₂>100
DX:
Pulmonary parenchymal disease or transposition of the great vessels
PaO₂>100
DX:
Dynamic pulmonary artery hypertension; consider:
■ hypoplastic left heart
■ coarctation of aorta with VSD
■ total anomalous pulmonary venous return
yes
DX:
Transposition of the great vessels

SUMMARY OF DELIVERY ROOM RESUSCITATION OF THE NEWBORN

I. Preparation
  A. Check equipment, especially suction, oxygen source, circuit, laryngoscope, endotracheal tubes, and airways.
  B. Check drugs and dilutions.
  C. Obtain multiple warm blankets.
  D. Turn on radiant warmer.

II. Anticipation
  A. Obtain maternal history: drugs and anesthesia, placental catastrophe, preeclampsia, etc.
  B. Obtain fetal history: gestational age and approximate weight, congenital anomalies, presence of meconium.

III. Immediate oropharyngeal suction after delivery of face

IV. Transfer to resuscitation table
  A. Quickly assess level of neonatal depression (usually by APGAR scoring).
  B. If thick meconium is present, immediately intubate and use suction before ventilating.
  C. If thin or no meconium is present:
    1. Dry and stimulate infant.
    2. Remove secretions from oronasopharynx.
    3. Begin resuscitation (see Table 2-4) if heart rate and respiratory efforts are inadequate.

V. Check temperature and maintain normothermia.

VI. Consider extubation in the vigorous stable infant after emptying the stomach.

VII. Transfer to nursery or intensive care nursery.

UMBILICAL VESSEL CATHETERIZATION

I. Indications
  A. Arterial (UAC): Blood pressure monitoring, serial arterial blood gases
  B. Venous (UVC): Emergency venous access, exchange transfusion, CVP monitoring

II. Complications
  A. Thrombosis
  B. Sepsis
  C. Hypertension
  D. Necrotizing enterocolitis
  E. Hemorrhage

III. Technique (Fig. 2-4)

The cord and abdomen are prepared and draped in a sterile fashion. The operators wear gowns, gloves and mask and the infant is restrained.
  A. The cord is constricted gently with an unknotted umbilical tape around the skin at the base.
  B. The cord is cut with a scalpel, 3 to 4 mm above the border of the skin (the longer the umbilical stump, the more difficult it may be to pass the catheter because of the helical descent of the vessels).

UMBILICAL VESSEL CATHETERIZATION—cont'd

C. The cord is stabilized with one or two hemostats.

D. The vessels are identified: arteries (2) are small and thick-walled, the vein is larger and often tortuous. Thrombus may need to be removed.

E. A closed iris forceps is used to dilate an artery (usually not necessary for the vein), by placing the closed tip inside the vessel and allowing the forceps to open gently—this maneuver and catheter placement may be facilitated by a second operator stabilizing the vessel walls with one or two fine forceps.

F. Choice of catheter: <2 kg: 3.5 French, >2 kg: 5.0 French (a difficult catheter passage may dictate use of the 3.5 French catheter in a >2 kg infant).

G. Catheters are flushed with saline with 1 U/ml heparin.

H. Determination of insertion length:

UAC length (cm) = (3 × kg) + 9 cm + umbilical stump length.
UVC length (cm) = (0.5 × UAC length) + 1 cm + umbilical stump length.
UVC length (cm) = (1.5 × kg) + 5.5 cm + umbilical stump length.

I. Catheter is passed into vessel using firm but gentle pressure.
   1. Resistance at 1-1.5 cm into lumen may be secondary to a tight umbilical tape. Resistance at 4-5 cm may indicate a "false lumen" and reassessment of placement is indicated.
   2. Gentle upward traction of the umbilical stump with the stabilizing hemostats often facilitates UVC passage, while moderate rostral traction may facilitate UAC passage.

J. Placement is confirmed by:
   1. Appropriate pressure wave.
   2. Free passage to the calculated length, with free blood flow.
   3. Chest x-ray. Except in the most dire situations, catheter tip location must be confirmed by x-ray. The formula listed above places the UAC catheter in the "high" position (T_7-T_8). A low position (L_3-L_4) also may be chosen (see Fig. 2-3).

   These positions are meant to avoid placement in the right atrium, or near the superior or inferior-mesenteric or renal arteries or the celiac axis.
   1. Cyanosis or mottling of a leg may occur with UAC placement, indicating passage into a femoral artery, vasospasm or hypovolemia. Severe symptoms dictate catheter removal.
   2. The UVC tip can be lodged within the liver or mesentery, indicated by limited passage and poor or no blood flow. In this position, instillation of hypertonic solutions or drugs may have catastrophic consequences.

K. Catheters are sutured to the umbilicus.

L. Crystalloid infusions usually contain 0.5 to 1 U/ml heparin to prevent thrombosis.

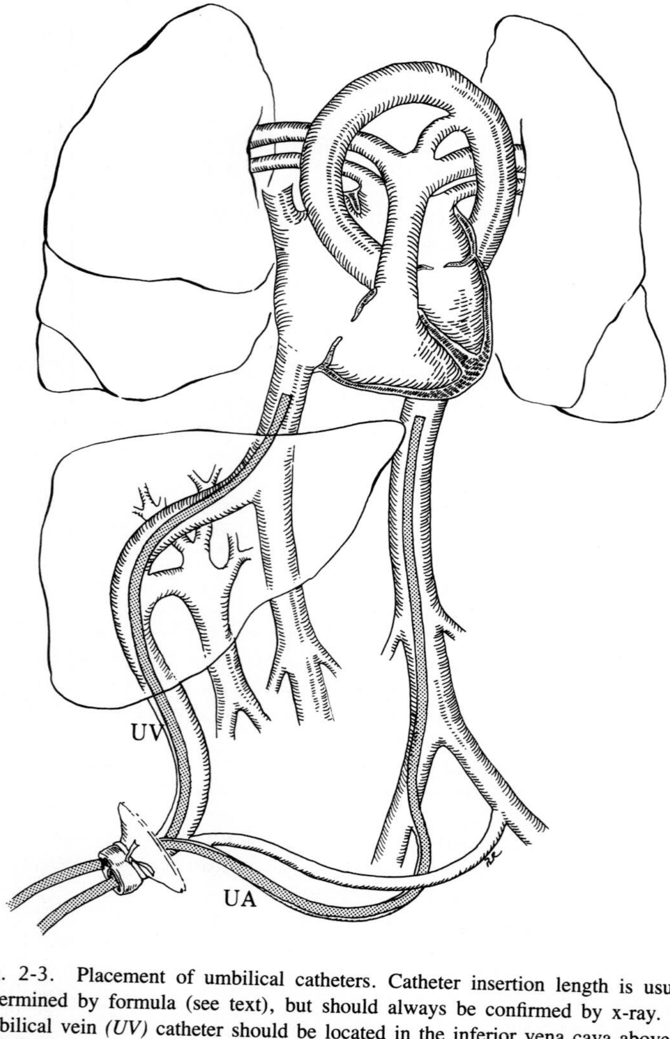

Fig. 2-3. Placement of umbilical catheters. Catheter insertion length is usually determined by formula (see text), but should always be confirmed by x-ray. The umbilical vein *(UV)* catheter should be located in the inferior vena cava above the ductus venosus and hepatic veins. The umbilical artery *(UA)* catheter can be placed in the low position above the aortic bifurcation ($L_{3\text{-}4}$) or high position above the diaphragm ($T_{6\text{-}9}$).

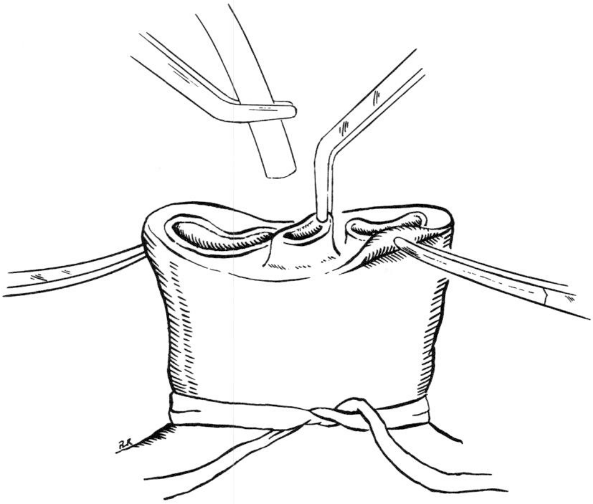

Fig. 2-4. Umbilical vessel catheterization. After placement of an umbilical tape at the base of the cord, the cord is cut with a scalpel 3 to 4 mm above the skin. Passage of the catheter will be facilitated by stabilizing the cord with hemostats and gentle dilatation of the artery with iris forceps.

REFERENCES

1. Ramanathan S: Obstetric anesthesia, Philadelphia, 1988, Lea & Febiger.
2. Brann AW and Cefalo RC, editors: Guidelines for perinatal care, ed 2, American Academy of Pediatrics and American College of Obstetrics and Gynecology, 1983.
3. Heyman MA: Pharmacologic use of prostaglandin E_1 in infants with congenital heart disease, Am Heart J 101:837-843, 1981.
4. Benitz WE and Tatro DS: The pediatric drug handbook, Chicago, 1981, Year Book Medical Publishers.
5. Apgar V: A proposal for a new method of evaluation of the newborn infant, Curr Res Anesth Analg 32:260, 1953.
6. Schnider SM and Gershon L: Anesthesia for obstetrics, ed 2, Baltimore, 1987, Williams & Wilkins.
7. Barash PG, Cullen BF, and Stoelting RK: Clinical anesthesia, Philadelphia, 1989, JB Lippincott Co.
8. Hodgkins R and others: Neonatal neurobehavioral tests following vaginal delivery under ketamine, thiopental, extradural anesthesia, Anesth Analg 56:548-553, 1977.
9. Barkin RM and Rosen P, editors: Emergency pediatrics, ed 3, St Louis, 1990, The CV Mosby Co.
10. Carlo WA and Martin RJ: Principles of neonatal assisted ventilation, Pediatr Clin North Am 33:221, 1986.
11. Stevenson DK and Benitz W: A practical approach to diagnosis and immediate care of the cyanotic neonate, Clin Pediatr 6:325, 1987.

BIBLIOGRAPHY

Bloom RS and Cropley C: Textbook of neonatal resuscitation. American Heart Association, 1987.

Brann AW and Cefalo RC, editors: Guidelines for perinatal care, ed 2, American Academy of Pediatrics and American College of Obstetrics and Gynecology, 1983.

Brooks TD and Gravenstein N: Pulse oximetry for early detection of hypoxemia in anesthetized infants, J Clin Monit 1:135, 1985.

Carlo WA and Martin RJ: Principles of neonatal assisted ventilation, Pediatr Clin North Am 33:221, 1986.

Cochran WD: Common Procedures. In: Cloherty JP and Stark AR, editors: Manual of neonatal care, Boston, 1985, Little, Brown & Co, Inc.

Falciglia HS: Failure to prevent meconium aspiration syndrome, Obstet Gynecol 71:349, 1988.

Frankel LR: The evaluation, stabilization, and transport of the critically ill child, Int Anethesiol Clin 5:77, 1987.

Gregory GA: Resuscitation of the newborn, ASA Refresher Courses in Anesthesiology 16:99, 1988.

Hackel A: An organizational system for critical care transport, Int. Anesthesiol Clin 25:1, 1987.

Heyman MA: Pharmacologic use of prostaglandin E_1 in infants with congenital heart disease, Am Heart J 101:837, 1981.

Linder N and others: Need for endotracheal intubation and suction in meconium stained neonates, J Pediatr 112:613, 1988.

McKlveen RE, Hunt CO, and Ostheimer GW: Neonatal resuscitation, Resident and Staff Physician 32:22, 1986.

Philipps AF: Resuscitation in the delivery room. In Barkin RM and Rosen P editors: Emergency pediatrics, ed 3, St Louis, 1990, CV Mosby Co.

Ramanathan S: Obstetric anesthesia, Philadelphia, 1988, Lea & Febiger.

Reid TJ: Transport of the high risk neonate. In Streeter NS, editor: High risk neonatal care, Rockville, Md, 1986, Aspen Books.

Sepkowitz S: Influence of the legal imperative and medical guidelines on the incidence and management of the meconium stained newborn, Am J Dis Child 141:1124, 1987.

Shnider SM and Levinson G: Anesthesia for obstetrics, ed 2, Baltimore, 1987, Williams & Wilkins.

Shukla H and Ferrara A: Rapid estimation of insertional length of umbilical catheters in newborns, Am J Dis Child 140:786, 1986.

Standards and guidelines for cardiopulmonary resuscitation and emergency cardiac care, JAMA 255:2905, 1986.

Stevenson DK and Benitz WF: A practical approach to diagnosis and immediate care of the cyanotic neonate, Clin Pediatr 6:325, 1987.

3

THE PREOPERATIVE EVALUATION OF THE PEDIATRIC PATIENT

Anne M. Savarese

There was an old owl who lived in an oak;
The more he heard, the less he spoke.
The less he spoke, the more he heard.
Why aren't we like that wise old bird?
ANON
A CHILD'S TREASURY OF POEMS

CONDUCTING THE INTERVIEW

Success in obtaining a medical history, performing a physical examination, and establishing rapport with the child and parents depends upon a relaxed, tactful, and professional approach. The objectives of this visit include:

1. Obtaining essential details of the child's present illness and medical history to formulate an anesthetic plan.
2. Providing information about the conduct of anesthesia for children and answering questions.
3. Securing informed consent.
4. Allaying anxiety and establishing trust and confidence with the parents and child.

Communicating in plain language and directing comments at the level of understanding of both parents and child will help to achieve these goals. Language barriers, developmental limitations in comprehension, and physical and mental handicaps may impede effective communication.

Planning the visit for the day or evening before surgery allows everyone time to digest the information provided and to prepare psychologically. Storybooks, brochures, slide shows, and videos targeted to specific age groups that explain anesthesia and surgery are recommended. Preparation for and understanding of the anesthetic experience contribute to a calm and cooperative child on the day of surgery, and well-informed parents can reinforce this preparedness.

It is important to emphasize that the child's safety and comfort are the highest priority when introducing the concepts of anesthetic risk and perioperative management. Issues that should be discussed with parents preoperatively include:

1. Dental risks of tracheal intubation (especially in children 6 to 12 years of age, with loose deciduous teeth).
2. Aspiration and the importance of adherence to NPO schedules.
3. Apnea in ex-premature infants and neonates.
4. Blood transfusion in children with anemias and those undergoing major surgery in which significant blood loss is anticipated.
5. Possible postoperative mechanical ventilation in children with significant respiratory dysfunction (e.g., respiratory distress syndrome, bronchopulmonary dysplasia, asthma, airway obstruction, epiglottitis) and those undergoing airway procedures (e.g., bronchoscopy, foreign body removal, tonsillectomy and adenoidectomy, tracheoesophageal fistula repair, thoracotomy).
6. Postoperative mechanical ventilation and intensive care for children undergoing major abdominal, neurosurgical, and open-heart procedures.

An explanation of monitors used to assess continuously the well-being of the child under anesthesia reassures parents (e.g., ECG, blood pressure cuff, pulse oximeter, stethoscope, capnograph, arterial and CVP catheters, Foley catheter, and temperature monitors). They also should be informed that the anesthesiologist will be in constant attendance until the child is in stable condition in either the recovery room or the intensive care unit.

It is necessary to provide a clear and honest description of events in the preinduction and induction periods. Laboratory tests requiring blood sampling, abstinence from food and fluids, injection of premedications, separation from parents, placement of an intravenous catheter, and application of an anesthesia mask proceed more smoothly when parents and child are prepared. Creative and appealing presentations of these events are encouraged to capture the child's interest and cooperation. For example, the anesthesia mask may become a "space mask" for an astronaut; an inhalation induction may become "blowing up a balloon with giggle gas" or "blowing out birthday candles"; the ECG and oximeter may become "TVs" or "video games." A knowledge of the child's developmental and perceptual level can guide the discussion. The child should be invited to bring a favorite toy or "security" object to the operating room to provide a sense of familiarity in the midst of a potentially fearful experience.

Children need reassurance that anesthesia is a special sleep during which the operation is performed without pain or awareness and from which they definitely will be awakened. An expected time frame from premedication to discharge from the recovery room is helpful to parents. An explanation should be provided of anticipated pain, nausea, grogginess, sore throat, and immobility from dressings on emergence and how these problems will be managed in the recovery room. An appropriate plan for postoperative analgesia should be outlined (e.g., regional techniques including nerve blocks, epidural, intrathecal, or parenteral narcotics, and patient-controlled analgesia for appropriately aged children).

TAKING A HISTORY

A thorough history of the pediatric patient includes an assessment of the chief complaint and proposed surgical or diagnostic procedure; details of the newborn period and subsequent health, growth, and development into childhood; prior hospitalizations, surgeries, and anesthetics; details of current and past medications, drug allergies or sensitivities, and immunization status; and a family history of anesthetic reactions and/or mishaps with particular attention to malignant hyperthermia susceptibility. Any abnormal conditions should be documented using a systematic approach as outlined in the box on p. 52.

Source

1. The relationship of informers to the patient and their reliability should be noted.
2. Information from present and old medical records should be documented.
3. Primary physician(s) for the child and availability of information from him or her should be recorded.

Chief Complaint and History of the Present Illness

A brief account of the ailment should be made, noting its onset and duration, principal clinical features and associated symptoms, precipitating, aggravating, and relieving factors, the course of the illness with attention to the functional limitations it imposes, and the child's response to therapy. The reasons for and expected outcome of the proposed surgical or diagnostic procedure for which the child is being anesthetized should be clarified.

REVIEW OF SYSTEMS

Inquiry should be directed to pertinent positives and negatives in relation to the present illness as well as the major organ system (see the box on p. 58).

THE PHYSICAL EXAMINATION

The child should be approached with a quiet, soothing voice and a slow, gentle manner that will indicate how he or she can expect to be handled during the induction of anesthesia. Infants and toddlers often can be examined in parents' laps; the baby will feel comfortable and secure, and this may facilitate the examination. School-age children may be more cooperative after a simple explanation of the examination; allowing them to see and touch instruments (e.g., stethoscope), and perhaps demonstrating that the examination will not hurt by first "practicing" on a doll or toy. Older children and adolescents are usually cooperative but may be modest or shy; closing the door or curtain gives them needed privacy. Warming the room, the examiner's hands, and the stethoscope are particularly important when examining small infants at risk for hypothermia. Some children will not cooperate despite the most disarming efforts, necessitating a calm, persistent, and systematic approach to obtain the needed examination. See the box on p. 60 for a description of what the anesthesiologist's limited physical examination should cover. Tables 3-1 and 3-2 list normal growth characteristics and vital signs that should be noted on the physical examination.

Text continued on p. 64

PAST MEDICAL HISTORY

Birth history	Gestational age	<38 weeks = premature 38 to 40 weeks = full term >40 weeks = postmature
	Condition at delivery	APGAR scores Resuscitation Presence of meconium
	Labor history	Condition of fetus Evidence for any fetal distress Results of fetal scalp pH tests Amniotic fluid quality and quantity Length of rupture of membranes Placental quality Bleeding
	Maternal health during pregnancy	Age Infections Diabetes Rh status Hypertension Toxemia Abnormal placentation (i.e., abruptio, previa, accreta) Outcome of previous pregnancies History of inherited diseases Maternal substance abuse (alcohol, narcotics, cocaine)

Neonatal history	Respiratory problems	Respiratory distress syndrome Bronchopulmonary dysplasia Meconium aspiration Retained fetal fluid Transient tachypnea of the newborn Apnea Congenital diaphragmatic hernia Tracheoesophageal fistula
	Cardiovascular problems	Murmurs Patent ductus arteriosus Cyanosis Congenital anomalies of the heart and great vessels Coarctation of the aorta Congestive heart failure Arrhythmias Heart block Hemodynamic instability Cardiotonic medications and response to therapy
	Neurological problems	Birth asphyxia Anoxic encephalopathy Hydrocephalus and elevated intracranial pressure Tremors Seizures Intraventricular hemorrhage in prematures Spasticity Hypotonia

Continued.

PAST MEDICAL HISTORY—cont'd

Neonatal history—cont'd	Neurological problems—cont'd	Congenital infections (e.g., cytomegalovirus (CMV), rubella, herpes simplex virus (HSV), and toxoplasmosis) Malformations: encephalocoele, meningomyelocele, Arnold-Chiari malformation, tethered spinal cord, and craniosynostosis
	Metabolic and endocrine problems	Hyperbilirubinemia Hypoglycemia (especially in infants of diabetic mothers) Hypocalcemia Hypomagnesemia Inborn errors of metabolism Acidosis Alkalosis Adrenal insufficiency Hypothyroidism Ambiguous genitalia
	Hematologic problems	Rh incompatibility Hemolytic anemia Hyperbilirubinemia Polycythemia Disseminated intravascular coagulation Hemorrhage Hemoglobinopathies (sickle cell, thalassemia)

	Renal problems	Renal agenesis Hydronephrosis Prune-belly syndrome Renal failure Genitourinary tract malformations/obstructions
	Infectious problems	Neonatal sepsis Meningitis Immunodeficiency syndromes (inherited and acquired) Congenital infections (TORCH) and hepatitis
	Gastrointestinal problems	Esophageal atresia and tracheoesophageal fistula Pyloric stenosis Duodenal bands or webs Intestinal atresia and stenoses Gut malrotations, duplications, and diverticula Omphalocele Gastroschisis Gastroesophageal reflux Malabsorption syndromes Bowel obstruction Failure to pass meconium Hirschsprung's disease Necrotizing enterocolitis
Childhood	Infectious diseases	Measles Mumps Varicella TB

Continued.

PAST MEDICAL HISTORY—cont'd

Childhood—cont'd	Infectious diseases—cont'd	Recent exposures or unusual travel history Sexually transmitted diseases in adolescents
	Immunization status	Routine immunization status (e.g., diphtheria-pertussis-tetanus, polio, measles-mumps-rubella, Hemophilus influenza Type b) Any special vaccinations for immunocompromised or splenectomized children (e.g., pneumococcal and meningococcal vaccines) Up-to-date complete immunization suggests that parent(s) has been compliant with routine pediatric care
	Growth and development	Percentiles documented for physical growth characteristics (weight, height, and head circumference from charts) Note normal growth or failure to thrive Appropriate psychomotor milestones or developmental delay (primarily mental, neurological, or physical disability) School performance
Hospitalizations/major illnesses		Location, reason, and when, duration of hospitalization, drugs given and response, chronicity, trauma, physical abuse, psychiatric disorders (autism, hyperactivity)

Previous surgical and anesthetic experiences		Previous operative procedures Type of anesthetic Previous blood transfusion Perioperative difficulties or complications, particularly airway problems Postoperative apnea Requirements for postoperative mechanical ventilation and/or intensive care Drug reactions
Medications		Current and past medications Responses to therapy Missed doses and compliance (Include over-the-counter medications and analgesics such as aspirin or acetaminophen, and oral contraceptives in adolescents)
Allergies/drug sensitivities		Anesthetic drugs and antibiotics which may be given perioperatively
Family history		Inherited diseases Details of anesthetic problems in blood relatives Any susceptibility to malignant hyperthermia or pseudocholinesterase deficiency
Time of last oral intake		What, how much, and when

REVIEW OF SYSTEMS

Respiratory

Asthma
Bronchiolitis
Croup
Epiglottitis
Tonsillitis
Recent upper respiratory tract infection
Nasal congestion
Pharyngitis/laryngitis
Cough
Pneumonia
History of apnea/bradycardia
Cystic fibrosis

Cardiovascular

Murmur
Palpitations
Cyanosis
Easy fatigability
Dyspnea
Peripheral edema
Hypertension
"Tetralogy spells"

Neurological

Seizures
Headache and vomiting (suggestive of elevated ICP)
Head trauma
Rhinorrhea
Otorrhea
Weakness
Spasticity
Hypotonia (suggestive of neuromuscular diseases)
Stroke
Intracranial hemorrhage
CNS malformations
CNS tumor(s)
Lead poisoning

Gastrointestinal

Reflux
Vomiting
Aspiration
Upper or lower GI bleeding
Malabsorption
Jaundice
Diarrhea
Obstructive symptoms

REVIEW OF SYSTEMS—cont'd

Renal

Pattern of urination
Time of last urination and urine specific gravity (to assess hydration status)
Urinary tract infections
Hydroureter and/or hydronephrosis
Renal failure
Dialysis
Nephritis/nephrosis
Wilms' tumor

Metabolic/endocrine

Polyuria
Polydypsia
Diabetes
Hypoglycemia
Hypothyroidism or hyperthyroidism
Inborn errors of metabolism
Neuroblastoma
Adrenal insufficiency
Steroid medications
Growth failure
Last menstrual period of adolescent females

Hematologic

Easy bleeding/easily bruised
Anemia
Iron deficiency
Sickle cell trait/disease
Thalassemia
G-6-PD deficiency
Hereditary spherocytosis
Leukemia/lymphoma
Solid tumors
Bone-marrow metastases from other malignancies
Splenectomy

Infectious

Recent upper respiratory tract infection
Pneumonia
Fever
Urinary tract infection
Meningitis
Otitis
Bacteremia/sepsis

Oral/dental

Age at eruption of teeth
Loose or missing teeth
Caries
Condition of soft and hard palates
Macroglossia
Micrognathia

PHYSICAL EXAMINATION

Vital signs	Routine	Tachycardia Bradycardia Hypotension Hypertension Hemodynamic instability Grunting Tachypnea Labored breathing Fever Four extremity blood pressures measured (in infants) Height, weight, head circumference, and percentiles for age
	Monitors	Pulse oximetry saturation Central venous pressures Intracranial pressure
General appearance	Color	Pale Cyanotic Plethoric Mottled
	Nutrition	Cachectic Obese
	Hydration	Skin turgor Mucous membranes moist or dry Tears Fontanelle/eyeballs sunken

		Edema Diaphoresis
	Distress	Does the child appear well or ill or in pain?
	Mental status/activity	Alert Active Obtunded Prostrate Sedated Neuromuscularly blocked
Head		Shape Asymmetry Size compared to age-related norms Fontanelle Sutures Craniofacial dysmorphisms, particularly of the nose, mouth, and jaw
Eyes/ears		Mongolian slant Nystagmus Strabismus "Sunset-eyes," suggestive of increased intracranial pressure Pupillary size and reactivity Active infections (e.g., conjunctivitis, otitis media)

Continued.

PHYSICAL EXAMINATION —cont'd

Nose/mouth		Patency of nares Choanal atresia Bleeding Oropharyngeal aperture Condition of soft and hard palates Dentition Size of tongue (macroglossia may predispose to difficult tracheal intubation) Adenotonsillar hypertrophy Dysmorphic mandible or maxilla (may predispose to difficult intubation)
Neck		Mobility Thyroid gland size Tracheal deviation External jugular veins for access
Chest		Shape and symmetry of the thorax Pectus excavatum Pattern and depth of spontaneous breathing Use of accessory muscles of respiration (e.g., neck muscles, intercostal retractions) Breath sounds (e.g., rales, stridor, wheezes, rhonchi, equality) Hyperresonance or dullness to percussion (may represent an emphysematous bleb or consolidation by mass or infiltrate, respectively)

Cardiovascular		Precordial bulges or heaves Palpate for the point of maximum impulse, note displacement Auscultate for S_1 and S_2, splitting of heart sounds, murmurs and their location, position in the cardiac cycle, intensity, pitch, and radiation Changes in these qualities with position, respiration, and exercise, note rubs or gallops Neck veins (distended, flat) Peripheral pulses and perfusion
Abdomen		Size Contour (scaphoid, flat, protuberant, distended) Palpate for masses, organomegaly, hernias Note tenderness and/or rigidity
Neurological		Direct examination to possible pathology indicated by history or review of systems Gait, muscle strength and symmetry of extremities, head control in infants, sensory examination to light touch, and function of cranial nerves If regional anesthetic planned, inspect back for vertebral landmarks, scoliosis/curvatures, flexibility, spina bifida or sacral dimple Review performance of child on psychomotor screening tests (e.g., Denver Developmental Screening Test, usually performed by the pediatrician

TABLE 3-1. Growth characteristics 50% for age values

	Weight (kg)		Height (cm)		Head circumference (cm)	
	male	female	male	female	male	female
Full term	3.4	3.2	51	50	35	34
1 to 6 mo	4	4	54	54	37	36
6 mo to 1 yr	8	7	68	66	44	43
1 to 2 yr	10	10	76	74	47	46
2 to 3 yr	13	12	88	86	49	48
3 to 6 yr	15-19	14-18	95-110	94-108	50	50
6 to 9 yr	21-25	20-25	116-127	115-127	52	51
9 to 12 yr	28-40	28-42	132-149	132-151	53	52
12 to 16 yr	45-62	46-56	156-173	157-163	55	54

Adapted from Hamill PVV and others: Physical growth: National Center for Health Statistics Percentiles, Am J Clin Nutr 32:607-629, 1979.

TABLE 3-2. Vital signs[1-3]

Age	HR	Systolic BP	RR
Preterm infant	120-180	40-60	55-60
Newborn	95-145	50-70	35-40
6 mo	110-180	60-110	25-30
1 to 2 yr	100-160	65-115	20-24
2 to 3 yr	90-150	75-125	16-22
3 to 5 yr	65-135	80-120	14-20
5 to 8 yr	70-115	92-120	12-20
9 to 12 yr	55-110	92-130	12-20
12 to 14 yr	55-105	100-140	10-14

PREOPERATIVE ORDERS

1. Specify NPO schedule (see Table 3-3).
2. Specify whether an IV should be established before coming to the operating room or by the anesthesiologist in the operating room, and what fluid and rate are desired.
3. Clarify what medications should be given the day of surgery, and by which route (e.g., PO with a sip of water, via NG tube, IV, rectal, etc.), and when (e.g., at 6 am; on call to the operating room).
4. Specify premedication: drug, dosage, route, and timing of administration.
5. Have vital signs recorded before coming to the operating room.
6. Give special orders (e.g., morning labs [glucose or dextrostix in prematures and neonates, spun hematocrit], and pulse oximetry saturation).
7. Obtain any special monitoring needed for transportation to the operating room (e.g., pulse oximeter, ECG, arterial/CVP waveforms, ICP monitor).
8. Request oxygen therapy for transportation.

TABLE 3-3. NPO timetable—hours NPO preinduction

Age	Milk/solids (hr)	Clear liquids (hr)
Preterm	4	2
Full term to 6 mo	6	4
6 to 36 mo	8	6
Over 36 mo	8	8

PREOPERATIVE LABORATORY EVALUATIONS

The child's age, illness, degree of debilitation, associated medical conditions, and proposed surgery are guides in deciding the extent of laboratory investigation required before safe conduct of anesthesia for that patient. Inflexible guidelines for "routine tests" are not recommended, except perhaps for a hemoglobin/hematocrit test. Further analyses that should be requested when the clinical situation dictates include the following:

1. Urinalysis
2. Serum electrolytes
3. Serum creatinine and BUN
4. Liver and/or thyroid function tests
5. Arterial blood gases
6. Pulmonary function tests
7. Chest x-ray
8. Electrocardiogram
9. Echocardiogram
10. Cardiac catheterization
11. Electroencephalogram
12. Head ultrasounds
13. Other diagnostic imaging studies such as CT, MRI, IVP, and barium studies of the GI tract

Table 3-4 provides age-related normal values for commonly requested laboratory data.

CHEST X-RAY

A chest x-ray may be useful in patients with congenital heart disease, prior thoracotomy, recent upper respiratory infection, intrathoracic masses, pneumonia, or chronic lung disease (e.g., bronchopulmonary dysplasia [BPD], cystic fibrosis, asthma, chronic aspiration). Evaluation of the radiograph should include:

1. Lung fields—air bronchograms, consolidation, foreign body, scarring, pulmonary edema
2. Costophrenic angles—pleural effusions, depth of inspiration, symmetry of diaphragmatic excursion
3. Mediastinum—thymic silhouette in infants, adenopathy
4. Heart size and shape—cardiomegaly, characteristic silhouettes for congenital heart disease
5. Pulmonary vascular markings—increased, decreased, pattern

TABLE 3-4. Common pediatric laboratory values[4-8]

Lab tests	Neonate		Infant		Child	
	Premature	Full term	1 mo	6 mo-2 yr	2-10 yr	11-15 yr
Hematologic						
Hgb g/dl	16-18	15-20	11-14	11-12	12-13	13-14
Hct %	45-47	46-62	31-41	35-36	36-37	39-40
White blood cells per mm^3 × 100	4-12	4-20	6-18	6-15	7-13	5-12
Platelets × 10^3 per mm^3	100-300	250-350	250-350	150-350	150-350	150-350
Serum chemistries						
Na^+ mEq/L	140	148	130-140	135-145	135-145	135-145
K^+ mEq/L	5.6	6.0	3.5-5.5	3.5-5.5	3.5-5.5	3.5-5.5
Cl^- mEq/L	108	102	94-105	94-105	94-105	94-105
HCO_3^- mEq/L	20	22	20-25	20-25	20-25	22-26
Total calcium mg/dl	6-10	7-12	8-11	8-11	8.5-10.5	8.5-10.5
Glucose mg/dl	40-65	40-110	60-105	60-105	60-105	60-105
BUN mg/dl	9	13	5-25	5-25	5-25	5-25
Cr mg/dl	≤0.5	≤0.5	≤0.5	0.5-0.6	0.5-0.9	0.5-1.2
Renal function						
GFR ml/min/1.73 m^2	13-58	15-60	40-60	60-120	120	120
Urine volume ml/24 hr	1-3 ml/kg/hr	15-60	250-400	500-600	600-800	800-1400
Maximal mOsm/L	400-600	400-600	400-800	1400	1400	1400
Arterial blood gases (room air)						
pH	7.35-7.39	7.38-7.41	7.35-7.45	7.35-7.45	7.35-7.45	7.35-7.45
PCO_2 mm Hg	37-44	34-35	35-45	35-45	35-45	35-45
PO_2 mm Hg	40-70	40-70	80-100	90-100	90-100	90-100
% SaO_2	90-99	90-99	95-100	95-100	95-100	95-100

6. Tracheal silhouette—diameter of airway, supraglottic or subglottic narrowing, deviation, evidence of tracheal compression

All findings should be confirmed by a radiologist skilled in the interpretation of pediatric radiographs.

THE ELECTROCARDIOGRAM IN THE PREOPERATIVE EVALUATION OF PEDIATRIC PATIENTS

The ECG should be obtained routinely in patients with known congenital heart disease, arrhythmias, electrolyte disturbances (such as are present in renal disease or bowel obstruction), or severe pulmonary disease that might predispose to cor pulmonale. The expertise of a pediatric cardiologist should be sought in its interpretation, although the following guidelines outline basic interpretation. The "three Rs" of the infant ECG are *r*apid rate, a *r*ightward QRS axis and *r*ight ventricular dominance.

Rate

With the paper speed set at 25 mm/second, each small 1-mm box represents 0.04 second, and each large 5-mm box represents 0.20 second. Regular heart rates are determined by the R-R interval between adjacent complexes (Fig. 3-1). Irregular heart rates are estimated by counting the number of complexes between 30 large boxes (6 seconds), and multiplying by 10.

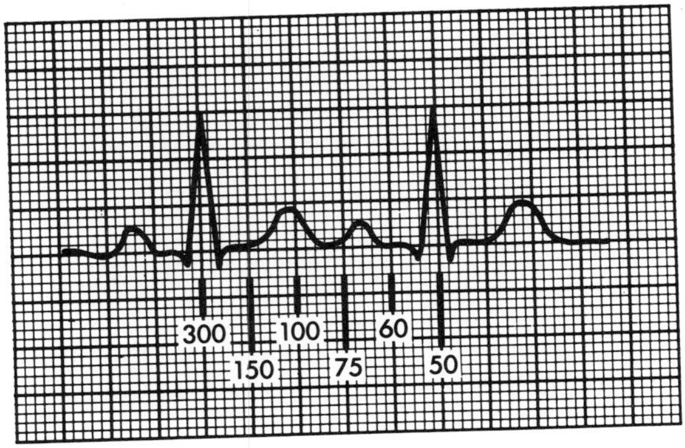

Fig. 3-1. Heart rate can be calculated by counting the number of large boxes between R-R intervals as illustrated.

Axis

To determine the frontal QRS axis (Table 3-5) the isoelectric lead is located; then the frontal axis is perpendicular to the isoelectric waveform (Fig. 3-2). A superior axis (LAD $\geq -30°$) is suggestive of serious congenital heart lesions such as double outlet right ventricle with ventriculoseptal defect, tricuspid atresia, transposition of the great vessels, and endocardial cushion defects.

Intervals

The P-R, QRS, and Q-T intervals should be determined and compared to the normal values given in Tables 3-6 and 3-7 and the box on p. 69. Heart

TABLE 3-5. Frontal QRS axis

Age	Mean	Range
0 to 24 hr	(+) 135	90-180
1 to 7 days	125	80-160
8 to 30 days	110	60-160
1 to 3 mo	80	40-120
3 to 6 mo	65	20- 90
6 to 12 mo	65	0-100
1 to 3 yr	55	20-100
3 to 5 yr	60	15- 90
5 to 8 yr	65	20-100
8 to 12 yr	65	20-100
12 to 16 yr	65	20-100

Adapted from Rowe PC, editor: Harriet Lane handbook, ed 11, Chicago, 1987, Year Book Medical Publishers, Inc.

Sachs EJ: Pediatric cardiology for the house officer, Baltimore, 1987, Williams & Wilkins.

TABLE 3-6. Maximum PR interval*

Age	Heart rate					
	< 70	71-90	91-110	111-130	131-150	151+
< 1 mo	–	–	0.11	0.11	0.11	0.11
1 to 9 mo	–	–	0.14	0.13	0.12	0.11
10 to 24 mo	–	–	0.15	0.14	0.14	0.10
3 to 5 yr	–	0.16	0.16	0.16	–	–
6 to 13 yr	0.18	0.18	0.16	0.16	–	–

*PR interval ≥ 0.20 second = first degree atrioventricular block.
Adapted from Rowe PC, editor: Harriet Lane handbook, ed 11, Chicago, 1987, Year Book Medical Publishers, Inc.

QRS INTERVAL

0.03 – 0.08 second

Adapted from Rowe PC, editor: Harriet Lane handbook, ed 11, Chicago, 1987, Year Book Medical Publishers, Inc.

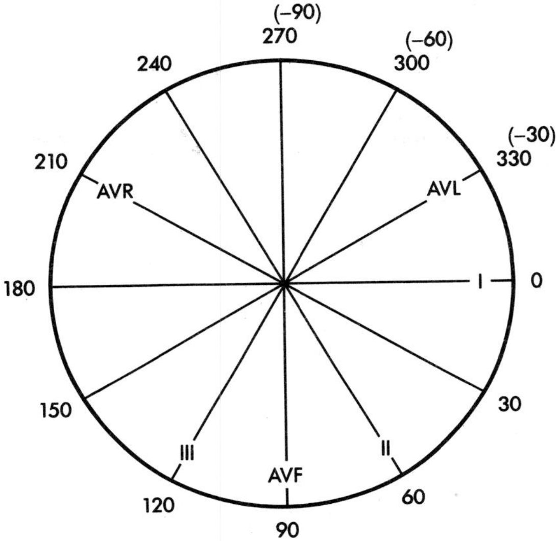

Fig. 3-2. Frontal (QRS) axis is located perpendicularly to the isoelectric waveform.

TABLE 3-7. QRS interval: maximum

Heart rate	Maximum Q-T*
300	0.19-0.20
250	0.20-0.22
150	0.25-0.28
125	0.28-0.30
100	0.31-0.34
88	0.33-0.36
75	0.36-0.39
60	0.40-0.44
50	0.44-0.48

$$*\text{Q-T corrected} = \frac{\text{measured Q-T interval}}{\sqrt{\text{RR interval}}}$$

QTC should not be $\geq$ 0.425 second

Adapted from Rowe PC, editor: Harriet Lane handbook, ed 11, Chicago, 1987, Year Book Medical Publishers, Inc.

blocks, preexcitation syndromes, acid-base disturbances, abnormalities of calcium metabolism, and drug effects of digoxin, quinidine, disopyramide, or β-agonists, may all be reflected in abnormalities of these intervals.

Rhythm

1. The presence of sinus rhythm usually can be confirmed by assessing P waves, and the relationship of P waves to QRS complexes should determine the pattern of atrioventricular conduction.
2. Unusual complex morphology with an irregular rhythm often indicates premature atrial or ventricular beats.
3. Potentially dangerous rhythms such as atrial fibrillation, atrial flutter, supraventricular tachycardia, junctional rhythms, second- or third-degree heart block, idioventricular rhythms, ventricular tachycardia, and ventricular fibrillation should be recognized immediately, investigated, and treated.

Morphology

The P wave, QRS complex, and T wave all have characteristic morphologies in standard leads, and any aberrations should be noted. Ventricular hypertrophy should be confirmed by standard charts that compare R and S wave amplitude and patient age.

REFERENCES

1. Ingelfinger JR, Powers L, and Epstein MF: Blood pressure norms in low–birthweight infants: Birth through four weeks. Pediatr Res 17:319A, 1983.
2. Kendig EL and Chernick V, editors: Disorders of the respiratory tract in children, Philadelphia, 1983, WB Saunders Co.
3. Nelson WE, editor: Textbook of pediatrics, ed 13, Philadelphia, 1987, WB Saunders Co.
4. Acharya PT and Payne WW: Blood chemistry of normal full-term infants in the first 48 hours of life, Arch Dis Child 40:430, 1965.
5. Meites S, editor: Pediatric clinical chemistry, ed 2, Washington, DC, 1981, The American Association for Clinical Chemistry.
6. Nathan D and Oski F: Hematology of infancy and childhood, Philadelphia, 1981, WB Saunders Co.
7. Royer P: Pediatric nephrology, Philadelphia, 1974, WB Saunders Co.
8. Thomas JL and Reichelderfer T: Premature infants: analysis of serum during the first seven weeks, Clin Chem 14:272, 1968.

ADDITIONAL READINGS

Park MK and Guntheroth WG: How to read pediatric ECGs, Chicago, 1987, Chicago Year Book Medical Publishers, Inc.

Sachs EJ: Pediatric cardiology for the house officer, Baltimore, 1987, Williams & Wilkins.

4

PREMEDICATION

Boonsri Kosarussavadi

One pill makes you taller
and one pill makes you small
And the ones that mother gives you
don't do anything at all.
GRACE SLICK
WHITE RABBIT

LEGEND OF FREQUENT ABBREVIATIONS FOR ROUTES OF ADMINISTRATION

IM = intramuscular
PO = per os (by mouth)
PR = per rectum
IV = intravenous
IN = intranasal
OT = oral transmucosal

GOALS OF PREMEDICATION

The primary goals of premedication in children are to facilitate a smooth separation from the parents and to ease the induction of anesthesia. Other effects that may be achieved by pharmacologic preparation of the patient include:

1. Providing amnesia
2. Providing analgesia
3. Prevention of physiologic stress (e.g., avoiding hypoxia in patients with cyanotic congenital heart disease)
4. Reduction of anesthetic requirements
5. Decreasing the probability of aspiration of acidic stomach contents
6. Vagolysis
7. Decreasing salivation and secretions
8. Antiemesis

TABLE 4-1. Premedications by route given

Intramuscular (IM)	Intranasal (IN)	By mouth (PO)	Rectal (PR)
Barbiturates		**Barbiturates**	**Barbiturates**
Pentobarbital Secobarbital	—	Pentobarbital Secobarbital	Pentobarbital Secobarbital Methohexital
Narcotics	**Narcotics**	**Narcotics**	
Morphine Meperidine	Sufentanil	Fentanyl (trans-mucosal)	—
Benzodiazepines	**Benzodiazepines**	**Benzodiazepines**	**Benzodiazepines**
Diazepam Midazolam	Midazolam	Diazepam Midazolam	Diazepam Midazolam
Dissociative anesthetic	**Dissociative anesthetic**	**Dissociative anesthetic**	**Dissociative anesthetic**
Ketamine	Ketamine	Ketamine	Ketamine
Antihistamines		**Antihistamines**	
Hydroxyzine	—	Hydroxyzine	—
Anticholinergics			
Atropine Scopolamine Glycopyrrolate	—	—	—
		H_2 antagonists/ gastric motility stimulants	
—	—	Cimetidine Ranitidine Metoclopramide	—

CONSIDERATIONS FOR PREMEDICATION

1. Should the drug be given as a premedication, or would the drug effect be achieved more predictably by intravenous injection? (e.g., atropine IM premedication *versus* IV preintubation. Is sufficient time predictably available for the drug to achieve the desired effect? Given a sufficiently large dose and enough time to work (60 to 90 minutes), most drugs will be effective.
2. Does the patient have any contraindications to receiving a sedative, such as altered mental status, increased intracranial pressure, a difficult airway, compromised respiratory function, or hypovolemia?
3. What route of administration (Table 4-1) will achieve the desired effect most effectively and be most acceptable to patient and parent?

4. Is the patient and/or parent able to participate in this decision? (e.g., selecting IM or PO).
5. Do the negative effects of the drug, such as respiratory or cardiovascular depression, tachycardia, or sedation lasting beyond the operation outweigh the relative benefits of the premedication?
6. Has the child's age been considered? Infants less than 6 months of age can be separated easily from their parents by cuddling, keeping them warm, and allowing them to suck a pacifier. The more difficult airway and decreased respiratory reserve present in this age group further add to the downside of using premedication.

Conversely, patients who probably will benefit from premedication include:

1. Toddlers and preschoolers in whom separation anxiety is paramount
2. Adolescents who are particularly sensitive about body image and loss of control
3. Patients with previous unpleasant hospital experiences
4. Patients who are unable to communicate or cooperate (e.g., mentally retarded)

BARBITURATES

Pentobarbital or Secobarbital

Pentobarbital or secobarbital produce sedation with minimal cardiovascular and respiratory depression and rarely cause nausea or vomiting. They have a bitter taste when taken by mouth and can cause persistent pain at the injection site if given by intramuscular injection. Paradoxical responses (agitation and disorientation instead of sedation) are not uncommon in children.

Dose: pentobarbital or secobarbital	2 to 3 mg/kg PO
	2 to 4 mg/kg PR
	3 to 4 mg/kg IM

Methohexital

Methohexital is an excellent agent for premedication/induction when given per rectum through a well-lubricated red rubber catheter. The child can be allowed to fall asleep in the parent's arms, which greatly reduces separation anxiety. Sedation occurs in 4 to 8 minutes and lasts 30 to 40 minutes. The anesthesiologist should be in attendance throughout the induction in an area well-equipped with suction and resuscitative equipment. Methohexital does not produce significant cardiovascular or respiratory depression. Dilution to a 10% solution may cause sufficient rectal irritation to precipitate defecation. For repeated administration (i.e., daily radiation therapy) a more dilute solution should be used to avoid proctitis.

Dose: methohexital 1% to 10% solution 20 to 30 mg/kg PR

NARCOTICS

Morphine or Meperidine

Morphine or meperidine given intramuscularly produce both analgesia and sedation. However, narcotics are potent respiratory depressants and can cause nausea, vomiting, pruritus, and dysphoria. In combination with barbiturates and/or scopolamine they produce excellent sedation and amnesia, particularly for patients with cyanotic congenital heart disease.

Dose:	morphine	0.1 to 0.2 mg/kg IM
	meperidine	1 to 2 mg/kg IM

Fentanyl

Fentanyl's lipid solubility makes it an ineffective premedication parenterally. However, oral transmucosal absorption in the form of the lollipop reportedly has produced good results.[1] It causes pruritus of the nose and eyes in most patients; postoperative nausea and vomiting is common. Administration of fentanyl lollipops potentially may increase gastric volume as well. Oxygen saturation is slightly but significantly lower (SaO_2 94%) in patients receiving oral transmucosal fentanyl.[2]

Dose: fentanyl 15 to 20 μg/kg OT

Sufentanil

Sufentanil has been given intranasally as a premedication.[3] Within 10 minutes of administration the patient should feel calm, cooperative, possibly euphoric, and easily separated from the parents. The majority of patients will have an oxygen saturation of less than 95%.[4] There is a high incidence of apnea and laryngospasm.[5]

Dose: sufentanil 1.5 to 3 μg/kg IN

BENZODIAZEPINES

Diazepam

Diazepam is given to allay anxiety and produce amnesia with minimal respiratory or cardiovascular depression. It rarely causes nausea or vomiting. Absorption from the gastrointestinal tract is more predictable than the intramuscular route. It also can be administered rectally. Paradoxical excitement and lack of inhibition often occur, particularly at lower doses. Onset is slow and duration of action long.

Dose: diazepam 0.1 to 0.5 mg PO, PR, IM

Midazolam

Midazolam produces similar effects to diazepam but with shorter duration. Given enterally it undergoes extensive first-pass hepatic extraction, so that the intranasal route may have a more predictable onset and effect.[6] Unlike most other benzodiazepines the intramuscular absorption of midazolam is reliable. It can be given per rectum, although this route may be objectionable to older children.

Dose: midazolam	0.2 mg/kg IN
	0.5 to 0.75 mg/kg PO[7]
	0.08 to 0.5 mg/kg IM
	0.3 to 1 mg/kg PR[8]

DISSOCIATIVE ANESTHETIC

Ketamine

Ketamine is used as a premedication/induction agent. It is the only rapidly acting agent that can be given intramuscularly, usually causing loss of consciousness in less than 5 minutes. It is very useful for extremely uncooperative patients. It stimulates the cardiovascular system (increasing heart rate and blood presure). It preserves airway reflexes, but secretions, blood, or gastric regurgitant can trigger laryngospasm. An antisialagogue should be given simultaneously to minimize secretions. Parents should be apprised of the appearance of the dissociative state produced by ketamine. The incidence of psychological sequelae from a single induction dose of ketamine is uncommon.

Dose: ketamine	2 to 5 mg/kg IM
	6 mg/kg PO[9]
	3 mg/kg IN[5]
	8 to 10 mg/kg PR

HYPNOTICS

Chloral Hydrate and Triclofos

Chloral hydrate and triclofos are converted in the body to trichloroethanol, an active hypnotic agent. These agents are relatively safe even in infants, producing minimal respiratory depression. Consequently they are used frequently by nonanesthesiologists when a child needs sedation. Chloral hydrate is the least palatable oral premedication and can cause gastric irritation.

Dose: chloral hydrate	25 to 50 mg/kg PO
triclofos	70 mg/kg PO

ANTIHISTAMINE

Hydroxyzine

Hydroxyzine produces mild sedation with antiemetic, antihistaminic, and antispasmodic effects. Sedation effects in combination with narcotics are additive.

Dose: hydroxyzine	0.5 to 1 mg/kg PO, IM

ANTICHOLINERGICS

Current inhalation anesthetics do not stimulate salivary or tracheobronchial secretions. Therefore, premedication with anticholinergic drugs is not routinely indicated, and may cause fever, confusion, flushing, or an extremely dry mouth. It can be given during the operative procedure for its antisialagogue effect (e.g., oral surgery, airway manipulation), or vagolysis (e.g., traction on peritoneum, strabismus surgery, or preceding succinylcholine administration). Atropine is a better vagolytic agent than scopolamine, however, scopolamine produces amnesia and a better drying effect. Glycopyrrolate is the only agent that does not cross the blood brain barrier, so it does not cause confusion. It is also more potent and its effect lasts longer than atropine.

Dose:	atropine	0.02 mg/kg IM, PO
		0.01 mg/kg IV
	scopolamine	0.02 mg/kg IM
		0.01 mg/kg IV
	glycopyrrolate	0.01 mg/kg IV, IM

H_2 ANTAGONISTS/GASTRIC MOTILITY STIMULANTS

Seventy-five percent of fasting children have a gastric volume greater than 0.4 ml/kg, a pH less than 2.5, and are therefore at risk of developing acid aspiration syndrome following inhalation of gastric contents. H_2 antagonists directly elevate gastric pH; metoclopramide decreases gastric fluid volume. This combination is effective when given by mouth 4 hours before operating.[10] These drugs usually are indicated in patients with gastrointestinal disorders.

H_2 antagonists dose:	cimetidine	7.5 mg/kg, PO IV
	ranitidine	2 mg/kg PO
		0.5 to 1 mg/kg IV
Gastric stimulants dose:	metoclopramide	0.1 mg/kg PO, IV

COMBINATIONS

The use of drug combinations has become very popular, particularly to ensure that the desired sedative effects will be achieved. Any of the following combinations can be given with atropine 0.02 mg/kg IM or PO.

Commonly used combinations include the following:

Narcotic and Barbiturate

1. Demerol 3 mg/kg + pentobarbital 4 mg/kg PO[11]
2. Morphine 0.1 to 0.2 mg/kg + secobarbital 4 mg/kg IM

Narcotic and Antihistamine

1. Demerol 1 mg/kg + hydroxyzine 0.5 mg/kg PO/IM
2. Morphine 0.1 mg/kg + hydroxyzine 0.5 mg/kg IM

Narcotic and Phenothiazine

1. Demerol 1 mg/kg or morphine 0.1 mg/kg + promethazine 0.5 mg/kg IM

Narcotic and Anticholinergics

1. Morphine 0.1 to 0.2 mg/kg + scopolamine 0.02 mg/kg IM

Narcotic and Benzodiazepine

1. Demerol 1.5 mg/kg + diazepam 0.2 mg/kg PO[12]

SUMMARY

See Table 4-2 for a summary of premedication pharmacology.

TABLE 4-2. Premedication pharmacology

Category/medication	Dosage/route	Onset	Elimination half-life	Side effects/contraindications
Barbiturates				
Pentobarbital or Secobarbital	2-3 mg/kg PO 2-4 mg/kg PR 3-5 mg/kg IM	60-90 min	17-50 hr	May cause paradoxical reaction; Bitter taste when taken PO; May cause persistent pain at IM injection site; Contraindicated in porphyria
Methohexital	20-30 mg/kg PR	4-8 min	1.5-4 hr	Unpredictable systemic bioavailability; May cause rectal irritation or defecation; Contraindicated in temporal lobe epilepsy or porphyria
Narcotics				
Morphine	0.1-0.2 mg/kg IM	45 min	2-4 hr	Potent respiratory depressant; May cause pruritis, nausea, vomiting
Meperidine	1-2 mg/kg IM	45 min	3-4 hr	
Fentanyl lollipop	15-20 μg/kg OT	5-20 min	3-3.5 hr	High incidence of itchy nose preoperatively; May cause respiratory depression, nausea, vomiting
Sufentanil	1.5-3 μg/kg IN	7.5 min	148 min	Profound respiratory depression (resuscitative equipment and personnel must be present); Can cause poor chest compliance, apnea, laryngospasm during anesthesia

Continued.

TABLE 4-2. Premedication pharmacology—cont'd

Category/medication	Dosage/route	Onset	Elimination half-life	Side effects/contraindications
Benzodiazepines				
Diazepam	0.1-0.5 mg/kg PO, PR, IM	60-90 min	21-37 hr	Slow onset and prolonged action; Insufficient doses may cause disinhibition and decrease patient cooperation
Midazolam	0.5-0.75 mg/kg PO 0.08-0.3 mg/kg IM 0.3-1 mg/kg PR 0.2 mg/kg IN	15-30 min 10 min 10 min 10 min	1-4 hr	May cause respiratory depression particularly in combination with narcotics
Dissociative anesthetic				
Ketamine	2-5 mg/kg IM 6 mg/kg PO 3 mg/kg IN 8-10 mg PR	30-40 sec 10 min <30 min 10 min	1-2 hr	Contraindicated in patients with increased intracranial pressure; Increases heart rate and blood pressure (not reported with oral routes); Accumulation of pharyngeal secretions may cause laryngospasm
Hypnotics				
Chloral hydrate	25-50 mg/kg PO	1-2 hr	8 hr	Gastric irritation
Triclofos	70 mg/kg PO	1-2 hr	8 hr	
Antihistamines				
Hydroxyzine	0.5-1 mg/kg PO, IM	1 hr	3 hr	Unpredictable level of sedation

Anticholinergics				
Atropine	0.02 mg/kg IM, PO 0.01 mg/kg IV	30 min 2-4 min	2-3 hr	Can cause fever, extremely dry mouth, flushing, tachycardia
Scopolamine	0.02 mg/kg IM 0.01 mg/kg IV	30 min 5 min	Decreased salivation—4-6 hr; Amnesia 2 hr; Mydriasis 8 hr	May cause confusion
Glycopyrrolate	0.01 mg/kg IV 0.01 mg/kg IM	1 min 15-30 min	Vagolytic effect 2-3 hr; Decreased salivation 7 hr	No CNS effects
H_2 antagonists				
Cimetidine	7.5 mg/kg PO, IV	60-90 min	1.5-2 hr	Decreases hepatic extraction of propranolol, diphenylhydantoin, diazepam; Avoid use in patients with thrombocytopenia, neutropenia
Ranitidine	2 mg/kg PO (given 4 hr preoperatively) 0.5-1 mg/kg IV	30-60 min	2-3 hr	Does not alter hepatic extraction of drugs; Fewer side effects than cimetidine
Gastric motility stimulants				
Metoclopramide	0.1 mg/kg PO (given 4 hr preoperatively) 0.1 mg/kg IV	40-120 min 15-30 min	2-4 hr	A single recommended dose does not cause extrapyramidal symptoms; Contraindicated in gastrointestinal obstruction and pheochromocytoma

REFERENCES

1. Streisand JB and others: Oral transmucosal fentanyl premedication in children, Anesth Analg 66:S170, 1987.
2. Ashburn MA and others: Clinical evaluation of oral transmucosal fentanyl citrate, OTFC, for use as a premedication in pediatric outpatient surgery, Anesthesiology 71:A1172, 1989.
3. Henderson JM and others: Preinduction of anesthesia in pediatric patients with nasally administered sufentanil, Anesthesiology 68:671-75, 1988.
4. Karl HW and others: Nasal midazolam or sufentanil for preinduction of anesthesia in pediatric patients: implications for intraoperative management, Anesthesiology 71:A1169, 1989.
5. Tasi SK, Wei CF, and Mok MS: Intranasal ketamine vs sufentanil as premedication in children, Anesthesiology 71:A1173, 1989.
6. Wilton NCT and others: Preanesthetic sedation of preschool children using intranasal midazolam, Anesthesiology 69:972-75, 1988.
7. Feld LH, Negus JB, and White PF: Oral midazolam: optimal dose for pediatric premedication, Anesthesiology 71:A1054, 1989.
8. Yaster M and others: Rectally administered midazolam for preinduction of anesthesia in children, Anesthesiology 71:A1043, 1989.
9. Gutstein HB and others: Oral ketamine premedication in children, Anesthesiology 71:A1176, 1989.
10. Lerman J, Christensen SK, and Farrow-Gillespie AC: Effects of metoclopramide and ranitidine on gastric fluid pH and volume in children, Anesthesiology 69:A748, 1988.
11. Nicolson SC and others: Comparison of oral and intramuscular preanesthetic medication for pediatric inpatient surgery, Anesthesiology 71:8-10, 1989.
12. Brzustowicz RM and others: Efficacy of oral premedication for pediatric outpatient surgery, Anesthesiology 60:475-77, 1984.

5

PEDIATRIC EQUIPMENT AND MONITORING

Richard A. DuBose

Martin knew monsters who crawled near his bed
They tickled his ankles and circled his head.
There were deep-throated dragons and silver snakes,
And they put him to sleep and kept him awake.

One day Martin listened and thought that he heard
In the monsters' strange language a kind-hearted word.
They were there for his comfort and to help him to mend
And Martin's old monsters became Martin's new friends.
RIVIAN BELL

The success of a pediatric procedure depends not only on the skill and knowledge of the anesthesiologist, but also on the possession and utilization of the proper equipment. The same method of pediatric anesthesia setup should be employed each time to avoid overlooking critical items and to ensure that all equipment is functioning properly. The mnemonic SCOMLADI serves this purpose and is easy to remember:

S = *S*uction
C = *C*ircuits
O = *O*xygen
M = *M*onitors
L = *L*aryngoscope
A = *A*irways
D = *D*rugs
I = *I*ntravenous equipment

SUCTION

Small flexible suction catheters should be used in conjunction with small endotracheal tubes. Numbers 8 and 10 French suction catheters are available commercially. A number 5 French feeding tube may be used for 2.5-mm endotracheal tubes. A large Yankauer-tip catheter should always be readily available in case of vomiting.

CIRCUITS

Circuits commonly used for children under 12 to 15 kg include Mapleson D, Bain, Jackson-Rees modification of an Ayre's T-piece, and a pediatric circle (Table 5-1).

The circuits used for pediatrics are designed specifically to:

a. Decrease the resistance to breathing by eliminating valves
b. Decrease the amount of dead space in the circuit
c. Help somewhat to decrease the amount of heat loss by means of a coaxial circuit with warm exhaled gas surrounding the fresh gas inflow

1. Semiopen systems (Mapleson) require high fresh gas flows to prevent rebreathing of exhaled gases. Several different methods of calculating fresh gas flow (FGF) exist, as follows:
   a. FGF = 2½ to 3 times minute ventilation
      Minute ventilation = 150 ml × kg
      or
      = Tidal volume (V_T) × Respiratory rate (RR)
   b. FGF = 1000 ml + 100 ml/kg
   c. FGF = minimum of 3 L/min for all children
2. The reservoir bag should contain a volume similar to that of the child's vital capacity. Use of the appropriate size is important; appropriate sizes, based on age, follow:

Age	Reservoir bag
Newborn	0.5 L
1-3 yr	1.0 L
3-5 yr	2.0 L
>5 yr	3.0 L

   The compliance of a child's respiratory system makes it more susceptible than an adult's to barotrauma caused by higher pressures and volumes in a reservoir bag that is too large.
3. Humidification is required when a nonrebreathing circuit is used to prevent excessive heat loss (high flows of cold gas can rapidly cool a small child), and to keep airway secretions moist. A small pediatric humidivent may be used for short procedures. A heated humidifier is necessary for longer procedures. Airway temperatures should not exceed 32° C. Condensed water should be drained periodically from the circuit. Fresh water drowning can result from obstruction of the endotracheal tube and airway by water.

OXYGEN

Oxygen must be available from more than one source and its availability checked before each procedure.

1. Wall oxygen delivered at 50 psi should be connected to the anesthesia machine and ventilator.

TABLE 5-1. Types of circuits: advantages and disadvantages

Circuit		Advantages	Disadvantages
Mapleson D (semiopen)	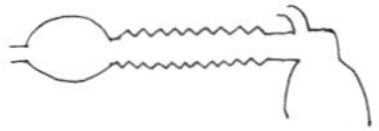	• Valveless (less work of breathing) • Minimal dead space • Short time constant for more rapid induction	• Requires high fresh gas flows • Increases heat and moisture loss • Breath sounds are often obscured by water condensation in tubing • Requires understanding of principles of nonrebreathing circuit
Bain (semiopen)	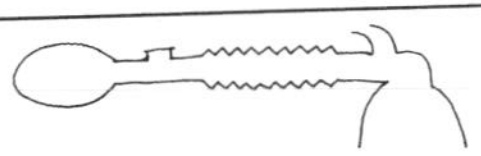	• Valveless (less work of breathing) • Minimal dead space • Compact, lightweight • Theoretically conserves heat because inspired gas tubing is surrounded by exhaled gas • Short time constant	• High fresh gas flows • Heat and moisture losses still occur • Cracks in coaxial tubing lead to re-breathing of expired gases • Requires understanding of principles of nonrebreathing circuit
Modified Ayre's T-piece (semiopen)	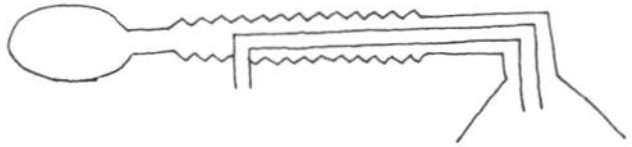	• Simplicity • Valveless • Less dead space • Short time constant	• Bulky because the reservoir bag is close to the airway • Requires high fresh gas flows • Heat and moisture loss
Pediatric circle (semiclosed)	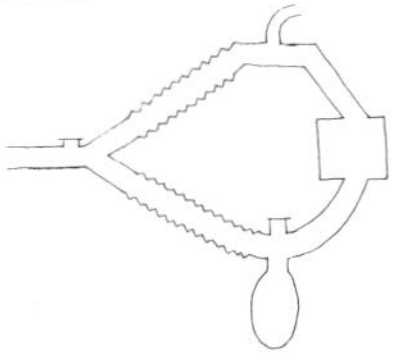	• Simplicity • Familiar system • No need to disassemble anesthesia machine for setup	• CO_2 absorber creates resistance • Valves create resistance and can malfunction

a. Oxygen via flow meters will be delivered at low pressure because of reducing values in the anesthesia machine.
b. Oxygen from the fresh gas inlet will flow at a rate of 35 to 75 L/min, depending upon the machine. Flushing the pediatric circuit with these flows can result in barotrauma.

2. A full oxygen reserve tank should be attached to every anesthesia machine and checked before each procedure. A free-standing E-tank with separate circuit is recommended for backup (e.g., power failure) and for transport.

MONITORS

The American Society of Anesthesiologists (ASA) put forth its standards of monitoring in 1986, and many states have followed with specific requirements (such as for oximetry and/or capnometry), which are rapidly becoming de facto standards as well. Monitoring standards must be age appropriate not only for the size of the patient but also for the specific physiologic factors of children (e.g., temperature monitoring in the neonate is more critical than ischemia monitoring). To limit morbidity, it is important that as much information as possible be obtained from noninvasive monitors.

Stethoscope

A precordial stethoscope is placed before induction and continuously monitors heart rate, quality of the heart tones, and breath sounds. It is placed over the left chest to optimize heart sounds and to help detect endobronchial intubation (more commonly, into the right main stem bronchus).

A regular stethoscope, preferably with a neonatal attachment, should always be available for auscultation.

ECG

ECG Capabilities

Although it is not specifically a monitor of cardiac output, the ECG has always been used to roughly estimate heart function, or cardiac output, the product of stroke volume and heart rate. The presence of ischemia in the adult compromises contractility and consequently stroke volume, making the detection of ischemia a valuable indicator of cardiac output. In the infant, however, stroke volume is fixed, and cardiac output is determined more by heart rate. Continuous monitoring of the pediatric ECG provides a determination of heart rate and rhythm abnormalities and of alterations in configuration of the complex.

Heart rate

1. The rapid heart rates of children (up to 3 or 4 Hz or 180 to 240 beats/min) require that the ECG have a digital rate meter with adjustable gain to eliminate artifact.
2. The T waves in infants are much larger, because the electrodes are situated much closer to the heart, and may be of the same amplitude as the QRS. This can lead to erroneous counting of heart rates, or double counting. The ability to remove this artifact is helpful.

Rhythm abnormalities

1. Monitoring lead II provides the best P wave configuration to help with dysrhythmia detection.
2. Variable sweep controls the speed at which the ECG is recorded. The standard speed for adults is 25 mm/sec, but faster rates are necessary for the rhythm analysis of children because they have more rapid heart rates. Rates of 50 mm/sec or 100 mm/sec will enable P-R, Q-T interval interpretation and arrhythmia detection.[1]

ECG complex configuration

1. Changes in the P wave or QRS configuration are usually the result of dysrhythmias.
2. Use of the monitor mode implies the presence of a low pass filter, which minimizes motion and respiratory artifact, high-frequency noise, baseline drift, and 60-Hz interference. It also distorts the S-T segment.[2]
3. To accurately determine if S-T segment changes are present, the diagnostic mode must be used.
4. S-T changes may indicate electrolyte imbalance (potassium and calcium), ischemia, pericarditis, or myocarditis or may represent nonpathologic early repolarization (J point elevation).[3]

Lead Placement

1. Leads placed on extremities (shoulders, thighs) will result in less movement artifact from breathing.
2. Smaller leads generate a higher current density in the presence of electrosurgical units (cautery), which can result in burns, particularly in older ECG units with grounded reference electrodes.
3. Leads should not be placed on bony protuberances.
4. To avoid trauma to fragile ribs, snap-on electrodes should be snapped to the lead before being stuck to the chest.
5. Leads for preterm infants should be changed as infrequently as possible to avoid skin trauma.
6. Leads placed on the nipple bud of preterm infants may cause permanent damage on removal.

Blood Pressure

Noninvasive Monitoring

Noninvasive measurement of blood pressure may be obtained in the following ways.

Auscultation. A blood pressure cuff and stethoscope are secured to the child's arm. The cuff is manually inflated and Korotkoff's sounds auscultated as the cuff is deflated 2 to 3 mm Hg at a time.

Oscillation. The systolic blood pressure is the pressure at which oscillations, or "bounces," of the needle occur on the manometer after the cuff is deflated.

Doppler. An ultrasound transducer is placed over an artery, distal to the blood pressure cuff. Systolic pressure is recorded when the sound of pulsatile flow is first appreciated.

Distal flow detection. Similar in use to the doppler, several other detectors of blood flow may be placed distal to the blood pressure cuff. Palpation, a

TABLE 5-2. Complications of arterial catheters

Complications	Comments
Hematoma	• More common if vessel is transfixed during cannulation. • Transfixation is not advised in small children.
Infection	• Seen when catheters are left in place for more than 4 days.[5]
Ischemia	• 51% of all children will have distal ischemia after percutaneous placement; the vessel will recanalize within 7 to 14 days.[6]
Embolization	• Retrograde embolization into the central circulation has occurred with aggressive flushing. Gentle flushing of the catheter by hand with a syringe is advised.[7]
NEC Renovascular hypertension Leg ischemia	• 95% of all umbilical artery catheters demonstrate clot formation.[8]

plethysmograph, and an oximeter probe are some of the more common techniques used.

Size of Cuff

1. The size of the blood pressure cuff must be correct for accurate readings. Use of too small a cuff is the number one cause of hypertension in children.[4] Several different cuff sizes should be available from which to select.
2. The bladder of the cuff should cover at least one half the circumference of the arm.
3. A cuff of the correct width will cover two thirds of the length of the upper arm (or will be 20% greater than the arm's diameter).

Invasive Monitoring

1. Placement of an intraarterial catheter is requisite for invasive monitoring of blood pressure. The use of nontapered teflon catheters (e.g., Jelco, Angiocath) is recommended.
2. A 22-gauge catheter is recommended for children under 5 years, and a 20 gauge for children over 5 years. The use of smaller catheters will provide greater accuracy and quality of monitoring but may be impractical for blood drawing purposes, often another important factor in placing the monitor. Larger catheters may predispose to distal ischemia (Table 5-2).
3. Because of intrauterine ductal presence, the site of the intraarterial catheter is highly important.
4. Preductal placement of an arterial catheter is optimal for:
   a. Infants with a patent ductus arteriosus (PDA)
   b. Coarctation repair
   c. Diaphragmatic hernia repair

5. The right radial artery is used for preductal monitoring. Use of the temporal arteries is not advised because of the possibility of cerebral hemispheric infarct if ischemia occurs.
6. The most commonly used arteries in children include the following:
   a. Radial
   b. Dorsalis pedis
   c. Posterior tibial
   d. Ulnar
   e. Axillary and femoral
   f. Umbilical (used in premature and newborn infants because of its accessibility)

Temperature

Temperature monitoring is crucial with children because they are more prone to heat loss than adults, the consequences of hypothermia are greater, and they have a higher incidence of malignant hyperthermia (1 per 15,000).

Methods of Monitoring Temperature

Thermistors. A thermistor is a thermal sensitive resistor placed in soft plastic tubing.
Thermocouples. Thermocouples are used for tympanic membrane monitoring.
Liquid crystal thermometers. Liquid crystal thermometers are placed on the forehead.

Preferred Sites for Temperature Monitoring

1. Core temperature is best recorded from within the distal third of the esophagus, rectum, or nasopharynx. Probes misplaced in the oropharynx or hypopharynx will record artificially low temperatures.
2. Rectal probes are not recommended in children under 3 kg because they may easily traumatize rectal mucosa. A nasopharyngeal probe may cause epistaxis.
3. Liquid crystal thermometers placed on the skin are noninvasive and allow temperatures to be easily monitored from induction onward. Although temperature readings are usually 3° C below core, trends can be followed.

Equipment for Maintaining Normothermia

Because the consequences of hypothermia are significant in the infant (see "Metabolism (Heat Production)" in Chapter 2 on p. 23), it is imperative that equipment to maintain the child's core temperature be readily available. This equipment includes the following:

1. Radiant heat lamps
2. Heating blanket on the operating table
3. Humidifier
4. Blood warmer
5. Variable thermostat to warm room temperature
6. Hats, plastic wrap for limbs, warm blankets, and irrigating solutions

Oximetry

Indications

Use of the oximeter is particularly important in pediatrics because of the greater tendency of the infant to develop a shunt with rapid desaturation and hypoxemia (because of low functional residual capacity, high closing capacity, and greater O_2 consumption). Care of critical infants requires the ability to closely follow arterial saturation in order to treat respiratory distress syndrome and congenital heart disease with minimal complications from oxygen usage (e.g., retrolental fibroplasia).

Characteristics

1. Pulse oximetry only *measures* functional hemoglobin:

$$\frac{\text{oxyhemoglobin (oxyHgb)}}{\text{oxyHgb} + \text{deoxyHgb}}$$

2. No oximeters can measure fractional hemoglobin:

$$\frac{\text{oxyHgb}}{\text{oxyHgb} + \text{deoxyHgb} + \text{dysHgb}}$$

3. Since most people have some percentage of dyshemoglobin (carboxyHgb, metHgb, sulfHgb, etc.), some oximeters *calculate* in a small percentage of dyshemoglobin to more closely approximate fractional hemoglobin.
4. Oxygen saturation in patients with large amounts of dyshemoglobin (e.g., burn patients with large percentages of carboxyhemoglobin, sickle cell patients) should be determined by cooximetry.
5. The presence of fetal hemoglobin or hemoglobin F will not interfere with the accuracy of pulse oximetry.
6. Table 5-3 lists sources of inaccurate saturations obtained from pulse oximetry.

Gas Monitoring

Capnometry

The measurement of CO_2 is mandated by law in some states (e.g., New York) for all patients under general anesthesia. The ASA strongly supports the use of capnometry.

1. Techniques of measuring CO_2 include the following:
   a. Infrared analysis
   b. Mass spectrometry
   c. Raman scattering
2. Adult flow-through devices for measurement are bulky, can increase dead space, and can easily cause circuit disconnections. Pediatric sampling chambers are smaller, have minimal dead space, and are reusable.
3. Side-stream or aspirated gas samples are affected by several factors:
   a. The size of the patient. The most accurate sampling of gas in children under 12 kg is thought to be from a distal port on the endotracheal tube.

TABLE 5-3. Sources of inaccurate saturations obtained from pulse oximetry

Type of interference	Cause	Solution
Excessive ambient light	• Operating room lights • Bilirubin lights • Bright fluorescent lighting • Infrared heating • Sunlight • Xenon surgical lamps	• Cover sensor with opaque material (e.g., blanket, foil).
Optical shunt	• Too large a sensor, which allows light to reach the sensor without passing through a pulsatile bed	• Sensor must completely adhere to skin and be the appropriate size.
Optical cross talk	• Multiple sensors too close to one another	• Cover each sensor with opaque material or separate sensors (one per extremity).
Movement artifact	• Spurious readings	• Pulse rate must correlate with displayed oximeter before credence can be given to oximeter reading. • Move the probe to a more central location (ear vs. finger). • Change the oximeter to a longer averaging time.
Absorption of light by non-oxyHgb or nondeoxyHgb sources	• IV dyes (methylene blue)[9] • Nail polish • Dyshemoglobinemia	• Remove nail polish. • Verify readings with cooximetry.
Electrical interference	• Usually caused by cautery; can be affected by 60 Hz interference	• 60-cycle interference may be improved by moving the plug to another outlet. • Some machines have built-in mechanisms to decrease interference by cautery.
Low perfusion	• Cold extremities • Decreased cardiac output	• Warm extremities. • Use inotropic agents or vasodilators. • Use a more central location for probe site (tongue or ear).
Active venous bed	• Right heart failure • Tricuspid regurgitation	• Using an oximeter with visual display of plethysmograph waveform may help interpretation.

TABLE 5-4. Examples of capnographs

Capnograph		Explanation
Normal	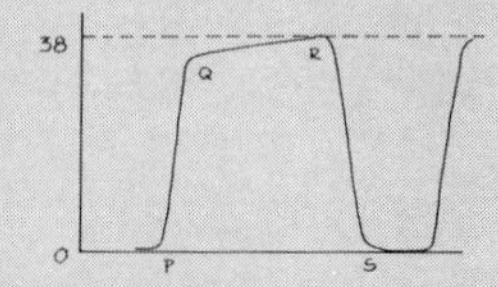	• Rapid increase P to Q • End tidal CO_2 is *only* equivalent to alveolar CO_2 when the plateau Q to R is nearly horizontal • End tidal = R • Rapid decrease from R to zero during inspiration
Pediatric	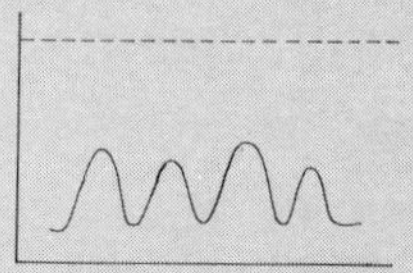	• Moderate rebreathing • Absence of plateau • Rapid rate
Obstruction: • Kinked tube • Asthma	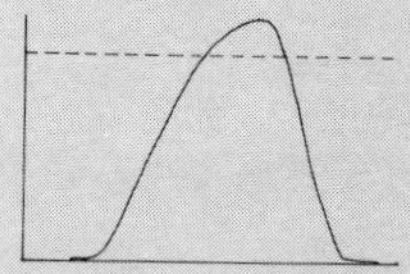	• Slowed expiratory phase • Poor plateau • Elevated CO_2
Curare cleft	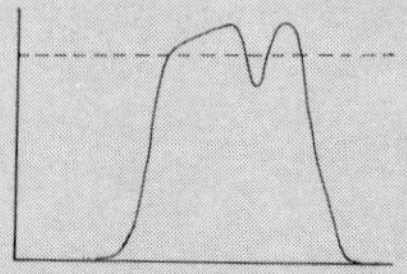	• Caused by lack of coordination between diaphragm and intercostal muscles with waning muscle relaxation • Cleft occurs in last third of plateau • Depth of cleft is proportional to degree of muscle relaxation

Camel capnogram	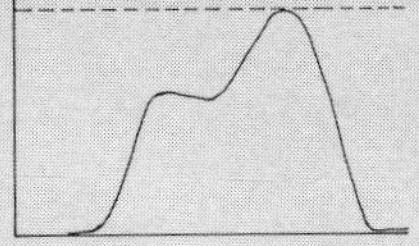	• Seen in patients in lateral position • Occurs during spontaneous or positive pressure ventilation
Patient breathing against ventilator	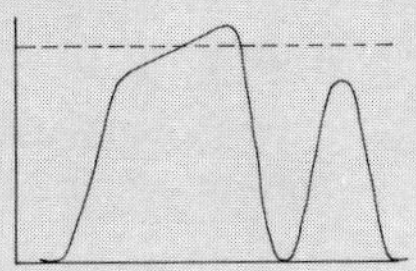	• Interrupts regular pattern of capnography • Capnography of ventilator and of spontaneous ventilation are merged

b. Dilution of expired gas by the high fresh gas flows needed with nonrebreathing circuits.
c. Amount of gas aspirated for sampling.[10]

Capnography provides additional information on airway dynamics, cardiac output, amount of rebreathing, patency of the endotracheal tube, and state of neuromuscular relaxation (Table 5-4).

Halogenated Agents

Measuring the concentration of halogenated agents in inspired or expired gases serves to monitor the accuracy of a vaporizer and can prevent accidental overdose or detect the use of an incorrect agent in the vaporizer.

Methods used to measure halogenated agents include the following:

1. Mass spectrometry
2. Raman scattering
3. Silicon rubber relaxation
4. Crystal oscillation

LARYNGOSCOPE

1. Use of a small pediatric handle is recommended. It is less bulky, allowing laryngoscopy to be performed while applying cricoid pressure with the fifth finger of the same hand.
2. In general, straight blades are used in infants to pick up the floppy epiglottis and expose the cords (Miller). The wider phlanged Wis-Hippel or Robert-Shaw blades are also useful in infants.
3. The following chart provides a list of the age-appropriate sizes of laryngoscope blades, according to type:

Laryngoscope blades	Age
Miller 0	Preterm, neonate
Miller 1	Neonate-age 2
Miller 2	Age 3 and older
Wis-Hippel 1.5	Age 2-5
Macintosh 2	Age 3-6

AIRWAYS

This section should remind the anesthesiologist to include not only oral and nasal airways but also masks and endotracheal tubes in the routine setup.

Oral Airway (See also Chapter 8—"Management of the Airway—Equipment" on p. 132)

The smooth Guedel airway is most commonly used in children. The appropriate size should be determined by placing the airway against the child's cheek with the blunt end at the mouth. The properly sized airway will just reach the angle of the mandible.

Sizes needed for an appropriate preoperative setup can be approximated from the following chart:

Age	Size	cm
Preterm	00,000	3.5, 4.5
Neonate-3 mo	0	5.5
3-12 mo	1	6.0
1-5 yr	2	7.0
>5 yr	3	8.0

Masks

A variety of masks are available:

1. The Rendell-Baker-Soucek and disposable Dryden masks are designed to conform to the face and reduce the amount of dead space. Made of clear plastic, they provide the added advantage of allowing for observation of the child's color, humidity from expired gases, and presence of secretions and vomitus.
2. Black rubber Ohio face masks and SCRAM masks may create a better seal in some children.

Endotracheal Tubes

Size (See also Chapter 8—"Management of the Airway—Endotracheal Tube" on p. 132)

A child's trachea is smaller than an adult's and funnel shaped. Even the slightest amount of edema from a tightly fitting endotracheal tube can result in significant airway obstruction from subglottic edema. Consequently, uncuffed endotracheal tubes are used in children under 8 years of age, and a leak is required around the tube (with less than 20 cm water inspiratory pressure). The following is a list of appropriate endotracheal tube sizes:

Age	Endotracheal tube size (inner diameter in mm)
Premature	
<2 kg	2.5
>2 kg	3.0
Neonate	3.5
0-6 mo	3.5
6-12 mo	4.0
12-18 mo	4.0-4.5
2 yr	4.5
2-3 yr	4.5-5.0
>4 yr	(Age + 16) ÷ 4

TABLE 5-5. Methods of verification of endotracheal tube depth

Method	Comment
X-ray	• Impractical in the operating room. • Useful in the ICU to confirm tube depth, but assumes child's position (neck extension) will remain constant.
Tube markings	• Requires controlled intubation by experienced individual. • The average distance from cords to carina in a neonate is 5 cm; placement of the tube with the first single line at the cords will put the tube midway in the trachea.
Age + 10 rule	• The centimeter mark at the lip should equal the age (in years) + 10 (e.g., a 1-year-old should have the tube inserted to a depth of 11 cm, a 2-year-old, of 12 cm, a 3-year-old, of 13 cm, etc.).
1, 2, 3, 4, 7, 8, 9, 10 rule for premature infants	• The weight of the child is used as a guide: **kg** — **cm at lip** 1 — 7 2 — 8 3 — 9 4 — 10

Positioning

The tip of the endotracheal tube should sit midway between the vocal cords and the carina. Correct placement will prevent endobronchial intubation or inadvertent extubation with either flexion or extension of the child's neck.

The correct tube depth may be verified by several methods (Table 5-5).

DRUGS

When preparing to anesthetize children under 10 kg, drugs should be administered from tuberculin (TB) syringes. These syringes are marked in increments of 0.1 ml allowing for more precise drug dosing. (Commonly used drugs are found in Table 5-6.)

INTRAVENOUS EQUIPMENT

Precise measurement of intravenous fluids for premature infants, neonates, and small children is crucial.

1. To prevent volume overload, a burette (150-ml capacity) should be used for fluid administration. Also useful is a minidrip (60 gtts/ml) or infusion pump to control the infusion rate over time.
2. Small-gauge nontapered teflon catheters are available for venous cannulation and are preferable to metal butterflies, which can easily perforate the vessel wall. Use of a 22-gauge catheter is suitable from neonate to 3 or 4 years. A 24-gauge catheter is reserved for use in small infants, and a 25- or 27-gauge catheter for very small premature infants.
3. Use of a T-piece connector directly attached to the venous catheter will limit the amount of dead space in tubing during drug adminis-

TABLE 5-6. Commonly used drugs

Drug	Dose
Atropine	0.01–0.02 mg/kg IV
Succinylcholine	(Preceded by atropine) 2 mg/kg IV 4 mg/kg IM
Nondepolarizing relaxants	Intubating dose:
Pancuronium	0.1 mg/kg
Vecuronium	0.1 mg/kg
Atracurium	0.5 mg/kg
Anticholinesterases	
Edrophonium	0.5–1.0 mg/kg
Neostigmine	0.4–0.7 mg/kg
Narcotics	Analgesic dose:
Morphine	0.1 mg/kg
Fentanyl	1 μg/kg

tration and provides almost instant access into the vasculature. Use of the T-piece connector is recommended for all children under 1 year of age.

4. Because of the possibility of an intracardiac shunt, all IVs in infants and children should have air bubbles scrupulously removed. Air filters in the IV tubing will assist in keeping the lines bubble-free. Air should also be aspirated from the needle or injection site before injection into any IV.

REFERENCES

1. Ward CF: Special considerations in monitoring children during anesthesia. In Saidman L and Smith NT, editors: Monitoring in anesthesia, ed 2, Boston, 1984, Butterworths.
2. McCloskey GF and Curling PE: Electrocardiography, Anesthesiology Clinics of North America 6:903-15, 1988.
3. Park MK and Guntheroth WG: How to read pediatric ECG's, Chicago, 1987, Year Book, 86-98.
4. Reitan JA and Barash PG: Noninvasive monitoring. In Saidman L and Smith NT, editors: Monitoring in anesthesia, ed 2, Boston, 1984, Butterworths.
5. Soderstrom CA and others: Superiority of the femoral artery for monitoring: a prospective study, Am J Surg 144:309-12, 1988.
6. Miyasaka K, Edmonds J, and Corm A: Complications of radial artery lines in the paediatric patient, Can J Anaesth 23:9-14, 1976.
7. Lowenstein E, Little JW, and Lott H: Prevention of cerebral embolization from flushing radial artery cannulas, N Engl J Med 285:414-15, 1971.
8. Neal WA and others: Umbilical artery catheterization: demonstration of arterial thrombosis by aortography, Pediatrics 49:6, 1972.
9. Eisenkraft JB: Pulse oximeter desaturation due to methemoglobinemia, Anesthesiology 68:279-82, 1988.
10. Badgwell JM and others: End-tidal pCO_2 measurements sampled of the distal and proximal ends of the endotracheal tube in infants and children, Anesth Analg 66:959-64, 1987.

6

FLUIDS, ELECTROLYTES, AND TRANSFUSION THERAPY

Charlotte Bell
Kevin S. Morrison

Was Ethan hungry as a bear?
No. He just looked at his plate.
He really didn't seem to care
whether or not he ate.
MARGUERITE RUSH LERNER, M.D.
DEAR LITTLE MUMPS CHILD

FLUIDS AND ELECTROLYTES

Parenteral fluid therapy is administered in the operating room with the following goals in mind:

1. As maintenance therapy to preserve hydration
2. To compensate for fluid and electrolyte deficits caused by patient disease or enforced preoperative fasting
3. To replace ongoing losses resulting from evaporation, insensible loss, or surgical bleeding
4. To compensate for acute changes in autonomic function that occur during anesthesia. Alterations in sympathetic and parasympathetic tone can markedly alter preload and afterload, with subsequent decreases in cardiac output and perfusion.

MAINTENANCE THERAPY: PERIOPERATIVE MANAGEMENT OF FLUIDS AND NUTRITION

Caloric Requirements

Age (yr)	kcal/kg/day
Preterm	120
0–1	90–100
1–7	75–90
7–12	60–75

1. Glycogen stores in the neonatal liver are limited and are rapidly depleted within the first few hours of life. Neonates tolerate fasting poorly because of their high metabolic demands and limited energy stores.
2. An infant is commonly placed on intravenous therapy of only 10% dextrose in water. At 100 ml/kg/day, this solution will provide only 40 Kcal/kg/day, or one third of the infant's basal metabolic requirements. Without further nutritional support, this infant will have a negative nitrogen and caloric balance.

Fluid Requirements

1. Water is necessary for growth, to replace evaporative and fecal losses, and for excretion of renal solute.
2. Preterm and small infants have a relatively high percentage of total body water (85% in a preterm and 75% in a full-term infant).
3. The minimal amount of water required to meet ongoing insensible losses is 60 to 100 ml/kg/day.

Electrolyte Requirements (See box on "Management of Electrolyte Imbalance")

Electrolyte	Daily requirement
Na^+	0.5–2.0 mEq/kg/day
K^+	0.5–2.0 mEq/kg/day
Cl^-	0.5–2.0 mEq/kg/day
Ca^{++}	20–100 mg/kg/day

Glucose Requirements

The intraoperative use of glucose-containing solutions for children continues to be controversial. An attempt must be made to balance the risk of hypoglycemia against the detrimental effects of hyperglycemia.

A. Patients at increased risk for *hypoglycemia* include the following:
   1. Children with depleted glycogen stores:
      a. Those in the lower percentiles of weight
      b. Those with chronic debilitating illness
      c. Those whose NPO period has been extensive
      d. Those who have been receiving total parenteral nutrition
   2. Neonates and infants in the following groups:
      a. Preterm infants
      b. Infants of diabetic mothers
      c. Infants small for gestational age
      d. Infants with erythroblastosis fetalis
   3. A small percentage of normal, healthy infants and children. These will exhibit asymptomatic or mildly symptomatic hypoglycemia pre- or intraoperatively even without an extended fast.

B. Intraoperative *hyperglycemia* in children seems to occur frequently when solutions containing glucose are given. Hyperglycemia is usually a result of the "stress response" to surgery. Increased sympathoadrenal activity results in:
   1. Decreased glucose tolerance

MANAGEMENT OF ELECTROLYTE IMBALANCE

Hyperkalemia—acute ($K^+ > 6.5$ mEq/L)

- Monitor ECG.
- Hyperventilation
- Sodium bicarbonate 1–2 mEq/kg (IV) (dilute 1:2 for infants)
- Calcium chloride 5–10 mg/kg (IV)
- Glucose (1 g/kg D_{50}) + regular insulin (1 unit/kg) (IV)

Hyperkalemia—chronic

- Monitor ECG.
- Sodium polystyrene sulfonate (Kayexalate), 1–2 g/kg/day, rectally or orally in 4 divided doses

Hypokalemia ($K^+ < 3.5$ mEq/L)

- Monitor ECG.
- Requires slow replacement because of potassium presence, primarily intracellularly.
- Potassium should not be administered before urine output has been established at 0.5 mEq/kg/hr.
- Total amount of K^+ to be replaced may be calculated as follows:

$$\text{wt} \times (C^+_D - C^+_M) \times 0.3 = \text{mEq required}$$

wt = weight in kilograms
C^+_D = serum concentration desired
C^+_M = serum concentration measured

Hypernatremia ($Na^+ > 160$ mEq/L)

- Gradual rehydration with isotonic solutions; rapid fall in intracellular sodium can cause cerebral edema.

Hyponatremia ($Na^+ < 130$ mEq/L)

- Can usually be replaced with isotonic solutions.
- 30% saline solution at the rate of 1 ml/min to a maximum of 13 ml/kg has been recommended for NA < 12 mEq/L with symptoms of cerebral edema (seizures, coma).

Hyperchloremia ($Cl^- > 109$ mEq/L)

- Usually seen with metabolic acidosis because of suppression of bicarbonate resorption by excessive chloride.
- Excess will usually self-correct when offending problem is resolved (e.g., diarrhea).

Hypochloremia ($Cl^- < 95$ mEq/L)

- Commonly seen in pyloric stenosis accompanied by metabolic alkalosis and hypokalemia
- Infusion of isotonic saline and potassium will correct Cl^- and K^+ deficits and therefore alkalosis
- Lactated solutions will worsen alkalosis by conversion of lactate to bicarbonate in the liver

MANAGEMENT OF ELECTROLYTE IMBALANCE—cont'd

Bicarbonate deficit/metabolic acidosis (base deficit of 10 mEq/L or greater)

- Correction of underlying problem (hypoxia, decreased perfusion, hypoglycemia, hypothermia, etc.)
- Initial dose 1–2 mEq/kg bicarbonate (dilute 1:2 for infants)
- Calculated dose:

$$\text{wt (kg)} \times \text{base deficit} \times 0.3 = \text{mEq bicarbonate required}$$

- Half of total dose is administered and a second pH or bicarbonate level obtained before completing the dose.

2. Decreased glucose utilization
3. Increased gluconeogenesis

C. The increased osmotic load caused by hyperglycemia may result in:
1. Osmotic diuresis when the renal threshold is exceeded, which may impair the determination of adequate cardiac output
2. Intraventricular hemorrhage in young infants

D. Recommendations for intraoperative glucose administration include:
1. Dextrose-containing solutions should be avoided in patients susceptible to complete cerebral ischemia (craniotomy, cardiac bypass). In these patients, dextrose infusions preischemia have been shown to correlate with worsened neurologic outcome. During hypothermic cardiopulmonary bypass, gluconeogenesis continues despite a dearth of insulin production, posing a threat of extreme hyperglycemia.
2. Glucose levels of patients receiving no intraoperative glucose must be closely monitored.
3. Glucose-containing solutions should be given intraoperatively to all other infants and children.
   a. Infants and chronically ill patients at greatest risk of hypoglycemia (or of adverse effects from hypoglycemia) should have frequent intraoperative blood glucose measurements.
   b. Use of dextrose concentrations of less than 5% is probably sufficient to prevent hypoglycemia and decreases the likelihood of hyperglycemia.

Protein Requirements

Age (yr)	g/kg/day
0–0.5	2.2
0.5–1.0	2.0
1–3	1.8
4–6	1.5
7–10	1.2

Infants and children who are briefly NPO in the perioperative period do not require parenteral protein so this problem is ordinarily not a concern of the anesthesiologist. Patients chronically unable to tolerate enteral feeding are maintained on total parenteral nutrition.

Perioperative Management of Total Parenteral Nutrition (TPN)

1. Peripheral TPN can provide up to 80 kcal/kg/day. The maximum allowable dextrose concentration by this route is 10%, and amino acids should not exceed 2%.
2. Central vein TPN is indicated when stresses are severe (burns, sepsis, major surgery), full growth and development are desired, or the bowel cannot be used for feeding.
   The maximum allowable concentration of dextrose given by central vein is 25% and of amino acids is 3%. Lipid emulsions can be administered as a source of fatty acids and calories. A 20% solution allows for a small volume relative to the amount of calories to be infused. Lipids should make up no more than 60% of the total daily caloric intake.
3. The development of glycosuria by a patient on a previously tolerated concentration of glucose may indicate sepsis.
4. The abrupt discontinuation of TPN should be avoided because it may result in rebound hypoglycemia.
5. There are several techniques for the intraoperative management of the patient on TPN. The stress of surgery alone is likely to cause hyperglycemia, and the concomitant administration of a concentrated glucose solution could induce severe hyperglycemia, glycosuria, an osmotic diuresis, and associated fluid and electrolyte derangements. A sudden withdrawal of TPN, on the other hand, could result in rebound hypoglycemia.
   a. An infusion of 10% dextrose should be started if TPN is to be discontinued intraoperatively.
   b. If large volumes of fluid must be administered intraoperatively (i.e., in a lengthy case involving evaporative losses), the TPN may be replaced by a less concentrated glucose solution. Large volumes of 5% dextrose solution can provide the same total caloric requirement as smaller infusions of 10% dextrose. The key to intraoperative management of the TPN, regardless of the glucose concentration chosen, is frequent glucose monitoring.
6. An additional peripheral IV should be started if the TPN line provides the only intravenous access. Third space losses and blood should be replaced through the peripheral line rather than the TPN line because of the risk of introducing infection. Drugs should be administered via the peripheral line because of possible drug incompatibilities.

FLUID AND ELECTROLYTE DEFICITS

Severity of Dehydration

The severity of dehydration (described as percent change in body weight secondary to dehydration) should be estimated on the basis of patient history and clinical observations (Table 6-1). Laboratory data are not useful in predicting severity.

TABLE 6-1. Severity of dehydration

Percent of body weight	Signs and symptoms
1%–5% (mild)	• History of 12–24 hours of vomiting and diarrhea • Dry mouth • Decreased urination
6%–10% (moderate)	• Tenting skin • Sunken eyes, fontanelle • Oliguria • Lethargy
11%–15% (severe)	• Cardiovascular instability: mottling, hypotension, tachycardia • Anuria • Sensorium change
20%	• Coma • Shock

Types of Dehydration

Dehydration is classified by its tonicity according to the concentration of serum sodium (Table 6-2). To differentiate among isotonic, hypotonic, and hypertonic dehydration, serum osmolarity can be calculated by the following formula:

$$\text{Serum osmolarity} = 2(Na^+ + K^+) + \frac{\text{BUN}}{2.8} + \frac{\text{Glucose}}{18}$$

If BUN and glucose are within normal ranges, then:

$$\text{Serum osmolarity} = 2(Na^+)$$

TABLE 6-2. Classification of dehydration

Type	Serum osmolarity	Serum sodium	Etiology
Isotonic	270–300	130–150	Hypotonic losses (fasting, thirsting, diarrhea, vomiting), replaced with hypotonic fluids
Hypotonic	<270	<130	Ongoing Na^+ loss with replacement by Na^+–poor beverages
Hypertonic	>310	>150	Inadequate replacement of free water

Replacement of Fluid Deficits

1. Selection of fluid (Tables 6-3 and 6-4)
   a. Generally either lactated Ringer's or normal saline is used for routine intraoperative fluid administration, because they closely resemble the intravascular fluids lost during surgery.
   b. Half normal saline is often used preoperatively for gradual (8- to 24-hour) replacement of dehydration deficits with frequent clinical and laboratory reassessment.

TABLE 6-3. Composition of intravenous crystalloid solutions

Solution	Glucose (g/L)	Na^+ (mEq/L)	K^+ (mEq/L)	Cl^- (mEq/L)	Lactate (mEq/L)	Ca^{+2} (mEq/L)	pH	Osm
5% Dextrose	50	—	—	—	—	—	4.5	253
Ringers	—	147	4	155	—	4	6.0	309
Lactated Ringers	—	130	4	109	28	3	6.3	273
D_5 lactated Ringers	50	130	4	109	28	3	4.9	525
D_5 0.22% NSS*	50	38.5	—	38.5	—	—	4.4	330
D_5 0.45% NSS*	50	77	—	77	—	—	4.4	407
0.9% NSS*	—	154	—	154	—	—	5.6	308

*NSS, Normal saline solution.

TABLE 6-4. Composition of intravenous colloid solutions

Solution	Composition	Indications	Comments
Dextran: D_{40} = low molecular wt D_{20} = high molecular wt	Branched-chain polysaccharides	Volume replacement in hypovolemic shock and burns	• Stays in intravascular compartment longer than crystalloid. • Interferes with platelet function, stimulates fibrinolysis, and may cause renal failure. • May cause anaphylactic reactions, fever, and rash. • Use of a filter is not necessary.
Hydroxyethyl starch (HES): 6% solution in NSS*	Starch composed of amylopectin with hydroxymethyl groups introduced to retard degradation by amylase	As for dextran	• Fewer side effects than dextran. • Can prolong PT/PTT—may cause pruritis. • Use of a filter is not necessary.
Albumin: 5% solution 25% solution	Donor plasma derived from whole blood by plasmapheresis 96% albumin 4% globulin Na^+ = 145 mEq/L	As for dextran except patients should also be hypoproteinemic	• 5% solution is osmotically equivalent to plasma. • No ABO testing or blood filter is required.

*NSS: Normal saline solution.

CALCULATION OF INTRAOPERATIVE FLUID REQUIREMENTS

1. Estimated fluid requirement (EFR) per hour (maintenance fluids)	0–10 kg = 4 ml/kg/hr + 10–20 kg = 2 ml/kg/hr + >20 kg = 1 ml/kg/hr (e.g., 23-kg child = 40 ml + 20 ml + 3 ml EFR = 63 ml/hr)
2. Estimated preoperative fluid deficit (EFD)	Number of hours NPO × EFR (e.g., 23-kg child NPO for 8 hrs, EFR = 23 × 8 = 184 ml) 1st hour = ½ EFD + EFR 2nd hour = ¼ EFD + EFR 3rd hour = ¼ EFD + EFR
3. Insensible losses (IL) (Add to EFR and EFD)	Minimal incision = 3–5 ml/kg/hr Moderate incision with viscus exposure = 5–10 ml/kg/hr Large incision with bowel exposure = 8–20 ml/kg/hr
4. Estimated blood loss (See section for calculation of blood replacement p. 106.)	Replace maximum allowable blood loss (ABL) with crystalloid 3:1.

c. Crystalloid (lactated Ringer's or normal saline) or colloid (hetastarch or albumin) can be used in cases of acute volume loss. While crystalloid is considerably less expensive, hetastarch may be more effective in acutely expanding the intravascular space.

2. Intraoperative replacement (for mild dehydration or to compensate for preoperative fasting):
   a. 50% of estimated deficit and hourly maintenance are replaced during the first hour.
   b. 25% of deficit and hourly maintenance are given during the second hour.
   c. 25% of deficit and hourly maintenance are given during the third hour.
3. Patients with moderate to severe dehydration require prolonged replacement over several hours to assure adequate intracellular volume and restoration of normal intracellular electrolytes. If possible, operative procedures should be delayed until the patient is rehydrated and electrolytes replaced.
4. Adequacy of replacement can be determined by the following:

EFFECTS OF ANESTHETICS ON FLUID AND ELECTROLYTE BALANCE

- Enforced preoperative fasting increases fluid deficit.
- Decreased energy expenditures during anesthesia decrease requirements for fluid, sodium, and potassium.
- Total peripheral resistance is decreased by isoflurane, enflurane, and morphine.
- Cardiac output is depressed by halothane, enflurane, and isoflurane.
- Decreased sympathetic tone caused by general or regional anesthetics increases venous capacitance with a resultant decrease in cardiac output.
- Baroreflexes are blunted.
- Decreased cardiac output decreases glomerular filtration rate and renal blood flow.
- Mechanical ventilation increases evaporative losses via the airway.
- Positive pressure ventilation and CPAP cause an increased secretion of atrial natriuretic factor (ANF), which increases sodium and water excretion.
- Hyperventilation causes a relative hypokalemia.
- Hypothermia increases oxygen consumption, thereby increasing caloric and water requirements.
- Hyperglycemia commonly results from the "stress response" (increased sympathoadrenal activity).
- Effectiveness of insulin is impaired and glucose tolerance is decreased.
- ADH secretion is increased by the sympathoadrenal axis (decreased excretion of sodium and water).
- Surgical trauma to tissues causes capillary leaks and tissue edema, decreasing intravascular volume.

   a. Patient's appearance and weight change
   b. Urine output (>0.5 ml/kg/hr)
   c. Urine specific gravity (1.010 or less if no proteinuria or glucosuria)
   d. Urine osmolality (for normal values, see Table 3-4)
   e. Central venous pressure monitoring

5. With cases involving acute intravascular volume loss, the rapid administration of 20 ml/kg of lactated Ringer's or normal saline may be warranted to restore cardiovascular stability and renal perfusion. If losses are ongoing, invasive monitoring will be necessary.

INSENSIBLE LOSSES

1. Insensible losses generally result from *evaporation,* either from the incision site and viscus exposure or from respiration. These losses increase with the size of incision and with increasing respiratory rate. (For replacement calculations see box on p. 104.)
2. The effects of anesthetics on *autonomic tone,* reflexes, and cardiac output may also increase fluid needs, even though an absolute fluid deficit does not exist. Fluids necessary to compensate for a relatively decreased preload due to autonomic effects should be given on a dose-response basis. (See box above.)

BLOOD REPLACEMENT

DETERMINATION OF BLOOD DEFICIT AND NEED FOR TRANSFUSION

Rapid Blood Loss

Rapid blood loss in the infant or child can lead to significant hemodynamic alterations more rapidly than in the larger adult.

1. Certain methods to quantitate blood loss, such as small traps in suction circuits and the weighing of bloody sponges, will help to determine blood loss intraoperatively.
2. If rapid or massive blood loss is anticipated, invasive monitoring (particularly the arterial tracing) will reveal acute hypovolemia.
3. The maximum allowable blood loss (ABL) before transfusion should be calculated preoperatively for any operation in which blood loss is anticipated.
4. Blood losses under the ABL can be replaced by crystalloid or colloid. Either of the following can be used to replace each ml of blood lost:
   - 2 to 3 ml of balanced salt solution
   - 1 ml of 5% albumin

   No conclusive studies have been done supporting the preferential use of either crystalloid or colloid in children. Albumin is considerably more expensive, however.

Calculating Allowable Blood Loss

1. The estimated blood volume (EBV) is calculated first.

Premature infant	90–100 ml/kg
Full-term infant	80–90 ml/kg
3 mo–1 yr	75–80 ml/kg
>1 yr	70–75 ml/kg

2. The preoperative hematocrit is then obtained and the lowest allowable hematocrit determined. Most commonly used as the minimum acceptable value is a hematocrit of 30% (0.30). However, in an effort to avoid transfusion-related illness, many anesthesiologists use a lower minimum if the child is basically healthy and if adequate perfusion and oxygenation can be maintained. Often the child can compensate for a lowered hematocrit by increasing cardiac output. Further compensation can be provided by decreasing oxygen consumption and increasing F_IO_2 during anesthesia.
3. Calculation by simple proportion:

$$ABL = EBV \times \frac{Hct_{pt} - Hct_{LA}}{Hct_{pt}}$$

where:

ABL = Allowable blood loss
EBV = Estimated blood volume
Hct_{pt} = Patient hematocrit (decimal)
Hct_{LA} = Lowest allowable hematocrit (decimal)

4. Calculation by estimating red cell mass loss (RCML):

$$EBV \times Hct_{pt} = ERCM_{pt}$$
$$EBV \times Hct_{LA} = ERCM_{LA}$$
$$ERCM_{pt} - ERCM_{LA} = ARCML$$
$$ARCML \times 3 = ABL$$

where:

EBV = Estimated blood volume
Hct_{pt} = Patient hematocrit (decimal)
$ERCM_{pt}$ = Estimated red cell mass (patient)
Hct_{LA} = Lowest allowable hematocrit (decimal)
$ERCM_{LA}$ = Estimated red cell mass (lowest allowable)
$ARCML$ = Allowable red cell mass loss (maximum)
ABL = Allowable blood loss (maximum)

5. The volume of whole blood to be transfused is calculated by:

$$RBV = AcBL - ABL$$

where:

RBV = Blood volume to be replaced
$AcBL$ = Actual measured or estimated blood loss
ABL = Calculated allowable blood loss

6. To convert the volume of whole blood to the volume of packed red blood cell transfusion necessary to increase the hematocrit to the desired level:

$$\frac{RBV \times Hct_{LA}\%}{Hct_{prbc}\%} = \text{ml necessary to achieve } Hct_{LA}*$$

where:

RBV = Blood volume to be replaced
Hct_{LA} = Lowest allowable hematocrit
Hct_{prbc} = Hematocrit of packed red blood cells to be transferred (CPDA blood: hematocrit 70%; ADSOL blood: hematocrit 55%)

BLOOD COMPONENTS
Red Blood Cells
Indications

The only reason for red cell transfusion is to increase oxygen carrying capacity in the normovolemic patient.

1. Preoperative: As more information becomes available on transfusion risks, anesthesiologists are increasingly hesitant to insist on a hemoglobin of 10 and a hematocrit of 30% prior to surgery.

*It is preferable to transfuse slightly more blood than required rather than expose the child to a second unit of blood in the perioperative period, which increases the risk of a transfusion reaction.

a. Although not proven conclusively, it appears that most healthy children can tolerate hematocrits of 25% or less without markedly increasing cardiac output and oxygen consumption.
b. The presence of coexistent disease (dyshemoglobinemia, chronic pulmonary or cardiac disease) and the anticipated surgical blood loss should be considered before transfusion.
c. Additional considerations exist for the full- or preterm neonate based on the presence of hemoglobin F and current medical problems. The decision to transfuse should be made with the pediatrician or neonatologist. Blood used for neonatal transfusion is frozen, deglycerolized, or less than 7 days old in order to preserve 2-3 DPG levels. It may also be irradiated to prevent graft vs. host disease.

2. Intraoperative: The need for intraoperative transfusion is based on preoperative calculations of allowable blood loss (see "Calculating Allowable Blood Loss" earlier) and the patient's ability to maintain adequate perfusion.

Categories of Red Blood Cell Components

Several different preparations of red blood cells are used. They are generally prepared by removing 200 to 250 ml of plasma from whole blood and are then stored in various preservatives and anticoagulants at 1° to 6° C (Table 6-5 on pp. 110-111 lists red blood cell transfusion preparations).

Administration of Red Cells

1. Requisite is the use of a standard 170-micron filter to trap debris. Microaggregate filters (20 to 40 micron) are used during cardiopulmonary bypass to prevent debris from directly entering the systemic circulation.
2. For pediatric patients, red cells are generally not diluted to ease administration because of the risk of hypervolemia.
3. Clinically significant hemolysis does not occur with infusions through 25- or 26-g catheters if the driving pressure is less than 300 mm Hg.

Alternatives to Homologous Red Cell Transfusion

1. Autologous transfusion of red blood cells (and supernatant plasma from the same unit, if necessary) has been used successfully in older, cooperative children. The risk of immunologic reactions and viral transmission is thereby eliminated.
2. In some situations, direct-donated blood may present less risk, although this subject remains controversial.
3. Intraoperative blood salvage, although commonly used in adult patients, is seldom used for pediatric patients but may be useful in large blood loss procedures.
4. Acute normovolemic hemodilution, controlled hypotension, and profound hypothermia with circulatory arrest have all been employed to reduce blood loss in children during procedures in which massive bleeding is anticipated.
5. Alternatives to red cell transfusion are currently unavailable. While both dextran and hetastarch are useful volume expanders, they do not carry

oxygen. Artificial perfluorocarbon emulsions have been disappointing thus far in their ability to carry oxygen.

Whole Blood

Description

Whole blood is approximately 450 ml of blood and 60 ml of anticoagulant preservative, which is from a single donor and not separated into components. Hematocrit is 36% to 44%. It is stored at 1° to 6° C.

Deficiencies

1. Few viable platelets or granulocytes exist after the first 24 hours.
2. 2-3 DPG levels decrease significantly after the first 7 days.
3. Factor V and VIII levels decrease according to storage time but are probably sufficient for normal clotting (>20% to 30%).

Indications

Whole blood is used for actively bleeding patients who require both an increased oxygen carrying capacity and expansion of blood volume. It is rarely available, however, because of widespread use of component therapy.

Fresh Frozen Plasma (FFP)

Description

FFP is the supernatant component of a single unit of blood consisting of water, protein, carbohydrates, and lipids. It is separated from the red cells and frozen within 6 hours of phlebotomy. All clotting factors are present.

Indications

1. For patients with active bleeding as a result of:
   a. Factor deficiency secondary to liver disease
   b. Disseminated intravascular coagulation (DIC)
   c. Dilutional coagulopathy from massive transfusion (more likely caused by platelet deficiency)
2. For patients with congenital factor deficiencies for which no coagulation concentrate is available
3. To reverse the effects of warfarin or coumadin in actively bleeding patients who cannot wait for reversal by vitamin K or when emergent surgery is necessary
4. Has been used in infants with immunodeficiency as a result of protein losing enteropathy
5. May be useful for the treatment of thrombotic thrombocytopenic purpura

Albumin

Description

Albumin is a plasma component containing 96% albumin and 4% globulin heated to 60° C for 10 hours. It is available in a 5% solution (Na^+ = 145 mEq/L) osmotically equivalent to plasma or in a 25% solution.

Plasma protein fraction (PPF) contains approximately 83% albumin and 17% globulins because it goes through less purification than albumin. It is

TABLE 6-5. Categories of red blood cell transfusion preparations

Type	Preparation	Indications for use	Comments
RBC/CPDA* preservative	Preserved with adenine to increase ATP, which results in a shelf life† of 35 days	• Treatment of anemia; improves oxygen carrying capacity	• Potassium 15-25 mEq/L • Decreased factors V, VIII • Absent platelets • Decreased 2-3 DPG • Hct approx. 70% (10 ml/kg raises Hct about 10%)
RBC/ADSOL preservative (adenine saline solution)	Preservative contains mannitol, dextrose, and adenine in a 100-ml volume (extends shelf life to 42 days)	• As above	• As above except Hct approx. 55% (10 ml/kg raises Hct about 7%)
Frozen thawed deglycerolized	Glycerol added to blood < 6 days old and frozen	• Depleted of leukocytes; safe for infants < 1,200 g at risk for CMV (decreases risk of seroconversion)	• Low potassium • Nearly normal 2-3 DPG • No fibrinogen • Contains less red cell mass • Contains almost no citrate (minimizes alkalosis because citrate is connected to bicarbonate in the liver)

Irradiated	Blood irradiated with cesium-137 (1-5 min with 1,500 rads) to eradicate lymphocytes	• To prevent graft vs. host disease in patients with immunodeficiency syndromes, bone marrow transplant, cytotoxic therapy, or for exchange transfusion in infants	• Functional components other than lymphocytes are not affected.
Leukocyte-poor (saline washed)	Blood centrifuged and filtered to remove "buffy coat" (leukocytes and platelets)	• Used in patients with recurrent or severe febrile nonhemolytic reactions due to alloimmunization to leukocyte antigens or plasma proteins	• After washing, shelf life is decreased to 24 hours because of possible bacterial contamination. • As much as 30% of red cell mass may be lost during washing.

*Citrate phosphate dextrose adenine preservative.

†Shelf life: Number of days during which blood cells maintain 70% viability 24 hours after infusion.

also available in a 5% solution. The presence of sodium acetate and Hageman factor may produce hypotension during rapid infusion.

Advantages

1. Cannot transmit viral disease because of the heating process.
2. Can be stored for up to 5 years at 2° to 10° C.
3. ABO antigens and antibodies are absent so blood typing is unnecessary.
4. Albumin does not need to be administered through a filter.

Indications

1. Hemolytic disease of the newborn (binds indirect bilirubin during exchange transfusion)
2. To support blood pressure in patients who are hypovolemic and hypoproteinemic (usual dose: 10 ml/kg of the 5% solution)

Platelets

Description

1. One unit of platelets is obtained by centrifuging a single unit of whole blood.
2. Each unit contains at least 5.5×10^{10} platelets in 50 to 70 ml of plasma.
3. Platelet concentrates are usually stored at 20° to 24° C for up to 5 days with constant gentle agitation to preserve cell survival.
4. Usual dose is 0.2 units/kg or 20 ml/kg.
5. Administration through a filter is necessary. Red cell compatibility testing is not.

Indications

1. Active bleeding:
   a. Platelet count of less than 50,000/μL
   b. Abnormal platelet function with template bleeding time greater than twice normal
2. Prophylaxis:
   a. Thrombocytopenia less than 20,000/μL
   b. Children with accelerated platelet destruction who are scheduled for splenectomy can be given platelet transfusions after the spleen is removed.
3. Dilutional thrombocytopenia associated with massive transfusion when active bleeding and documented thrombocytopenia are present
4. *Not* indicated for routine prophylaxis after cardiac surgery

Risks of Platelet Transfusion

1. Alloimmunization to platelets or leukocytes may occur in patients receiving repeated transfusions (e.g., oncology patients). Antibodies to subsequent transfusion platelets may result in platelet destruction.
2. Infection:
   a. Viral risk increases by pooling concentrates from multiple donors.
   b. Bacterial risk is increased by storage at 20° to 24° C.

3. Graft vs. host disease can be prevented by irradiation of platelets for immunocompromised patients.

Granulocytes

Description

1. Usually prepared by centrifugation electrophoresis of a single donor.
2. Must be infused within 24 hours of collection.
3. Neonatal granulocyte transfusions use "buffy coat" preparations.

Indications

Severe neutropenia, fever or sepsis unresponsive to antibiosis, and hypoplastic bone marrow with reasonable chance of recovery.

Plasma Derivatives

Several plasma derivatives are now available to replace congenital deficiencies. Although their use is rarely required intraoperatively, the anesthesiologist may need to discuss these options with the hematologist to adequately prepare the patient before surgery (see box below).

PLASMA DERIVATIVES

Cryoprecipitate

- Contains concentrated factor VIII: C, factor VIII: vWF (von Willebrand factor), fibrinogen, factor XIII.
- Useful for hemophilia A, von Willebrand's disease, congenital or acquired fibrinogen deficiency, factor XIII deficiency, and consumptive coagulopathy.

Factor VIII concentrate

- Indicated for the treatment of hemophilia A.
- Prepared from pooled plasma with techniques that reduce (*not* eliminate) viral transmission.

Factor IX concentrate

- Factor IX complex (prothrombin complex) contains factors IX (1%–5%), II, VII, X.
- Coagulation factor IX contains factor IX (20%–30%), trace II, VII, X.
- Useful for patients with Christmas disease (factor IX deficiency).
- Heat treated to reduce (*not* eliminate) viral transmission.

Antithrombin III concentrate

- Fraction of pooled plasma used to treat congenital deficiency of antithrombin III with associated thrombosis and to restore response to heparin.
- Heat treated to reduce (*not* eliminate) viral transmission.

Alpha$_1$ proteinase inhibition concentrate (alpha$_1$ antitrypsin)

- Fraction of pooled plasma used for patients with severe alpha$_1$ antitrypsin deficiency and demonstrable emphysema.
- Heat treated to reduce (*not* eliminate) viral transmission.

TRANSFUSION REACTIONS

Acute Hemolytic Reactions

ABO Incompatibility (Intravascular Hemolysis)

1. Usually the result of clinical errors
2. Caused by activation of complement to C_9 by anti-A or anti-B with resultant intravascular hemolysis
3. Clinical symptoms
   a. Chest, back pain
   b. Fever
   c. Hemodynamic instability and cardiorespiratory failure
   d. Disseminated intravascular coagulation (DIC)
   e. Renal damage from renovascular thrombus, prolonged hypotension, or vasoconstriction of renal microcirculation. (Renal dysfunction is probably not due to inspissation of hemoglobin in renal tubules.)
4. Treatment
   a. Transfusion is immediately stopped.
   b. Blood bank is notified and samples of patient blood sent for Coombs test to verify transfusion reaction.
   c. Crystalloid is infused; furosemide can be used to maintain urine output and increase renal cortical blood flow.
   d. Low-dose dopamine also increases renal circulation and supports pressure (3 to 5 μg/kg/min).
   e. An anticoagulated blood sample should be centrifuged and assessed for hemolysis.
   f. Baseline coagulation profile, BUN, and creatinine should be obtained.

Extravascular Hemolysis

1. Usually seen when antibodies other than ABO (Kell, Duffy, Kidd) are present.
2. No activation of C_9 occurs.
3. Clinical symptoms
   a. Fever
   b. Anemia
   c. Increased bilirubin
   d. Positive direct antiglobulin test
4. These reactions may occur up to 14 days after transfusion and usually require only supportive care.

Febrile Reactions

1. Characterized by chills and a rise in temperature without other signs of transfusion reaction.
2. Usually result from antibodies against leukocytes or platelets.
3. Repeat reactions are uncommon but can be prevented by using leukocyte-poor red cells.
4. Fever can be treated with acetaminophen. Meperidine may be used to stop shaking chills in older children.

Nonimmune Hemolysis

May be caused by:

1. Exposure to hypotonic solutions
2. Exposure to dextrose
3. Warming of blood products to more than 45° C
4. Cardiopulmonary bypass
5. Prosthetic valves

Allergic Reactions

Urticaria

1. Caused by antibodies to plasma proteins.
2. Transfusion may continue.
3. Antihistamines alleviate symptoms once it is determined that an intravascular hemolytic reaction is not occurring.

Anaphylaxis

1. Seen in patients with IgA deficiency who have anti-IgA antibodies as a result of a previous transfusion.
2. No fever is present.
3. Blood is discontinued and epinephrine administered.
4. Diagnosis is confirmed by measuring IgA levels in patient.

Noncardiogenic Pulmonary Edema

1. Onset: minutes to hours after transfusion
2. Symptoms: pulmonary edema and hypoxemia
3. Etiology: antigen/antibody reaction causing increased microvascular lung permeability (plasma and cells)
4. Treatment: ventilatory support

Hypervolemia

1. Etiology: rapid transfusion in normovolemic patients
2. Symptoms: pulmonary edema and hypertension
3. Treatment: diuresis and ventilatory support indicated.

Immunosuppression

It appears that red cell transfusions before kidney transplants result in immunosuppression probably related to lymphocyte depression. This effect may improve homograft survival.

Bacterial Sepsis

1. Etiology: transfusion of a contaminated unit of blood component
2. Symptoms: fever, signs of sepsis, and possible collapse soon after onset of transfusion. Diagnosis is differentiated from hemolytic reaction by negative Coombs test and absence of hemolysis.
3. Treatment: transfusion should be discontinued and hemodynamic support provided as needed.

COMPLICATIONS OF MASSIVE TRANSFUSION

Depletion of Factors V and VIII

Indications

Indications are coagulopathy when 2 to 3 blood volumes are lost and replaced with citrated blood.

Treatment

Treatment is to administer FFP in a dosage of 20% to 30% of each blood volume lost or 10 to 20 ml/kg.

Platelet Depletion

Indications

These include a platelet count less than 50,000 μL or abnormal bleeding time (indicating nonfunctional platelets).

Treatment

Treatment is to administer platelets in the amount of 0.2 units/kg or 20 ml/kg.

Caveats of Platelet Infusion

1. Platelets should never be refrigerated.
2. Large-pore filters must be used; micropore filters adsorb platelets.
3. Frequent platelet transfusions may increase antibody production and decrease the half-life of future platelet transfusions (alloimmunization).

Hyperkalemia

1. As blood ages, the K^+ concentration can increase by 17 to 27 mEq/L, although it usually averages 3 to 6 mEq/L.
2. K^+ in transfused blood moves into the intracellular compartment and is not usually a problem unless active hemolysis is occurring.
3. Frozen red blood cells have a low K^+ content and may cause hypokalemia.
4. Serum K^+ should be monitored frequently and hyperkalemia treated if necessary (see box on p. 98).

Hypocalcemia

1. Hypocalcemia occurs when citrate in FFP or blood chelates calcium, lowering serum-ionized calcium.
2. No treatment is indicated unless hemodynamic deterioration is present and consistent with ECG changes (prolonged Q-T, decreased S-T segment, flattened T waves), or ionized serum calcium levels are lowered.
3. Treatment: calcium chloride 2.5 mg/kg (should be given centrally) or calcium gluconate 7.5 mg/kg. Dosages may be repeated as necessary.

Acid-Base Changes

1. Acidosis is usually the result of decreased tissue perfusion and/or hypoxia.
2. Alkalosis caused by the conversion of citrate to bicarbonate in the liver may occur with massive transfusion.

Pulmonary Injury

1. Embolization may occur as a result of microaggregates of nonviable cells or debris.
2. Noncardiogenic pulmonary edema may occur from an inflammatory reaction in the pulmonary microvasculature, leading to increased vascular permeability.

Infection

Hepatitis

Incidence is approximately 10%. Over 90% of cases are non-A non-B type.

Human Immunodeficiency Virus (HIV)

Incidence is approximately 1 in 200,000 patients transfused.

Cytomegalovirus (CMV)

Incidence of transmission by transfusion to the neonate can be decreased by the use of leukocyte-depleted blood.

Hypothermia

1. Blood products have a temperature of 4° to 6° C. Massive transfusion without warming can easily result in hypothermia.
2. Energy must be expended by the infant or child to warm the infused blood. This process greatly increases oxygen consumption.
3. Warming blood to more than 45° C may result in hemolysis.

Oxyhemoglobin Dissociation

Shifting the oxyhemoglobin dissociation curve to the left decreases hemoglobin's capacity to release oxygen to tissue. The following factors are responsible for the leftward shift:

1. Hypothermia caused by unwarmed blood products
2. Alkalosis caused by conversion of citrate to bicarbonate in the liver
3. Decreased 2-3 DPG, which is minimally present in CPDA- or ADSOL-preserved cells.

Frozen red cells contain no citrate and normal amounts of 2-3 DPG and should cause a minimal shift in oxyhemoglobin dissociation.

BIBLIOGRAPHY

Adzick NS and others: Major childhood tumor resection using normovolemic hemodilution anesthesia and hetastarch, J Pediatr Surg 20:372-75, 1985.

Bikhazi GB and Cook DR: Perioperative fluid therapy and blood replacement. In Motoyama EK and Davis PJ, editors: Smith's anesthesia for infants and children, ed 5, St Louis, 1990, The CV Mosby Co.

Christensen RD and others: Granulocyte transfusions in neonates with bacterial infection, neutropenia, and depletion and mature marrow neutrophils, Pediatrics 70:1-6, 1982.

Cote CJ: Blood replacement and blood product management. In Ryan JF and others, editors: A practice of anesthesia for infants and children, Orlando, 1986, Grune & Stratton, Inc.

Lanier WL and others: The effects of dextrose infusion and head position on neurologic outcome after complete cerebral ischemia in primates: examination of a model, Anesthesiology 66:39-48, 1987.
Lattanzi WE and Siegel NJ: A practical guide to fluid and electrolyte therapy. In Lockhart JD, editor: Current problems in pediatrics, Chicago, 1986, Year Book Medical Publishers, Inc.
Lindahl SGE: Energy expenditure and fluid and electrolyte requirements in anesthetized infants and children, Anesthesiology 69:377-82, 1988.
Liu LMP: Pediatric blood and fluid therapy, ASA Refresher Courses, American Society of Anesthesiologists 12:109-20, 1984.
Milligan NS and others: Excision of giant haemangioma in the newborn using hypothermia and cardiopulmonary bypass, Anaesthesia 40:875-78, 1985.
National Institute of Health Consensus Development Conference: Fresh frozen plasma: indications and risks, JAMA 5:551-53, 1985.
National Institute of Health Consensus Development Conference: Perioperative red cell transfusion, JAMA 7:2700-03, 1988.
National Institute of Health Consensus Development Conference: Platelet transfusion therapy, JAMA 6:1777-80, 1986.
Payne K and Ireland P: Plasma glucose levels in the perioperative period in children, Anaesthesia 39:868-72, 1984.
Pisciotto PT, editor: Blood transfusion therapy, ed 3, Arlington, VA, 1989, American Association of Blood Banks.
Sieber FE and others: Glucose: a reevaluation of its intraoperative use, Anesthesiology 67:72-81, 1987.
Stehling LC: Recent advances in transfusion therapy. In Stoelting RK, Barash PG, and Gallagher TJ, editors: Advances in anesthesia, vol 4, Chicago, 1987, Year Book Medical Publishers, Inc.
Tremper KK and others: The preoperative treatment of severely anemic patients with a perfluorochemical oxygen-transport fluid, fluosol-DA, N Engl J Med 307:277-83, 1982.
Welborn LG and others: Perioperative blood glucose concentrations in pediatric outpatients, Anesthesiology 65:543-47, 1986.

7

THE POSTANESTHESIA RECOVERY ROOM

Jody Lynn Shapiro

> Fly away, fly away, over the sea
> Sun-loving swallow, for summer is done.
> Come again, come again, come back to me,
> Bringing the summer and bringing the sun.
>
> CHRISTINA GEORGINA ROSSETTI
> **THE SWALLOW**

THE GOALS OF THE RECOVERY ROOM

See Table 7-1 for a summary of goals.

Primary Goals of Recovery

The primary goal of the recovery room is to provide a safe environment (with presence of skilled nurses, appropriate monitoring, and resuscitative equipment), where patients can return to their preanesthetic homeostasis. Children often require more attention and observation in the recovery period because of their specific anatomy and physiology.

Ventilation

Upon arrival to the recovery room, attention should be focused on patency of the airway and adequacy of ventilation. Presence or absence of cyanosis, chest excursion, grunting, retractions, nasal flaring, stridor, and wheezing should be noted. The chest always should be auscultated by the nurse as well as the physician. If there is any doubt about the adequacy of ventilation the airway should be supported and an arterial blood gas obtained.

TABLE 7-1. Goals of recovery

Goals	Indicators
PRIMARY GOALS	
Adequate ventilation	Patent airway Clear breath sounds by auscultation Good chest excursion No stridor, retractions, or nasal flaring No wheezing Normal respiratory patterns without apnea or periodic breathing
Oxygenation	$SpO_2 > 90\%$ on room air Acyanotic
Recovery of wakefulness	Return of cardiorespiratory reflexes: • Ability to prevent soft tissue airway obstruction • Ability to cough • Presence of baroreceptor and chemoreceptor reflexes Conscious; responds to verbal stimuli
Achieve normothermia	Temperature of 36° to 37° C
Reversal of neuromuscular blockade	Return of muscle strength; assess by peripheral nerve stimulation or clinical indices: • Inspiratory force > -20 cm H_2O • Vital capacity > 15 ml/kg • Ability to protrude tongue and lift head for more than 5 seconds • Knee flexion in infants
SECONDARY GOALS	
Relief from pain	Treatment should ablate physiologic responses that may indicate presence of pain especially with preverbal children (i.e., tachycardia, hypertension, nausea, vomiting, agitation)
Relief from nausea and vomiting	Possibilities of raised intracranial pressure, swallowed blood from posttonsillectomy bleeding, or severe gastric distention must be considered before treating
Reduction of psychologic stress	Calming the child with warm blankets, rocking, pain relief may help decrease long-term psychological and behavioral sequelae

Oxygenation

Oxygenation usually goes along with ventilation. The pulse oximeter has become a de facto standard in many recovery rooms. Children recovering from general anesthesia are at greater risk for hypoxia caused by decreased functional residual capacity (FRC), higher closing volumes, and greater oxygen consumption. Supplemental oxygen should always be administered and SpO_2 continually monitored.[1]

Awakening

Wakefulness depends upon many factors. The most important aspect of awakening is the return of cardiorespiratory reflexes—the ability to gag and cough to protect the airway, the return of baroreceptor reflexes to support perfusion, and the return of chemoreceptor responses to hypercarbia and hypoxia. The presence of a safe airway in children may be predicted by spontaneous eye opening in the immediate postanesthetic period.[2] The child also needs to achieve a certain level of consciousness that will allow the appropriate assessment of pain.

Normothermia

Both hypothermia and hyperthermia are common intraoperative problems, particularly in infants. The inability to regulate body temperature under general anesthesia, cold operating rooms, and continued heat loss are major reasons for hypothermia. Similarly, hyperthermia may be caused by dehydration, atropine administration, and overaggressive attempts to warm the child. On rare occasions malignant hyperthermia may be present. The etiology of the aberrancy in body temperature must be sought and corrected.

Reversal of Neuromuscular Blockade (NMB)

Adequate oxygenation and ventilation can only be accomplished with adequate reversal of neuromuscular blockade. NMB in toddlers and school-age children can be assessed by the same clinical indices as adults; full train of four and sustained tetany on NMB monitor, inspiratory force greater than -20 cm H_2O, and a vital capacity of at least 15 ml/kg. Small infants will demonstrate brisk flexion of the hips and knees when adequate muscle strength has returned.[3]

Secondary Goals of Recovery

The secondary goals are not concerned with the basic survival needs, but are directed towards the comfort and psychological well-being of the child.

Analgesia

Preverbal children cannot convey their perceptions of pain. However, prompt treatment of pain is urged, both for physiologic and psychologic well-being. Crying is not always an indication of pain, but physiologic responses such as tachycardia, hypertension, nausea, vomiting, and agitation are interpreted as signs that pain may exist.

TABLE 7-2. Treatment of pain in the PARR

Degree of pain	Drugs	Techniques of administration
Moderate-to-severe	Morphine: 0.1-0.2 mg/kg IV* Demerol: 1-2 mg/kg IV Fentanyl: 1-2 μg/kg IV Codeine: 0.5-1.0 mg/kg IV	Start with ¼ of dose and titrate to effect Observe child for 30 min after a narcotic is given Administer naloxone 1-2 μg/kg for respiratory depression and observe child for at least one hour before discharge
Moderate	Acetaminophen PR*: 0-3 months 40 mg 4-11 months 80 mg 12-24 months 120 mg > 24 months 5-10 mg/kg/dose	Anticipate onset approximately 30 min after administration

*IV, intravenous.
*PR, per rectum.

Intravenous narcotics are used most commonly to treat moderate to severe pain. The intravenous route allows quicker onset, a more predictable and earlier peak effect than intramuscular injections, and facility of titrating dose to response. Carefully titrated intravenous narcotics present few untoward effects (Table 7-2).

Control of Nausea and Vomiting

Nausea and vomiting occur commonly after eye or ear surgery but can occur after any procedure or anesthetic. The mechanism may be central as seen after the administration of narcotics or caused by a specific GI malfunction such as ileus or gastric distension. More serious causes include raised intracranial pressure (ICP) or swallowed blood from posttonsillectomy bleeding. Before any antiemetic is given these more serious etiologies should be ruled out.

Drugs commonly employed in the treatment of nausea and vomiting include phenothiazines (droperidol),[4] antihistamines (diphenhydramine, promethazine), and metoclopramide (see the box below).

TREATMENT OF NAUSEA AND VOMITING

Droperidol	50-100 μg/kg IV/IM
Diphenhydramine	0.75-1.0 mg/kg IV/IM
Promethazine	0.25-0.5 mg/kg IM
Metoclopramide	0.1-0.15 mg/kg IV

Psychologic Stress

Many children are terrified in the recovery room. They awaken in a strange place with unfamiliar people and may be disoriented from the residual effects of the anesthesia. Some children may experience nightmares, develop enuresis, or have behavioral problems after a surgical procedure.[5] Measures taken to calm and comfort the child may reduce the incidence of these sequelae and aid in the overall recovery.

An agitated child will not return to physiologic baseline as quickly as a calm child. Increased catecholamines can result in poor perfusion and increased shunting. A crying child can easily reverse intracardiac shunts and become hypoxic. Comforting the child with warm blankets, rocking him, and having a familiar toy available can be reassuring.

Attempts should be made to recover children in a quiet area of the recovery room. Some institutions allow parents in the recovery area when the child's condition is stable.

TABLE 7-3. Common problems in the Postanesthesia Recovery Room (PARR)

Problem	Predisposing factors	Therapy
Hypoxia	High metabolic requirements Increased right-to-left intracardiac shunting Decreased FRC, with increased closing volume causing atelectasis and shunts May manifest as bradycardia All factors leading to hypercarbia can also lead to hypoxia: airway obstruction, central hypoventilation, splinting from pain or tight dressings	• Pulse oximetry for early recognition of hypoxia • Oxygen therapy for at least 30 min after general anesthesia • Correction of predisposing factor • Intubation if indicated
Hypercarbia	Hypoventilation caused by: Residual anesthetic and narcotics Airway obstruction Incomplete reversal of NMB Atelectasis Splinting secondary to pain Casts Tight dressings Malignant hyperthermia	• Suspect hypercarbia in the restless, agitated, or overly narcotized patient • Stimulate child • Analgesics when indicated • Reversal of neuromuscular blockade if indicated • Assist ventilation with bag and mask • Reintubation if necessary
Cardiovascular problems		
Bradycardia	Hypoxia Vagal response Drugs (fentanyl, neostigmine, edrophonium) Increased intracranial pressure	• Administer oxygen, atropine • Neurologic evaluation

Tachycardia	Hypoxia and/or hypercarbia Hypovolemia Sepsis Hyperthermia Heart failure Pain Drugs (atropine/epinephrine) Psychologic stress	• Administer oxygen • Assist ventilation as needed • Evaluate fluid and cardiac status • Use analgesics and/or sedatives
Hypotension	Cuff of inappropriate size Hypovolemia Cardiac failure	• Cuff of appropriate size (⅔ length of upper arm) • Fluid resuscitation (10 ml/kg isotonic crystalloid) • Inotropic agents or vasopressors
Hypertension	Cuff of inappropriate size Pain, stress Hypercarbia Drugs (epinephrine, ketamine) Bladder distension	• Cuff of appropriate size • Assist ventilation • Analgesics and sedatives • Foley catheter • Vasodilators
Subglottic edema (post-intubation croup)[6]	Age 1-4 yr Traumatic intubation Tight fit of endotracheal tube (air leak > 25 cm H_2O) Coughing with the endotracheal tube in place Change in position while intubated Surgery of head and neck Duration of surgery >1 hr	• Humidified oxygen (cold steam) • Nebulized racemic epinephrine (0.05 ml/kg/dose diluted to 3 ml with saline, not more frequently than every 2 hr (maximum dose 0.5 ml) • Dexamethasone 0.1-0.2 mg/kg • Calm the child with judicious use of narcotics or parents' presence • Consider overnight admission for outpatients; edema may rebound after racemic epinephrine • Reintubation if airway is severely compromised

Continued.

TABLE 7-3. Common problems in the Postanesthesia Recovery Room (PARR)—cont'd

Problem	Predisposing factors	Therapy
Edematous upper airway; macroglossia[7]	Surgery around the airway Prone position Craniofacial abnormalities Trauma from clamps/retractors in the mouth Common procedures: • Cleft palate repair • Resection of cystic hygroma • Tonsillectomy • Adenoidectomy • Tongue resection	• Stimulate patient • Support airway by head tilt and jaw displacement • Nasal/oral airway • Early reintubation if severe compromise of airway • Emergency cricothyroidotomy if failed reintubation • Upper airway obstruction may rarely result in pulmonary edema caused by the transudation of fluid from large negative intrathoracic pressures generated when inspiring against a closed glottis[8] • Negative pressure pulmonary edema can be managed by intubation and positive pressure ventilation and usually resolves within hours
Bleeding tonsil[9]	Inadequate surgical hemostasis Severe coughing Bleeding diathesis Presentation may be insidious because of swallowed blood from persistent oozing; tachycardia may be presenting sign	• Intravenous placement and hydration is desirable but not always possible; treatment consists of swift surgical ligation • Cross-matched blood available in OR • No premedication • Rapid sequence induction is preferable, but not always possible if there is no IV access and bleeding is life-threatening; in this situation an immediate awake intubation and surgical ligation is indicated • In rare situations it may be necessary to proceed with an inhalation induction without IV access (with patient in the head down lateral position); spontaneous ventilation is maintained with cricoid pressure—positive pressure ventilation can precipitate vomiting of swallowing blood • Have two large-bore suction catheters, forceps, two laryngoscopes, and several endotracheal tubes on hand

PARR SCORING SYSTEM AND CRITERIA FOR DISCHARGE

A variety of criteria for discharge from the PARR have been developed; however, decisions must be based ultimately on clinical judgment (Table 7-4). Discharge criteria for outpatients tend to be more strict because these patients will not be supervised by medical personnel and will not have access to intravenous hydration and parenteral analgesics.

Both Aldrete[10] (Table 7-5) and Steward[11] (Table 7-6) have developed scoring systems to help quantitate recovery from anesthesia.

TABLE 7-4. Criteria for discharge[2]

Inpatients	Recovery of protective airway reflexes
	Hemodynamic stability and control of bleeding
	Absence of any anticipated instability in respiration or circulation
	Reasonable control of pain and vomiting
	Appropriate duration of observation after administration of narcotics (a minimum of 30 min for an intravenous dose)
Outpatients	All criteria as for inpatients
	Return of consciousness to near-baseline level
	Return of stable gait (age-appropriate)
	Control of pain such that oral analgesics may be used
	Control of nausea and vomiting, to allow for oral hydration

TABLE 7-5. Aldrete PARR score[10]

Activity	
Moves four extremities	2
Moves two extremities	1
Moves no extremities	0
Respiration	
Deep breathing and cough	2
Limited breathing, good airway	1
Apneic/obstructed	0
Circulation	
SBP* $< \pm$ 20% preoperative level	2
SBP* $\pm$ 20-50% preoperative level	1
SBP* $\geq \pm$ 50% preoperative level	0
Consciousness	
Awake, answers questions	2
Arousable by name	1
Nonresponsive	0
Color	
Pink	2
Pale, dusky, blotchy, jaundiced	1
Cyanotic	0

Using this scoring system, Aldrete suggests that a total score of eight out of ten is necessary for discharge.

*SBP, systemic blood pressure.

TABLE 7-6. Steward PARR score[11]

Consciousness	
Awake	2
Responds to stimuli	1
Not responding	0
Airway	
Cough on command or crying	2
Maintains good airway	1
Airway requires maintenance	0
Movement	
Moving limbs purposefully	2
Moving limbs nonpurposefully	1
Not moving	0

Steward suggests that scoring be done at frequent intervals to evaluate the progression of recovery from anesthesia. No absolute score is recommended as a criteria for discharge.

REFERENCES

1. Motoyama EK and Glazener CH: Hypoxemia after general anesthesia in children, Anesth Analg 65:267-72, 1986.
2. Berde CB and Todres ID: Recovery from anesthesia and the postoperative recovery room. In Ryan JF and others, editors: A practice of anesthesia for infants and children, Orlando, Fla, 1986, Grune & Stratton.
3. Mason LJ and Betts EK: Leg lift and maximum inspiratory force, clinical signs of neuromuscular blockade reversal in neonates and infants, Anesthesiology 52:441, 1980.
4. Abramowitz MD and others: The antiemetic effect of droperidol following strabismus surgery in children, Anesthesiology 59:579-83, 1983.
5. Eckenhoff JE: Relationship of anesthesia to postoperative personality changes in children, Am J Dis Child 86:587, 1953.
6. Koka BV and others: Post-intubation croup in children, Anesth Analg 56:501-05, 1977.
7. Bell C, Oh TH, and Loeffler JR: Massive macroglossia and airway obstruction after cleft palate repair, Anesth Analg 67:71-74, 1988.
8. Lee KWT and Downes JJ: Pulmonary edema secondary to laryngospasm in children, Anesthesiology 59:347, 1983.
9. Montgomery JN, Watson CB, and Mackie AM: Anesthesia for tonsillectomy and adenoidectomy, Otolaryngol Clin North Am 20(2):331-44, 1987.
10. Aldrete JA and Kroulik D: A postanesthetic recovery score, Anesth Analg 49:924, 1970.
11. Steward DJ: A simplified scoring system for the post-operative recovery room, Can Anaesth Soc J 22:111, 1975.

8

THE PEDIATRIC AIRWAY

Michael D. Ho

Christopher Robin
Had wheezles
And sneezles,
They bundled him
Into
His bed.
They gave him what goes
with a cold in the nose,
And some more for a cold
In the head.

A.A. MILNE
NOW WE ARE SIX

ANATOMY AND PHYSIOLOGY—UPPER AIRWAY (Fig. 8-1)

Tongue

The infant tongue is large in relation to the oral cavity, predisposing to airway obstruction.

Larynx

The infant larynx is higher in the neck (C-3 to C-4) than it is in the adult (C-5 to C-6).

1. This high position allows swallowing to occur simultaneously with nasal breathing but also places the tongue against the soft palate during quiet respirations, causing oral airway obstruction.
2. Infants are obligate nasal breathers until the age of 3 to 5 months.
3. The acute angulation of the infant larynx at the base of the tongue makes intubation difficult by creating the impression of an anterior larynx. The larynx is not anatomically more anterior but is anterior to the line of view of the laryngoscope.

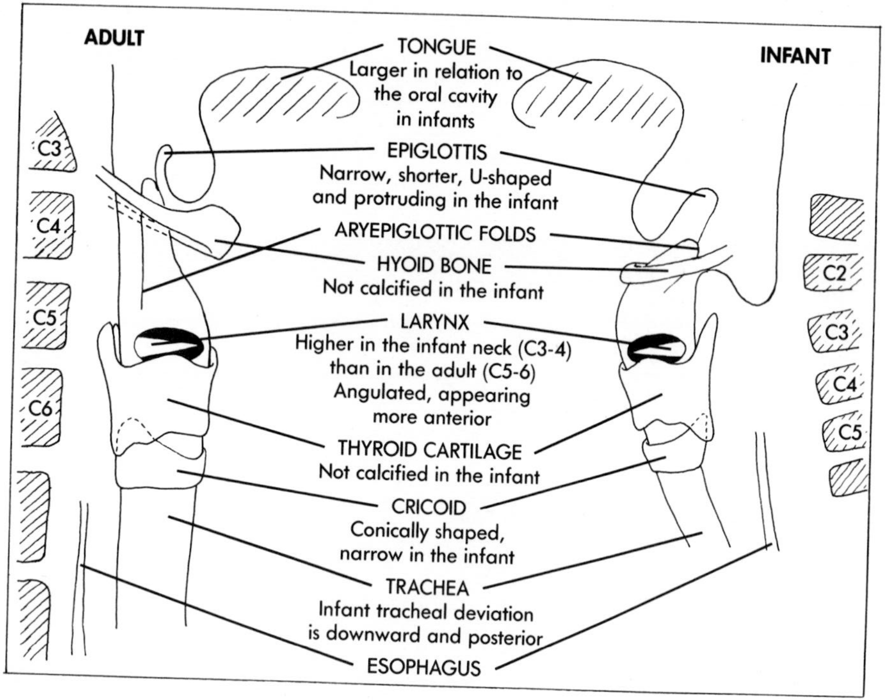

Fig. 8-1. Anatomic differences between the infant and adult airway. (Adapted from Cote CJ and Todres ID: The pediatric airway. In Ryan JF and others, editors: A practice of anesthesia for infants and children, Orlando, 1986, Grune & Stratton, Inc.)

4. External laryngeal pressure during intubation helps push the larynx into view. A straight blade also makes it easier to lift the base of the tongue and epiglottis to visualize the larynx.

Epiglottis

The infant epiglottis is narrow, short, U-shaped, and protrudes posteriorly over the larynx at a 45° angle.

Vocal Cords

The anterior attachment of the vocal cords is more caudal in infants. This slant in the vocal cords predisposes toward catching the tip of the endotracheal tube in the anterior commissure during intubation.

Cricoid Cartilage

The narrowest part of the upper airway in the infant is at the conically shaped cricoid cartilage.

1. Rather than selecting an endotracheal tube (ETT) size to fit between the cords, the pediatric ETT must fit through the cricoid cartilage.
2. This narrowing assumes special importance because the resistance to laminar air flow is proportional to the fourth power of the radius. For example, 1 mm of circumferential edema in a 4-mm infant airway will reduce cross-sectional area by 75% and increase the resistance 16 times. The same amount of edema in an 8-mm adult airway will decrease the cross-sectional area by 44% and increase the resistance 3 times.
3. The cricoid narrowing and angulation of the cords generally disappear by 10 to 12 years of age.

Tonsils

The tonsils and adenoids are small in a neonate but grow during childhood to achieve their maximal size by 4 to 7 years of age, after which they gradually recede.

Large Occiput

The relatively large size of the infant head and the short cords-to-carina distance (4 to 5 cm) can cause the tip of the endotracheal tube to move down the trachea with head flexion and up with head extension by as much as 2 cm.

A small rolled towel beneath the neck when the infant is lying supine will prevent neck flexion caused by the large occiput.

Angulation of Trachea

The infant tracheal deviation is downward and posterior. In the adult, it is straight downward. Cricoid pressure is thus more effective in aiding endotracheal intubation in infants.

MANAGEMENT OF THE AIRWAY

General Approach

In the history and physical examination, particular attention should be paid to past or recent problems (e.g., snoring, upper respiratory infections, history of croup) and physical findings (e.g., congenital anomalies, obesity, degree of respiratory distress, loose teeth) that may affect airway management.

Positioning

1. The axes of the mouth, oropharynx, and trachea should be aligned. Placement of a folded sheet or towel under the occiput will align the pharyngeal and tracheal axes. Extension of the head at the atlanto-occipital joint brings the oral axis into line with the other two, achieving a "sniffing position."
2. The relatively large occiput in patients under 3 years of age allows alignment of the airway without elevating the head. A folded towel beneath the shoulders will usually suffice.
3. Overextension may cause anterior displacement of the glottis and tracheal compression.

Equipment

Oral Airway

To fit properly, the tip of the oral airway should align just before the angle of the mandible when held against the side of a patient's face with the opening against the mouth. An airway that is too large can push the epiglottis down. One that is too small can push the tongue against the posterior oropharynx.

Nasal Airway

Care must be used in placing a nasal trumpet to avoid injuring the hypertrophied adenoids and causing bleeding. The presence of any airway (nasal or oral) near the glottis can precipitate laryngospasm in the lightly anesthetized patient.

Endotracheal Tube (See boxes on p. 133 for complications and sequelae of intubation)

1. The following formulas can be used to estimate appropriate tube size:

$$\text{Size} = \frac{\text{age(yr)} + 16}{4}$$

or

$$= \frac{\text{age(yr)}}{2} + 12$$

or

$$= \frac{\text{wt(kg)}}{5} + 12$$

2. Small-diameter endotracheal tubes increase airway resistance and work of breathing.
3. An oversized endotracheal tube can injure the narrow cricoid area. The resultant edema predisposes to postintubation croup.
4. Cuffed tubes increase the potential for cricoid damage and reduce the

COMPLICATIONS OF INTUBATION BASED ON TIME OF OCCURRENCE

Laryngoscopy

- Cardiovascular changes (HTN, tachycardia)
- Dental and soft tissue damage
- Aspiration
- Laryngospasm

Tube in situ

- Obstruction or kinking of tube
- Endobroncheal intubation
- Inadvertent extubation
- Increased resistance to breathing
- Bronchospasm
- Tracheal mucosa ischemia

Postintubation

- Laryngospasm
- Laryngitis
- Granuloma formation
- Tracheitis
- Tracheal stenosis
- Vocal cord paralysis
- Arytenoid cartilage dislocation

COMMON SEQUELAE OF INTUBATION IN CHILDREN

Endobronchial intubation

- Occurs typically into right main stem bronchus.
- Difficult to detect in neonates because breath sounds are well transmitted.
- Initially detected by a decrease in SaO_2, unequal breath sounds, or wheezing.

Croup

- Incidence of postintubation croup in children is 1% to 6%.
- Risk factors include age (6 mo–4 yr), length of intubation, lack of leak around tube, and increased head movement.
- Treatment includes cold mist tent and nebulized 2.25% racemic epinephrine (0.05 ml/kg/dose in 3 ml of normal saline).
- Use of steroids to reduce edema is controversial.

Laryngospasm

- Defined as approximation of true vocal cords or both true and false cords.
- Commonly caused by inadequate depth of anesthesia with sensory stimulation (secretions, manipulation of airway, surgical stimulation).
- Treatment includes removal of stimulus, 100% oxygen, continuous positive pressure by mask, and muscle relaxants if necessary.

maximum tube size allowable. They are generally not used for patients under age 8.

5. Ultimately, the proper tube size is confirmed by the ability to generate positive pressure greater than 30 cm H_2O and the presence of a leak at less than 20 cm H_2O.
6. The tube should be secured at the point where the second mark on the ETT tip just passes through the cords. Tube-to-lip taping distances are as follows:

Preterm infant	8–9 cm
Neonate	10 cm
1 year	11 cm
2–3 years	12 cm
5 years	13–14 cm
10 years	16–17 cm

Laryngoscope

A straight laryngoscope blade is preferred to a curved one in infants and small children to retract the epiglottis and directly expose the larynx. Sizes and choice of blades vary according to age.

DISORDERS OF THE AIRWAY
General Considerations

Signs of airway obstruction in an infant are often nonspecific and may be indicative of many other problems. Tachypnea, retractions, tachycardia, nasal flaring, restlessness, obtundation, cyanosis, wheezing, stridor, use of accessory muscles, and paradoxical breathing are indications that airway patency needs to be evaluated.

Infections and Immunologic Disorders
Epiglottitis

1. Epiglottitis is an acute, life-threatening infection of the supraglottic area, usually due to *Hemophilus influenza*. The region becomes edematous and inflamed, leading to the sudden onset of sore throat, fever, inspiratory stridor, and respiratory distress. Typically, the child will be leaning forward to breathe, drooling, and appearing quite toxic. The age of onset is usually 2 to 8 years of age. There is no seasonal predilection.
2. The patient should be kept calm and comforted by the parents. Radiographic studies and physical examination, including attempts to visualize the epiglottis, should be deferred because of the potential for laryngospasm and irrevocable loss of the airway.
3. A physician with the ability to perform emergent tracheostomy in children should be in attendance.
4. The patient is brought into the operating room under the supervision of an experienced anesthesiologist and surgeon.
5. The induction may be done with the child sitting upright, possibly on a parent's lap to keep the patient calm. Forcing the child into a supine position may precipitate acute airway obstruction.

6. Anesthesia is induced with halothane and oxygen. After obtaining a deep plane of anesthesia, an intravenous line is started and atropine administered. Airway obstruction will increase the amount of time necessary to produce deep anesthesia using an inhalation induction.
7. Direct laryngoscopy and oral endotracheal intubation is performed using a tube one size smaller than normal with a stylet in place. Spontaneous ventilation is maintained and muscle relaxants are avoided.
8. Replacement of the oral tube with a nasal one is recommended when prolonged intubation is anticipated and the change can be accomplished easily. If the initial intubation was difficult, the tube should be well secured and no further airway instrumentation attempted ("the enemy of Good is Better").
9. The patient is transferred to the intensive care unit where maintenance on intravenous sedatives will allow spontaneous ventilation via T-tube until defervescence and the presence of an air leak indicate improvement (usually 36 to 48 hours). "Second look" direct laryngoscopy with atropine, sedation, and succinylcholine is performed to evaluate readiness for extubation.

Laryngotracheobronchitis (Croup)

1. A common wintertime illness of the subglottic area in children, croup occurs between 6 months and 6 years of age and is usually of viral origin.
2. Symptoms include an insidious onset of low-grade fever, a croupy or seal-bark cough, inspiratory stridor, retractions, and if severe, cyanosis.
3. Differentiation from epiglottitis may be difficult because the development of respiratory distress and stridor can be the final common pathway of both. Pathologic conditions that can have similar symptoms include bacterial tracheitis, laryngeal foreign body, retropharyngeal abscess, and diphtheria.
4. Basic guidelines for care include keeping the patient calm and administering oxygen in cold steam (croup tent).
5. The use of aerosolized racemic epinephrine may produce temporary improvement of symptoms, but rebound hyperemic obstruction may result after its use.
6. The use of steroids as a treatment option remains controversial, although recent data seem to favor its use.
7. Intubation or tracheostomy is seldom needed but may be necessary in cases of severe respiratory compromise. The usual duration of intubation is longer than for epiglottitis (3 to 5 days), perhaps because of the lack of specific antibiotic treatment for the viral pathogens.

Peritonsillar Abscess (Quinsy)

1. Peritonsillar abscess tends to occur in older children or young adults. Incision and drainage is required if the response to antibiotic therapy is inadequate.
2. Severe pharyngeal swelling, trismus, distortion of pharyngeal anatomy (shifted uvula), and airway obstruction can occur. Dehydration results from swallowing difficulty and hyperventilation.

3. Aspiration during incision and drainage is best avoided in an older child by keeping the patient awake. A rapid sequence induction is performed in young children if no airway difficulty is suspected (peritonsillar abscesses rarely obstruct the airway). Alternatively, if significant trismus or a difficult intubation is anticipated, an inhalation induction with spontaneous ventilation can be performed. On rare occasions, an extremely critical airway will require tracheostomy under local anesthesia before general anesthesia.
4. Bleeding can be profuse from the hyperemic, infected area. Perforation of an abscess calls for rapid suctioning and immediate placement of the patient in the Trendelenburg position to prevent aspiration.

Ludwig's Angina

Ludwig's angina is a submandibular, sublingual cellulitis. Because the molars are usually the origin of infection, this disease occurs primarily in older children and young adults. Fulminant edema of the mouth, tongue, neck, and deep cervical fascia can occur, making oral intubation impossible. Tracheostomy under local anesthesia is usually indicated to avoid airway obstruction.

Angioneurotic Edema

1. Angioneurotic edema is an autosomal dominant disorder of the complement pathway. Deficiency of C esterase inhibitor allows unopposed activity of the early complement pathway components.
2. Clinically, episodic swelling of the extremities, face, and bowel wall is seen. Involvement of the larynx is associated with a mortality of up to 30%.
3. Prophylactic use of purified C1 inhibitor has proven effective in preventing the swelling. Prophylactic fresh frozen plasma (FFP) can supply adequate amounts of C1 inhibitor but may also adversely fuel further pathway activation. Danazol, an androgen, can prevent attacks by stimulating production of the deficient C1 esterase inhibitor.
4. The local trauma of intubation has been known to trigger attacks of edema. Normal levels of C1 inhibitor and C4 should be demonstrated preoperatively before any airway manipulation. Symptomatic airway edema warrants either intubation or tracheostomy.

Congenital Anomalies

Choanal Atresia

1. Choanal atresia occurs in varying degrees, ranging from a unilateral membranous obstruction located between the nasal cavity and nasopharynx to bilateral bony obstruction. Often an inability to pass a catheter into the nasopharynx at birth is the first sign.
2. Immediate steps to relieve the obstruction include making the infant cry, securing the tongue with a tongue blade, or placing an oral airway.
3. Corrective surgery is usually not performed until the infant is several months old.
4. There has been renewed interest in primary endonasal puncture in newborns with the use of stenting tubes to prevent orifice closure.

Macroglossia

1. The term *macroglossia* broadly describes a tongue too large for the oral cavity, due to either a large tongue or a small mouth. Primary macroglossia is a benign condition, generally not requiring surgical correction until later in childhood for orthodontic or speech problems.
2. Secondary macroglossia arises from several causes, the most common of which is congenital lymphangioma (cystic hygroma).
   a. Extension of a cystic hygroma is a rare but troublesome condition with severe pharyngeal obstruction manifested at birth or when a hemorrhage causes its sudden enlargement (see section on "Cystic Hygroma," p. 138).
   b. A lingual thyroid, another cystic tumor, occurs as an incomplete migration of thyroid tissue from its original position at the base of the tongue. More common in females, the mass may cause dysphagia and bleeding, although small tumors can be asymptomatic. Following thyroid function tests and radionuclide scanning, thyroid supplementation usually shrinks the gland.
   c. Salivary, dermoid, and epidermal cysts are either treated with marsupialization or removed.
   d. Solid tumors such as hemangiomas, fibromatosis, and fibrolipomatous dysplasia are rare in children, as are childhood malignant tumors such as lingual carcinoma and rhabdomyosarcoma.
3. Awake intubation is the safest approach to airway management. Occasionally, primary tracheostomy with local anesthesia is necessary. Lesions involving the neck make preoperative tracheostomy difficult if not impossible to perform.
4. Intraoperative blood loss may be significant.
5. Pharyngeal packing during surgery may obstruct the airway or kink the endotracheal tube.
6. Postoperative edema and swelling, particularly if the operation involved the posterior tongue, require prolonged intubation or tracheostomy.

Cleft Lip and Palate

1. Isolated cleft palates have a greater association with umbilical hernias, club feet, ear defects, and syndromes such as Pierre Robin and Klippel-Feil.
2. Cleft lips are repaired surgically in early infancy. The repair of cleft palates is delayed until age 1 or later.
3. An inhalation induction is typically employed.
4. Placement of a gauze into the cleft can prevent the laryngoscope blade from becoming lodged there.
5. Careful stabilization of the endotracheal tube with tape is particularly important because the tube will be present in the operative site.
6. Blood loss is usually not excessive, although the performance of a pharyngeal flap increases its likelihood.
7. Removal of pharyngeal packs before extubation allows for examination of pooled blood and secretions before extubation.
8. Awake extubation reduces the chances of postextubation airway collapse and damage to the repair from subsequent oral or nasal airway placement.

9. Macroglossia and airway obstruction have been reported after lengthy use of oral retractors and necessitate prolonged postoperative intubation.

Cystic Hygroma

1. Cystic hygroma is a congenital dysplasia of the lymphatics, consisting of multiple cavernous cysts that contain serous, serosanguinous, or bloody fluid. They are usually located in the posterior triangle of the neck (60% to 70%) or in communication with the axilla (20% to 30%). They can also be found, although rarely, in the anterior triangle of the neck with intraoral involvement.
2. Present at birth, these hygromas can rapidly enlarge as a result of bleeding, infection, or fluid accumulation.
3. The extent of the lesion and the existence of any mediastinal or oral involvement are determined during the preoperative evaluation.
4. If possible, surgery is delayed until age 18 to 24 months because spontaneous regression can occur in the interim. Surgery is necessary at an earlier age if the airway is obstructed by either direct involvement of the airway or compression of surrounding tissues.
5. Neonates are given atropine and intubated while awake. Older patients may undergo inhalation induction, spontaneous ventilation being maintained until intubation is accomplished. Tracheostomy may be warranted if oropharyngeal masses are prominent or if substantial oropharyngeal edema is anticipated.
6. The prognosis is poor for neonates with massive hygromas.

Laryngomalacia

1. Laryngomalacia results from flaccid supraglottic laryngeal cartilages (epiglottic and aryepiglottic), which infold with inspiration.
2. High-pitched inspiratory stridor usually appears within the first few days or weeks of life. Crying aggravates the symptoms; a prone position alleviates them.
3. The condition usually resolves spontaneously between 12 and 24 months.
4. Head extension, jaw thrust, and continuous positive airway pressure can help alleviate acute episodes of obstruction. The flexible nasopharyngoscope for bedside diagnosis has reduced the anesthesiologist's role in the management of laryngomalacia, although tracheostomy or suturing of the epiglottis to the base of the tongue is occasionally required.

Tracheomalacia

1. Tracheomalacia is an uncommon anomaly, leading to collapse of the trachea during expiration and stridor.
2. Rarely found as a primary deficit, it is more commonly associated with tracheoesophageal fistulas, extrinsic compression by vascular anomalies or mediastinal masses, Ehlers-Danlos syndrome, or following prolonged tracheal intubation.
3. The trachea stiffens with age, obviating the need for surgery in most cases. Occasionally tracheostomy, vascular suspension of the aorta or innominate arteries, or implantation of a splint are necessary.

Laryngeal Web, or Laryngeal Atresia

1. Complete laryngeal atresia requires immediate tracheostomy or bronchoscopy and may be an unrecognized cause of stillbirths. Diagnosis is made by direct laryngoscopy. A weak cry or aphonia at birth may be indicative of partial obstruction.
2. Simple membranous webs can be treated by surgical endoscopic division. Thicker webs tend to recur and may require tracheostomy or laryngofissure with insertion of a prosthetic implant.

Vocal Cord Paralysis

1. Unilateral paralysis is more frequent than bilateral and suggests peripheral nerve injury. It is more common on the left vocal cord because of the long course of the recurrent laryngeal nerve under the aortic arch. Left-sided paralysis may be indicative of cardiac, pulmonary, or esophageal anomalies.
2. The occurrence of right-sided vocal cord paralysis following right-sided carotid artery cannulation for extracorporeal membrane oxygenation has also been described.
3. Bilateral paralysis is associated with central nervous system disease such as hydrocephalus, Arnold-Chiari malformation, intracerebral hemorrhage, encephalocele, and dysgenesis of the nucleus ambiguous.
4. Symptoms of unilateral paralysis include a weak cry, occasional choking, stridor, and coughing. Marked stridor, cyanosis with feeding, and intermittent aspiration are more common with bilateral paralysis. The diagnosis is made by direct laryngoscopy. If obstruction or aspiration are persistent, arytenoidectomy or tracheostomy may be necessary.

Tumors

Mediastinal Masses

1. Anterior mediastinal masses include Hodgkin's and non-Hodgkin's lymphoma, teratoma, thymoma, and angiomatous tumors.
2. Middle mediastinal masses include lymphoma, tuberculosis, bronchogenic cysts, and esophageal duplications.
3. Posterior mediastinal masses are primarily neurogenic in origin (neuroblastomas), with diaphragmatic hernias occurring in a small group of patients.
4. Cardiorespiratory arrest and death on induction of anesthesia in patients with anterior mediastinal masses is well recognized. Compression and distortion of the trachea may make intubation extremely difficult even with fiberoptic visualization. Compressed small airways are often stented open only by the normal negative intrathoracic pressure in the chest during spontaneous ventilation. In this situation, conversion to positive pressure ventilation may result in complete stoppage of flow through the airway. Intubation will not relieve this problem because obstruction is distal to the trachea. Compression of the superior vena cava or pulmonary artery by tumor can also precipitate rapid demise in the supine position.
5. A diligent preoperative evaluation for signs of airway obstruction or vessel compression, including computerized tomography of the chest and flow-

volume loops, is essential. Preoperative radiation therapy to shrink the tumor may be required to maintain ventilation, even before a diagnostic biopsy is performed.

6. Intraoperative management usually includes awake fiberoptic intubation with maintenance of spontaneous ventilation in a semi-Fowler's position throughout the procedure, avoidance of all relaxants, readiness to turn the patient quickly to a lateral or prone position, and availability of rigid bronchoscopy and standby femoral-to-femoral bypass.

Papillomatosis

1. Juvenile papillomatoses are multiple tumorous growths found in the larynx, pharynx, trachea, and occasionally the lung tissue of children.
2. Although classified as benign entities, the nature of these tumors is aggressive and recurrent. The disease is self-limited, and most cases enter remission in puberty.
3. Hoarseness is usually the first symptom, and progressive respiratory obstruction often occurs.
4. Frequent endoscopic removal is required, often by laser excision (Table 8-1 and box on p. 141 for types and principles of lasers). Spontaneous ventilation should be maintained to avoid pushing polypoid lesions into an already compromised airway. A protected endotracheal tube for use

TABLE 8-1. Types of lasers*

Type	Active media	Properties and uses
CO_2	Gas	Emits invisible infrared energy absorbed by all tissue traversed; therefore damages all surface tissue (continuous wave mode).
Helium-neon	Gas	Emits a visible beam of low energy, which does not affect tissue. Used to direct invisible laser beams (CO_2) and to focus X rays.
Argon	Gas	Emits visible radiation highly absorbed by hemoglobin or pigment and poorly absorbed by water. Used on the retina or to photocoagulate large areas (continuous wave mode).
Ruby	Crystalline Solid	Pulsed emission absorbed by hemoglobin or melanin. Also used primarily on the retina.
Neodynium yttrium aluminum garnett (NdYAG)	Glass	Pulsed emission preferentially absorbed by hemoglobin or melanin (not water), which can be directed via fiberoptics to tracheobronchial lesions.

*Lasers (*l*ight *a*mplification by *s*timulated *e*mission of *r*adiation) are classified according to the active media used to produce the intense beam (gases, liquid solids, crystalline solids, or glasses).

with laser equipment should be selected, often several sizes smaller than that predicted because of laryngeal narrowing by papillomas. Tracheostomy may be required for severe obstruction but involves the risk of papilloma virus seeding the trachea.

Hemangiomas

1. Congenital hemangiomas occur in the laryngeal and subglottic regions of young infants. This diagnosis is suspected in those with a fluctuating pattern of respiratory obstruction, inspiratory stridor, and cutaneous hemangiomas on the body.
2. Spontaneous regression by the age of 2 years is typical. Resection with a CO_2 laser or cryoprobe, with concurrent use of systemic steroids, may become necessary.

Angiofibromas

1. Angiofibromas are the most common benign tumor of the nasopharynx in children. The usual sign is episodic epistaxis in adolescent males.
2. Controlled hypotension with nitroprusside is a useful technique to minimize bleeding during excision of this tumor. Intraoperative monitoring

PRINCIPLES OF LASER USE

Advantages of laser use

- Precision
- Lack of bleeding
- Complete sterility
- Reduced tissue reactions (edema)

Hazards of laser use

- Operating room personnel are susceptible to eye injury and must wear protective goggles designed to absorb energy of the wavelength emitted by the laser in use.
- Direct laser ignition of the endotracheal tube with resultant airway fire, thermal burns, and smoke inhalation is possible.
- Normal tissue can be damaged by reflected or misdirected laser beams.

Anesthetic techniques for laser microsurgery of the airway

- An ETT smaller than the calculated size is used.
- If a cuffed tube is used, the cuff is filled with water, not air.
- The tube is spirally wrapped with aluminum or copper tape, or manufactured tubes of silicone and metal can be used.
- Muscle relaxants are used to assure an immobile surgical field.
- The patient's eyes are protected with moist pads.
- The use of O_2 and N_2O is minimized; they are replaced with air to decrease fire hazards.
- The use of highly reflective instruments and mirrors is avoided in the surgical field.
- If a fire occurs, the flow of O_2 is discontinued, the ETT removed, the fire extinguished with saline, and tissue damage assessed with bronchoscopy.

of central venous pressure, arterial pressure, and hematocrit is essential during controlled hypotension (see Chapter 14).

3. Surgery is usually staged with initial devascularization followed by later transpalatal excision. Since the tumor is thought to be androgen dependent, preoperative estrogens have also been employed.

Sleep Apnea

Classification

Sleep apnea can be classified as central, obstructive, or mixed. During REM sleep, brief periods of apnea lasting less than 10 seconds are frequently seen in normal children. Pathologic apnea, however, is of longer duration and occurs frequently throughout the sleep cycle.

Obstructive Sleep Apnea

1. The definition of obstructive sleep apnea syndrome may vary from institution to institution, but it is usually defined as multiple apneic periods, each occurring for more than 10 seconds, during several consecutive hours of sleep. Other symptoms of the syndrome include excessive daytime sleepiness, enuresis, hyperactivity, declining school performance, and behavioral changes.
2. The majority of apneas in children (except premature neonates) are obstructive. Causes include enlarged tonsils and adenoids, choanal atresia or stenosis, nasal hamartomas or tumors, enlarged tongue, cleft palates, temporomandibular joint (TMJ) dysfunction, and facial anomalies. Two thirds of children with obstructive sleep apnea respond to tonsillectomy and adenoidectomy. Tracheostomy is avoidable in all but the most refractory cases.
3. Changes in respiratory physiology are often seen in patients with obstructive sleep apnea. It is not uncommon to see a decreased CO_2 ventilatory response with CO_2 retention and dependence on hypoxic ventilatory drive. These changes involve a central component in the pathogenesis of obstructive apnea, perhaps implying mixed etiologies.

Anesthetic Management

1. Children with chronic obstructive apnea are prone to pulmonary hypertension and cor pulmonale. Preoperative echocardiography is useful in identifying this population. Patients with pulmonary hypertension are more susceptible to the development of negative pressure pulmonary edema if airway obstruction occurs during anesthesia.
2. All patients with a history of sleep apnea require perioperative apnea monitoring and oximetry, even after surgical correction. Although the reasons are unclear, apnea and obstruction often continue into the perioperative period after tonsillectomy or adenoidectomy.

Routine ENT Procedures

Tonsillectomy

In addition to airway obstruction, recurrent infection may be an indication for tonsillectomy. Patients with chronic tonsillitis do not necessarily exhibit signs of sleep apnea and airway obstruction.

1. An inhalation induction followed by a narcotic technique is commonly used to provide postoperative analgesia.
2. Extubation
   - A deep extubation may minimize trauma to the open surgical wound (tonsillar bed) that can result from coughing or "bucking" on the tube.
   - Conversely, many anesthesiologists feel the patient should have reflexes intact before extubation because of the presence of blood and secretions in the airway. In either case, it is best to minimize airway trauma that may be caused by vigorous suction or airway placement.
   - Extubation in the lateral position helps to visualize secretions and bleeding and prevent aspiration.
   - In this position pooled secretions can be removed by suction of the buccal sulcus (cheek) rather than along the tonsil beds.
   - Posttonsillectomy bleeding usually occurs either in the first 8 hours postoperatively or approximately 1 week later when the eschar retracts (see Chapter 7, Table 7-3).

Pressure Equalizing Tubes (PETs)

Myringotomy with placement of pressure equalizing tubes prevents recurrent otitis media in children. The very short time required by this procedure often precludes the need for IV placement.

Ear Operations

Children with complications of chronic otitis may require more complex ear surgery, including mastoidectomy, middle ear exploration, or tympanoplasty.

1. These procedures are generally performed using microsurgical techniques. Muscle relaxation is useful to maintain a quiet operative field.
2. Use of nitrous oxide during reconstruction of the tympanic membrane (TM) may result in expansion of the middle ear space and disruption of the TM repair. Nitrous oxide should be discontinued for approximately 10 minutes before replacement of the TM or graft.

Trauma

Maxillofacial Trauma

1. Lacerations, bleeding, edema, and fractures of the maxillofacial area make airway management extremely difficult. Blood, vomitus, secretions, and broken teeth or bony fragments can occlude the airway.
2. In general, awake intubation or intubation with spontaneous ventilation is preferred.
3. Intraoperatively, the use of halothane can trigger dysrhythmias if large amounts of epinephrine have been used to minimize bleeding during surgical repair.

Laryngeal and Tracheal Trauma

1. Open or closed injuries to the larynx and trachea can occur from direct trauma but are unusual in children. Closed injury, because it is easily overlooked, can be the more dangerous of the two.
2. Subcutaneous emphysema, dyspnea, hoarseness, cough, hemoptysis,

and, in particular, voice changes indicate the possibility of laryngeal damage. Computerized tomography is useful in identifying specific injury.

3. Excessive positive pressure by face mask, coughing, struggling, and nitrous oxide all increase subcutaneous emphysema, which can worsen the obstruction.
4. Overzealous attempts at intubation can result in further laryngeal or tracheal damage and create a false passage through a mucosal tear.
5. Cricoid pressure is not used with laryngeal trauma, because it can collapse an incompetent larynx. Blind nasotracheal intubation is also to be avoided because of potential trauma to the larynx.
6. One of the safest approaches to securing the airway is the use of fiberoptic bronchoscopy, especially when the anatomy is grossly distorted. Tracheostomy under local anesthesia below the level of injury may be necessary.

Foreign Body Aspiration

1. Foreign body aspiration is common in children between 1 and 4 years of age. Most foreign bodies (95%) lodge in the right mainstem bronchus.
2. The obstruction can be partial, producing wheezing that is unresponsive to bronchodilators. A greater degree of obstruction can result in a ball-valve phenomenon, leading to gas trapping and hyperinflation. Atelectasis results from more complete distal obstruction.
3. The remaining 5% of foreign bodies lodge in the trachea, usually prevented from further passage through the trachea by their large size. Cough, voice change, drooling due to painful swallowing, and partial or complete obstruction can result.
4. Chronic cough and recurrent pneumonia are often the manifestations of a foreign body when there is no known history of aspiration.
5. Urgent removal is indicated when a sharp object has been aspirated and in the presence of hemoptysis, dyspnea, or cyanosis. A peanut, because it releases inflammatory mediators, frequently causes pneumonitis and should also be urgently removed.
6. Any recent aspiration of a foreign body is considered an emergency because of the possibility of obstruction, edema, or dislodgement.
7. Esophageal foreign bodies can produce obstruction at the level of the aortic arch or cricopharyngeus, producing drooling and dysphagia.
8. Most foreign bodies (90%) are radiolucent. Expiratory films looking for air trapping on the obstructed side or fluoroscopy is used in the diagnosis.
9. Anesthetic management of foreign body aspiration involves inhalation induction with maintenance of spontaneous ventilation. Avoidance of nitrous oxide is advised to prevent expansion of trapped gas. Induction may be prolonged depending on the degree of airway obstruction.
10. Rigid bronchoscopy with removal of the foreign body is performed once the patient is anesthetized. Lidocaine spray provides additional topical anesthesia. The use of muscle relaxants during removal of a foreign body from the airway is controversial. Positive pressure ventilation can

convert partial to complete obstruction and precipitate disaster. Conversely, it is difficult to maintain adequate depth of anesthesia with spontaneous ventilation in partially obstructed patients, resulting in coughing or movement. The use of short-acting muscle relaxants has been advocated when attempting to grasp the foreign body via the bronchoscope because coughing during the procedure can cause fragmentation.

11. Fragmentation of the object can occur during the extraction, resulting in occlusion of the trachea or bronchus. Pushing the object back into the bronchus may be necessary. A Fogarty embolectomy balloon catheter can also be used to pull back a foreign body that has become impacted and is inextricable. If all measures are unsuccessful, emergency thoracotomy and bronchotomy may be required.
12. The use of medical management with bronchodilators, postural drainage, and chest physiotherapy has been largely abandoned. Dislodging the foreign body can result in complete obstruction of the trachea with subsequent respiratory arrest.

Special Techniques of Airway Management

Macroglossia, micrognathia, glossoptosis, and the myriad pathologic conditions encountered in pediatric airway management (see Table 8-2 for pediatric syndromes with airway involvement) can present a formidable challenge to even the most experienced anesthesiologist. It is not inappropriate to consider every pediatric airway a potentially difficult intubation so that a contingency plan is always available.

Inhalation Induction

Indications

1. Isolated lesion obstructing the airway (epiglottitis, croup, foreign body aspiration, tumors)

Technique

1. Mask induction using high gas flows, maintaining spontaneous ventilation.
2. N_2O is contraindicated in situations of severe hypoxia, pneumothorax, subcutaneous emphysema, burns, or acute abdomen.
3. An intravenous line is started and atropine administered before induction.
4. Intubation is accomplished during spontaneous ventilation under deep inhalation anesthesia.
5. Muscle relaxants are given only after the ability to ventilate the child has been demonstrated.

Awake Intubation

Indications

1. Critical airway lesions (trauma, large tumors, craniofacial defects)
2. Neonates, infants

Technique

1. The child is positioned with the head slightly extended and the neck supported (shoulder roll).

TABLE 8-2. Syndromes or conditions causing difficult intubation

Syndrome or condition	Associated anomalies: Maxillary hypoplasia or high arched palate	Macrognathia	Macroglossia	Microstomia	Cleft palate	Choanal atresia	Short neck	Comments
Achondrodysplasia		F						
Achondrogenesis	F							
Aniridia Wilms tumor association		F						
Apert	F					O		
Arthrogryposis		F			O			
Beckwith Wiedemann			F					
Bloom	F	F						
CHARGE association		O			O	F		
Cornelia de Lange	F	F			O	O		
Cri du chat		F						
Crouzon	F		O		O	O		Narrow nasopharynx, oropharynx
DiGeorge		O				O		
Down			F	F			F	Atlantoaxial instability
Fetal alcohol syndrome	F	O			O		O	
Goldenhar	F	F			O			Hypoplasia of ramus, condyle of mandible and TMJ; cleft tongue, cervical fusion

Hallerman Streiff	F	F		F				Hypoplasia of ramus, anterior displacement of TMJ
Hemifacial microsomia						O		Lateral cleft lip
Homocystinuria	O							
Hurler			O				F	
Hypothyroidism	O							
Juvenile rheumatoid arthritis								TMJ fusion, mandibular hypoplasia, cricoarytenoid arthritis, atlantoaxial subluxation
Klippel-Feil					O			Fused cervical vertebrae
Larsens		O			O			Floppy epiglottis, arytenoids, and tracheal cartilage
Marfan	F							
Maternal PKU fetal effects	F	F						
Meckel Gruber		F			F		F	
Noonan	O							
Oral facial digital	F	O			F	O		
Pierre Robin		F			F	O		
Pompe (GSDIII)			F					
Progeria	F							
Retinoic acid embryopathy		F			F			
Rubinstein Taybi	F	O						
Russel Silver		F						
Smith Lemli Opitz		F			O			
Treacher Collins	F	F		O	O	O		
Trisomy 13		O			F			
Trisomy 18		F		F	O	O		
Turner	F	F						

F = Frequent; O = Occasional

2. 100% oxygen is insufflated near the child's airway.
3. Atropine (0.2 mg/kg) IM or IV is given before instrumentation of the airway.
4. The ETT is placed under direct laryngoscopy (see Table 10-3 for detailed procedure).
5. Placement is verified by auscultation of breath sounds, aphonia, presence of end-tidal CO_2, and water vapor in ETT.

Blind Nasal Intubation

Indications

1. Spontaneously ventilating patient
2. Critical airway lesions
3. Older child able to comply with procedure (if awake)
4. Operations in the oropharynx

Technique

1. IV access is secured before instrumentation of nasopharynx.
2. Topical anesthesia is applied to nares (if awake, older child).
   a. 4% cocaine (dose of 1.5 mg/kg, solution contains 2 mg/drop)
   b. 1% lidocaine ointment or jelly
   c. 0.25% neosynephrine drops or oxymetazoline hydrochloride 1% (Afrin)
3. Alternatively, anesthesia may be induced by mask and spontaneous ventilation maintained.
4. Nares are dilated with increasing sizes of well-lubricated nasal trumpets.
5. The ETT is inserted gently into the nares and advanced 1 to 2 cm with each inspiration.
6. Trauma to Kiesselbach's triangle (anterior septum) or the area beneath the inferior turbinate may precipitate epistaxis.
7. Once the ETT is in the pharynx, turning the tube 180 degrees may improve the angle of entry into the trachea and minimize deflection off the anterior commissure (see Fig. 8-2).
8. If necessary, the tube may be placed in the larynx under direct laryngoscopy, using McGill forceps. This technique can be used in the non-spontaneously ventilating patient.
9. Gently closing the opposite nostril and the mouth will augment the passage of air through the tube and amplify breath sounds.
10. Auscultation of bilateral breath sounds, presence of end-tidal CO_2, aphonia, and water vapor in the ETT will verify proper placement.

Lighted Stylet

Indications

1. Used when the airway cannot be visualized directly
2. Can be used in the presence or absence of spontaneous ventilation
3. Can only accommodate an ETT size of 5.5 mm or greater

Technique

1. Anesthesia can be induced by intravenous or inhalation technique and ventilation maintained.

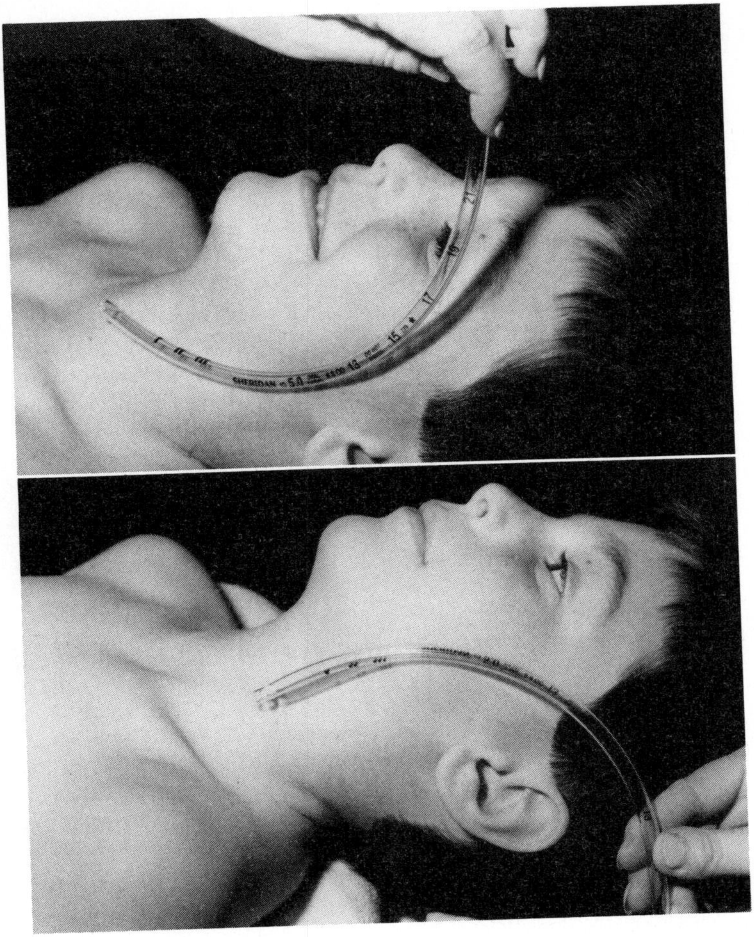

Fig. 8-2. Nasal intubation. With the endotracheal tube (ETT) in the pharynx, rotation of the tube 180° may improve the angle of entry into the trachea and minimize deflection at the anterior commissure. The angle of entry may also be improved by flexing the neck when the ETT is at the level of the larynx.

2. A flexible lighted stylet can be used to transilluminate the airway as the ETT is blindly passed together with the stylet inside.
3. In a darkened room, the tip of the lighted tube provides a diffuse area of illumination in the hypopharynx, epiglottis, and larynx.
4. Once through the cords, a brighter area several cm in diameter is visualized directly beneath the skin.

5. The ETT is then advanced over the wand into the trachea.
6. Position is confirmed by auscultation, capnography, aphonia, etc., as previously discussed.

Fiberoptic Bronchoscopy

Indications

1. Critical airway lesions
2. Lesions involving the neck that distort airway anatomy
3. Failed orotracheal or nasotracheal intubation

Technique

1. An antisialagogue/anticholinergic is used for premedication.
2. The oral approach will accommodate a larger ETT, but the acute angle between the oropharynx and trachea makes threading the tube more difficult.
3. The nasal approach more readily guides the endotracheal tube into the larynx but limits the size of the tube and is contraindicated in patients with coagulopathy.
4. The airway is anesthetized with topical anesthesia or deep inhalation anesthesia after inhalation induction, using one of the following:
   a. Nebulized 4% lidocaine
   b. Aerosol sprays
   c. Field blocks of airway
5. The largest endoscope that will easily fit into the ETT should be used:
   a. A 5.8-mm bronchoscope fits a 6.5-mm internal diameter ETT.
   b. A 3.2-mm bronchoscope fits a 4.5-mm ETT.
   c. A 2.7-mm bronchoscope fits a 3-mm tube ETT.
6. Common causes of failed fiberoptic intubation are inexperience and insufficient planning.
7. A trained assistant must be available to monitor the child while the anesthesiologist performs the procedure.

Percutaneous Cricothyroidotomy

Indications

1. Emergency technique when attempts at mask ventilation and intubation have failed.
2. Infants are poor candidates for this procedure because of the small length of the cricothyroid (1 mm), small diameter trachea, and potential for glottic injury.

Technique

1. The trachea is exposed by positioning the patient with a rolled towel beneath the shoulders and the head extended.
2. The cricothyroid membrane is punctured with a 14-gauge intravenous catheter in caudal direction. A small incision in the vertical plane may facilitate cricothyroid puncture.
3. Aspiration of air will confirm placement.
4. The inner needle is removed from the plastic catheter, and the catheter advanced into the trachea.
5. A 3-ml syringe is attached; aspiration of air confirms position.

6. The plunger is removed from inside the syringe.
7. An 8-mm ETT adapter is attached to the barrel of the 3-ml syringe (Fig. 8-3).
8. A 3.5-mm ETT adapter can also be directly attached to the catheter hub and decreases dead space.
9. Transtracheal jet ventilation is now possible by delivering intermittent bursts of oxygen at 50 psi.
10. Bag ventilation is also possible but often results in hypercarbia.
11. The plastic catheter is easily kinked and not easily secured. Ultimately, conversion to tracheostomy is advised.

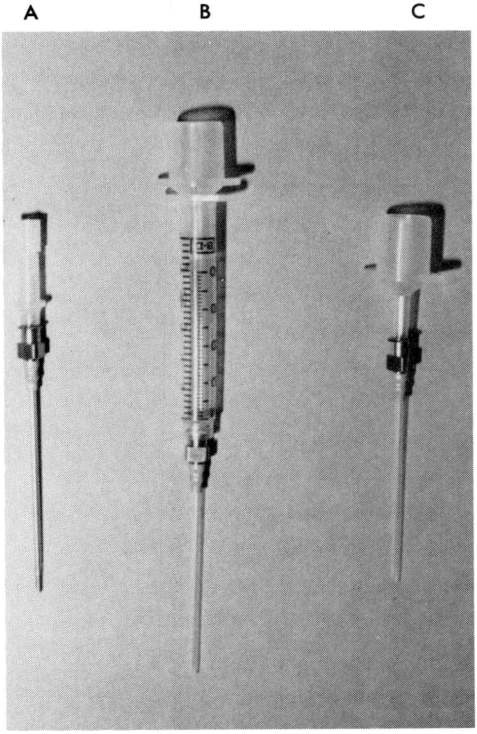

Fig. 8-3. Percutaneous cricothyroidotomy. In an emergency, a 14g intravenous catheter **(A)** can be converted for tracheal ventilation. A 3 ml syringe attached to the catheter allows for confirmation of placement in the trachea by aspiration of air. An anesthesia circuit or jet ventilator can be attached to the syringe by removing the plunger and adding an 8-mm ETT adaptor **(B).** A 3.5-mm ETT adaptor can be attached directly to the 14g catheter (after the needle is removed) **(C)**. Elimination of the 3 ml syringe decreases deadspace and makes it easier to hold the catheter securely with one hand without kinking or dislodging.

Rigid Bronchoscopy

Indications

1. Examination of airway while under general anesthesia.

Technique

1. The size of the scope refers to its internal lumen with the smallest having a 4-mm external diameter and a 3.2-mm internal diameter (e.g., Storz).
2. General anesthesia is induced and IV access secured.
3. Spontaneous ventilation is maintained and allows examination of vocal cord function.
4. A ventilating bronchoscope has a side port, which connects to the anesthesia circuit, allowing the continued delivery of oxygen and anesthetic gases.
5. 100% oxygen should be used while the bronchoscope is in the trachea because hypoxia is a constant threat during instrumentation and suctioning.
6. Higher concentrations of halogenated agents may be needed both during instrumentation of the airway and while on 100% oxygen.
7. Hypercarbia frequently occurs because passive ventilation is difficult as a result of the high airway resistance caused by the narrow bronchoscope. Capnography can be obtained at the side port, although the increased dead space caused by the bronchoscope will affect the accuracy of the capnogram.
8. Insertion of the telescope worsens airway resistance. Resultant air trapping can lead to pneumothorax or impede venous return. The surgeon will need to remove the telescope at intermittent intervals so that the patient can be ventilated.
9. An open bronchoscope delivers oxygen through a high-pressure source. Room air is entrained by the Venturi effect. The actual delivered F_IO_2 depends on the amount of entrained room air. The amount of gas delivered will decrease in less compliant lungs. Spontaneous or assisted ventilation through a ventilating bronchoscope is preferred to jet ventilation through an open bronchoscope in pediatrics because of the risk of barotrauma, air trapping, and hypoxia.

BIBLIOGRAPHY

Backofen JE and Rogers MC: Emergency management of the airway. In Rogers MC: Textbook of pediatric intensive care, 1987, Baltimore, Williams & Wilkins.

Bivins HG and others: The effect of axial traction during orotracheal intubation of the trauma victim with an unstable cervical spine, Ann Emerg Med. 17:25-29, 1988.

Cote CJ and Todres ID: The pediatric airway. In Cote CJ and others, editors: A practice of anesthesia for infants and children, Orlando, 1986, Harcourt, Brace, Jovanovich, Publishers.

Feinstein R and Owens WD: Anesthesia for ENT. In Barash PG, Cullen BF, and Stoelting RK, editors: Clinical anesthesia, Philadelphia, 1989, JB Lippincott Co.

France NK and Beste DJ: Anesthesia for pediatric ear, nose and throat surgery. In Gregory GA, editor: Pediatric anesthesia, ed 2, New York, 1984, Churchill Livingstone.

Jones KF: Smith's recognizable patterns of human malformation, Philadelphia, 1988, WB Saunders Co.

Karotkin EH: Physiological principles. In Goldsmith JP and Karotkin EH: Assisted ventilation of the neonate, Philadelphia, 1988, WB Saunders Co.

Morray JP and Krane EJ: Anesthesia for thoracic surgery. In Gregory GA, editor: Pediatric anesthesia, ed 2, New York, 1989, Churchill Livingstone.

Morrison JD: Otolaryngological diseases. In Katz J and Steward DJ, editors: Anesthesia and uncommon pediatric diseases, Philadelphia, 1987, WB Saunders Co.

Neuman GG and others: The anesthetic management of the patient with an anterior mediastinal mass, Anesthesiology 60:144-47, 1984.

O'Rourke PP and Crone RK: The respiratory system. In Gregory GA, editor: Pediatric anesthesia, ed 2, New York, 1989, Churchill Livingstone.

Palmisano BW: Anesthesia for plastic surgery. In Gregory GA, editor: Pediatric anesthesia, ed 2, New York, 1989, Churchill Livingstone.

Richardson MA and Cotton RT: Anatomic abnormalities of the pediatric airway, Pediatr Clin N Amer 31:821-33, 1984.

Schumacher RE, Weinfeld IJ, and Bartlet RH: Neonatal vocal cord paralysis following extracorporeal membrane oxygenation, Pediatrics 84:793-96, 1989.

Sibert KS, Biondi JW, and Hirsch NP: Spontaneous respiration during thoracotomy in a patient with a mediastinal mass, Anesth Analg 66:904-7, 1987.

Stoelting RK: Endotracheal intubation. In Miller RD: Anesthesia, New York, 1986, Churchill Livingstone.

Todres ID: Diseases of the respiratory system. In Katz J and Steward DJ, editors: Anesthesia and uncommon pediatric diseases, Philadelphia, 1987, WB Saunders Co.

Ward CF: Pediatric head and neck syndromes. In Katz J and Steward DJ, editors: Anesthesia and uncommon pediatric diseases. Philadelphia, 1987, WB Saunders Co.

Weller RM: Anesthesia for cystic hygroma in a neonate. Anaesthesia 29:588-94, 1974.

Woods AM: Pediatric bronchoscopy, bronchography and laryngoscopy. In Berry FA, editor: Anesthetic management of difficult and routine pediatric patients. New York, 1986, Churchill Livingstone.

9

THE PEDIATRIC PULMONARY SYSTEM

Anne M. Savarese
Howard A. Zucker

Then Michael sneezed and wheezed and coughed.
Dr. Paul said, "You just sit and rest
while I take my stethoscope
and listen to your chest."
MARGUERITE RUSH LERNER
MICHAEL GETS THE MEASELS

BASIC PULMONARY MECHANICS

Mechanics of Breathing

Quiet tidal breathing occurs when there is active inspiratory contraction of the diaphragm and intercostal muscles, followed by relaxation and passive expiration from elastic recoil of the lungs and chest wall. Contraction of the accessory muscles of respiration (strap muscles of the neck, sternocleidomastoid, anterior serratus, and external intercostals) augments forced inspiration. This effect, however, is diminished in the neonate, who has a "floppy," highly compliant chest wall and poorly developed musculature. Consequently, attempts at forceful inspiration in neonates appear as chest and sternal retractions with tracheal "tugging." Forceful expiration is equally difficult for neonates because of their poorly developed abdominal and internal intercostal musculature. These features illustrate why the only significant means for enhancing alveolar minute ventilation in neonates is by increasing respiratory frequency. The cost includes increased work of breathing, increased oxygen consumption, increased dead-space ventilation, ventilation/perfusion ($\dot{V}/\dot{Q}$) mismatching, and susceptibility to fatigue and respiratory failure.

After approximately 6 months of age, the chest wall begins to stiffen, the elastic recoil of the lungs increases, overall compliance decreases, and the ventilatory musculature develops. These developments allow for increased tidal volume (V_T), decreased respiratory frequency, and improved performance of forced inspiratory and expiratory maneuvers (e.g., sigh and cough). (See Table 9-1 for normal values of pulmonary function.)

Surfactant

1. Surfactant acts essentially as a detergent, forming a monomolecular interface between alveolar fluid and alveolar gas. Produced by type II pneumocytes, it is composed primarily of dipalmitoyl lecithin, as well as sphingomyelin, phosphatidyl inositol, and phosphatidyl dimethyl ethanolamine. The hydrophobic fatty acid portions of these molecules project into the gas phase, while the hydrophilic glycerol base portions project into the alveolar lining fluid. LaPlace's law explains why the pressure *inside* a bubble (alveolus) is greater than the surrounding pressure (pleural pressure), by an amount determined by (1) the surface tension of the liquid, and (2) the radius of curvature of the bubble:

$$P = \frac{2T}{r}$$

where:
P = Pressure within the bubble (dyne/cm^2)
T = Surface tension of the liquid lining the bubble (dyne/cm)
r = Radius of the bubble

Thus, to maintain alveolar patency, intraalveolar pressure and the transmural gradient must be preserved throughout the respiratory cycle as the alveolar radius changes with inspiration and exhalation. This is accomplished by the variable surface tension exerted by surfactant. The con-

TABLE 9-1. Pulmonary function: normal values

Components of pulmonary function	Neonate 0-3 days	Infant 1 year	Child to adult
Weight (kg)	3.3-3.5	10	20-80
Resting oxygen consumption ($\dot{V}O_2$) (ml/kg/min)	5-8	5	3-4
Minute ventilation (V_E) (ml/kg/min)	150-170	175-185	80-100
Respiratory frequency (bpm)	30-50	20-30	12-16
Tidal volume (V_T) (ml/kg)	6-8	6-8	7-8
Dead space (V_D) (ml/kg)	2-2.5	2-2.2	2-2.2
V_D/V_T ratio	0.3	0.3	0.3
Vital capacity (VC) (ml/kg)	35-40	45-50	50-60
Functional residual capacity (FRC) (ml/kg)	22-25	25-30	30-45
Lung compliance (C_L) (ml/cm H_2O)	5-6	15-20	130-150
Airway resistance (R_{AW}) (cm H_2O/L/sec)	25-30	10-15	1.5-2
Peak flow rate (L/min)	10		350-450
Number of alveoli (saccules × 10^6)	30	130	300

Adapted from: Motoyama EK: Respiratory physiology in infants and children. In Motoyama EK and Davis PJ, editors: *Smith's Anesthesia for infants and children,* ed 5, St Louis, 1990, The CV Mosby Co; and O'Rourke PP and Crone RK: The respiratory system. In Gregory GA, editor: *Pediatric anesthesia,* ed 2, New York, 1989, Churchill Livingstone.

centration of surfactant at the interface is proportional to its surface tension.

- During inspiration, the alveolar radius is large, the surfactant molecules are spread thinly ("loosely packed"), and surface tension increases.
- During exhalation, the alveolar radius is small, the surfactant molecules are spread thickly ("tightly packed"), and surface tension decreases.

2. Surfactant, with a surface tension much less than water, functions to:
   - Maintain alveolar patency, even at a small radius
   - Prevent pulmonary edema by counteracting the hydrostatic and oncotic driving pressure for transudation of capillary water into the alveolus
   - Prevent obstructive or resorption atelectasis by delaying absorption of gas from small radius alveoli
3. The concentration of surfactant is reduced in the following conditions:
   - Neonatal respiratory distress syndrome (RDS)
   - Cardiopulmonary bypass
   - Pulmonary embolism
   - Normobaric oxygen toxicity from hyperoxia exposure

Administration of surfactant suspensions (from bovine lung tissue or human amniotic fluid) to premature neonates may prevent or ameliorate the course of RDS.

Lung Volumes and Capacities (See Fig. 9-1)

1. *Functional residual capacity (FRC)* as it relates to overall respiratory reserve is critical to the anesthetic management of the pediatric patient. FRC is the volume of gas in the lung at the end of tidal expiration, when there is zero gas flow and alveolar pressure equals ambient pressure (when the forces of inward retraction by the lungs are balanced by those of the outward expansion of the thoracic cage).
2. FRC *decreases* under the following conditions:
   - General anesthesia with either spontaneous or controlled ventilation; increasing depth of anesthesia changes compliance as the outward recoil of the thorax decreases with muscle relaxation:

$$\downarrow \text{Compliance} \rightarrow \text{Airway closure} \rightarrow \downarrow \text{FRC}$$

   - Neuromuscular blockade, from loss of residual end-expiratory muscle tone
   - Pulmonary edema
   - Pulmonary fibrosis
   - Neonatal RDS
   - Kyphoscoliosis
   - Restrictive lung disease
   - Obesity
   - Pregnancy
   - Lateral decubitus or Trendelenburg position
   - The first 24 hours of the newborn period

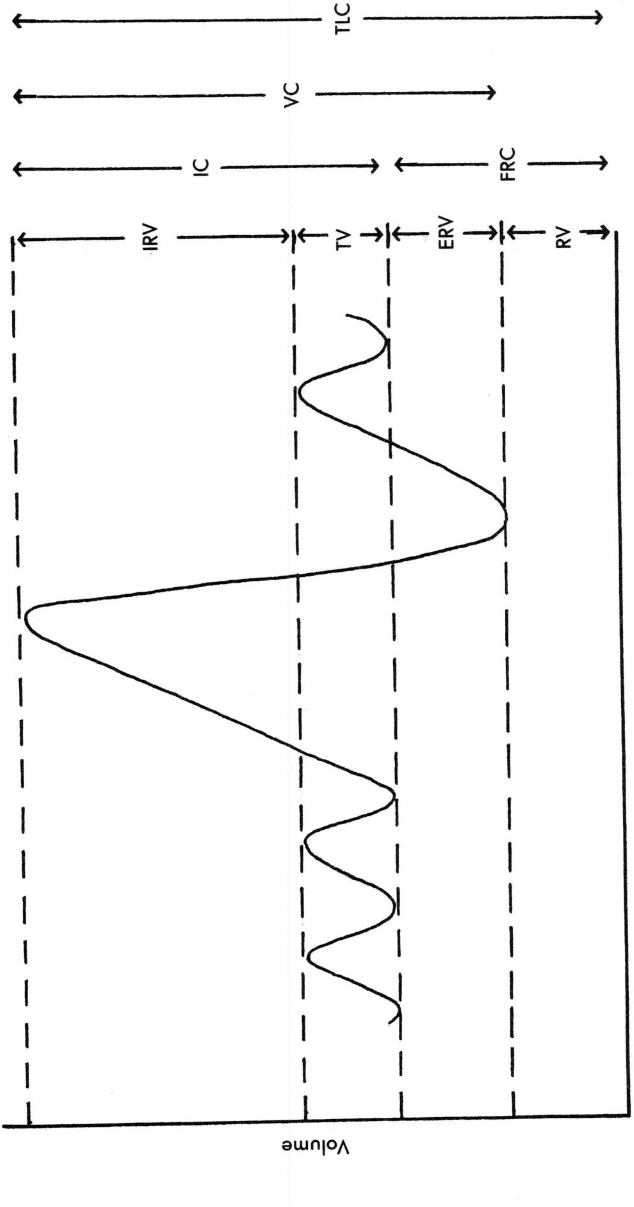

Fig. 9-1. Lung volumes. IRV = Inspiratory reserve volume, TV = Tidal volume, ERV = Expiratory reserve volume, RV = Residual volume, IC = Inspiratory capacity, FRC = Functional residual capacity, VC = Vital capacity, TLC = Total lung capacity.

3. FRC *increases* with the following:
   - Increasing height (a linear relationship)
   - Male sex
   - Erect body position (versus supine)
   - Positive end-expiratory pressure (PEEP) or continuous positive air pressure (CPAP)
   - Chronic obstructive pulmonary disease (COPD) because of decreased elastic recoil of the lungs (this has a salutary effect because at higher lung volumes airway resistance decreases and gas flow increases)
4. FRC does *not change* with age.
5. The adverse consequences of diminished FRC include:
   - Small airway closure
   - Uneven distribution of ventilation
   - $\dot{V}/\dot{Q}$ mismatching
   - Hypoxemia

   Preserving or restoring FRC is a major goal of clinical interventions such as chest physiotherapy, diuretic and bronchodilator therapy, PEEP/CPAP, and positive-pressure mechanical ventilation, as well as adequate postoperative analgesia and early ambulation following major thoracic and abdominal surgery.
6. The *dynamic FRC* in spontaneously breathing infants is maintained at about 40% of total lung capacity (as in the supine adult) by three mechanisms:
   a. Premature cessation of the expiratory phase by glottic closure; also referred to as "laryngeal braking"
   b. Forced expiration against a partially closed glottis; also referred to as "grunting" or "auto-PEEP"
   c. Maintenance of continuous, tonic inspiratory muscle tone in the diaphragm and intercostals, thereby stiffening the chest wall to oppose the elastic recoil of the lungs, which improves compliance and diminishes airway closure

Application of distending airway pressure during controlled ventilation under anesthesia or with mechanical ventilation mimics grunting and laryngeal braking. PEEP and CPAP increase expiratory resistance, thereby increasing end-expiratory lung volume, because only at higher lung volumes is the elastic recoil of the lung sufficient to overcome this applied resistance and permit exhalation. Increased end-expiratory lung volume (increased FRC) contributes to decreased airway resistance and airway collapse, and therefore to improved $\dot{V}/\dot{Q}$ matching.

Airway Closure

1. *Airway collapse* may be either *volume related* or *flow related*. Except at total lung capacity, airways and alveoli are smaller in dependent lung regions than in the top regions. The *closing capacity* (CC) is the lung volume above the residual volume at which airways in dependent lung zones begin to close. In most patients, closing capacity is less than FRC. Closing capacity approaches FRC with aging, the supine position, and anesthesia. When tidal breathing occurs within the closing capacity range

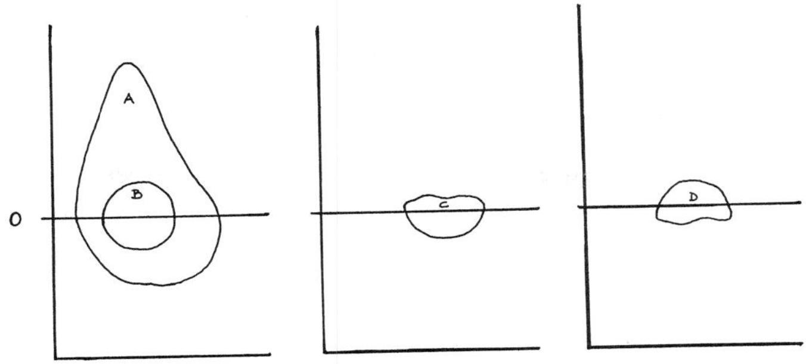

Fig. 9-2. Flow volume loops. *A*, Schematic tracing of an adult flow volume curve demonstrating maximum expiratory and inspiratory flow. *B*, Schematic tracing of a flow volume loop in a child using a face mask to diagram tidal breathing (requires virtually no patient cooperation). *C*, Intrathoracic obstruction in an infant demonstrated during tidal breathing. *D*, Extrathoracic obstruction in an infant during tidal breathing. (Adapted from Abramson AL and others: The use of the tidal breathing flow volume loop in laryngotracheal disease of neonates and infants, Laryngoscope 92:922, 1982.)

of lung volume, then some pulmonary blood flow goes to areas of low ventilation, leading to increased $\dot{V}/\dot{Q}$ mismatching, increased shunt, and hypoxemia.

2. Collapse of the airway also occurs at high flow rates, as with forced expiratory maneuvers. Examination of spirometrically obtained flow-volume loops (Fig. 9-2) reveals that maximal or peak expiratory flow rates depend on initial lung volume; the higher the lung volume, the lower the airway resistance and the greater the peak expiratory flow rate. In the midportion of the expiratory curve, maximum flow rate is limited by *dynamic airway collapse*. The normal transmural pressure gradient during the respiratory cycle that maintains peripheral airway patency consists of relative positive pressure inside the airway lumen and negative or subatmospheric intrathoracic pressure. With forced expiration, intrathoracic pressure becomes positive or supraatmospheric, and this positive pressure is transmitted to the airways and alveoli. Since this forced expiration also generates high gas flow rates, an increased pressure drop occurs along the airways, and eventually the *equal pressure point* (EPP) is reached, where airway luminal pressure equals surrounding pleural pressure and there is zero transmural pressure gradient to maintain airway patency. *Dynamic compression* of the airway between the EPP and proximal trachea occurs so that airways collapse downstream from the EPP. As total lung volume decreases, the EPP moves progressively toward smaller airways, and flow-related airway collapse occurs even more readily.
3. Measurement of maximum midexpiratory flow rate (MMEFR) using spirometry detects dynamic obstruction and/or the collapse of distal small airways and increased airway resistance because this portion of the curve is (a) independent of patient force or effort and (b) not affected by upper airway resistance between the EPP and mouth. Maximum flow rate in

this portion of the curve is determined by the airway resistance between the alveoli and EPP (known as the upstream segment) and the elastic recoil pressure of the lung:

$$V_{MAX} = \frac{P_{LUNG}}{R_{UPSTREAM\ SEGMENT}}$$

The MMEFR is an important tool in assessing the severity of obstruction in bronchospastic diseases such as asthma, bronchiolitis, and cystic fibrosis, as well as response to bronchodilator therapy.

4. Application of positive end-expiratory pressure by grunting, pursed-lip breathing, or CPAP/PEEP tends to preserve the normal transmural gradient (airway lumen more positive than surrounding pressure), move the EPP proximally, and therefore minimize or eliminate flow-related airway collapse, preserving FRC and $\dot{V}/\dot{Q}$ matching, and diminishing shunt.

Compliance

Compliance is an expression of the elastic properties of the lung and chest wall (see Table 9-2 for equations of respiratory function), specifically the transmural gradient between the airway and pleural pressures required to produce a given tidal volume:

$$C_{LUNG} = \frac{\Delta V}{\Delta P}$$

1. *Specific compliance,* defined as C_{LUNG}/FRC, is fairly constant across age, sex, and size. Normal is 0.04-0.07 ml/cm H_2O.
2. *Static lung compliance* is defined by the following equation:

$$C_{STAT} = \frac{\Delta V}{\textit{Ultimate}\ \text{transmural pressure gradient}}$$

   C_{STAT} is proportional to lung stiffness. The ultimate transmural pressure gradient is usually 20% to 30% less than the *initial* transmural pressure gradient. It is measured at extremes of V_T when there is no flow or during interrupted mechanical ventilation (1 to 1.5-second inspiratory pause).
3. *Dynamic lung compliance* is defined by the following equation:

$$C_{DYN} = \frac{\Delta V}{\textit{Initial}\ \text{transmural pressure gradient}}$$

where the initial transmural pressure gradient is measured at peak inflation pressure. C_{DYN} is proportional to airway resistance.

The time dependency of pulmonary elastic behavior is reflected in the difference between static (C_{STAT}) and dynamic (C_{DYN}) compliance. During quiet tidal breathing, C_{STAT} is equal to C_{DYN}. With increased respiratory

CAUSES OF INCREASED COMPLIANCE

- Increased lung volume
- COPD (loss of elastic forces)
- The cartilaginous (nonossified) chest wall of the neonate

CAUSES OF DECREASED COMPLIANCE

Decreased lung volume

- Consolidation
- Atelectasis
- Vascular engorgement
- Pleuritic disease

Increased elastic forces

- Pulmonary fibrosis
- Adult respiratory distress syndrome (ARDS)

Increased alveolar surface tension

- Neonatal RDS
- Oxygen toxicity

Restriction of chest wall expansion

- Kyphoscoliosis
- Scleroderma
- Burns
- Scar contractures

rate or bronchospasm, C_{DYN} becomes less than C_{STAT}, reflecting airway closure and increased airway resistance.

Airway Resistance and Gas-Flow Properties

1. Resistive properties are of two types:
   a. Tissue-viscous properties (e.g., the resistance of lung tissues to deformation)
   b. Airflow resistive properties (e.g., the resistance within air passages)
2. *Airway resistance* is defined by the following equation:

$$R_{AW} = \frac{P}{V}$$

where
R_{AW} = Airway resistance
P = Driving pressure
V = Flow
(See also Table 9-2 for equations of respiratory function.)

TABLE 9-2. Important equations relevant to respiratory function

Name	Description	Equation	Variables	Normal values
Alveolar gas equation	Describes composition of alveolar gas	$P_AO_2 = P_B - P_AH_2O - P_ACO_2 - P_AN_2$ For any F_IO_2: $P_IO_2 = F_IO_2(P_B - P_AH_2O)$ $P_AO_2 = P_IO_2 - \frac{P_ACO_2}{R} + \left(P_ACO_2 \times F_IO_2 \times \frac{1-R}{R}\right)$	P_AO_2 = Partial pressure of alveolar O_2 P_B = Barometric pressure P_AH_2O = Vapor pressure of water P_ACO_2 = Partial pressure of alveolar CO_2 (equiv. to $PaCO_2$) P_AN_2 = Partial pressure of alveolar nitrogen F_IO_2 = Fractional inspired oxygen P_IO_2 = Partial pressure of inspired oxygen R = Respiratory quotient	Room air at 37°C: P_AO_2 = 103-105 mm Hg P_B = 760 mm Hg P_AH_2O = 47 mm Hg P_ACO_2 = 40 mm Hg P_AN_2 = 570 mm Hg F_IO_2 = 0.21 R = 0.8
Alveolar-arterial oxygen tension difference (A-a DO_2)	Measures degree of shunt	$A - aDO_2 = P_AO_2 - PaO_2$	$P_AO_2 = P_IO_2 - \frac{P_ACO_2}{R}$ PaO_2 = Partial pressure of arterial O_2	5-10 mm Hg at F_IO_2 = 0.21 and 20-35 mm Hg at F_IO_2 = 1.0
Oxygen content	Measures adequacy of oxygenation, used to determine best PEEP	O_2 content = (% Sat) (Hgb g/dl) (1.39 ml O_2/g Hgb) + (.003 vol %/mm Hg) (PaO_2 mm Hg)	% Sat = Oxygen saturation Hgb = Hemoglobin concentration PaO_2 = Partial pressure of arterial O_2	20-21 ml O_2/dl
Shunt equation	Measures % right-to-left shunt, or the inefficiency of oxygenation	$\frac{Q_s}{Q_T} = \frac{CcO_2 - CaO_2}{CcO_2 - C_VO_2}$	Q_s = Shunt flow; Q_T = Total flow CcO_2 = Pulmonary capillary O_2 content (equivalent to C_AO_2) CaO_2 = Arterial oxygen content C_VO_2 = Mixed venous oxygen content	3-5%

V_D/V_T ratio	Measures the inefficiency of ventilation	$\frac{V_D}{V_T} = \frac{P_ACO_2 - P_{expir}CO_2}{P_ACO_2}$ *or* $\frac{PaCO_2 - P_{expir}CO_2}{PaCO_2}$	V_D = Dead space volume V_T = Tidal volume P_ACO_2 = Partial pressure of alveolar CO_2 $P_{expir}CO_2$ = Partial pressure of average expired CO_2 $PaCO_2$ = Partial pressure of arterial CO_2	0.3-0.4
Compliance	Change in lung volume divided by the pressure gradient change	$1/C_T = 1/C_L + 1/C_{cw}$ (obeys the law of capacitance in series) $C_{EFF} = \frac{V_T - V_{compression}}{P_{plateau} - P_{end\text{-}expir}}$	C_T = Total compliance C_L = Lung compliance C_{CW} = Chest wall compliance C_{EFF} = Effective compliance V_T = Tital volume $V_{compression}$ = Circuit compressible volume $P_{plateau}$ = Plateau inspiratory pressure $P_{end\text{-}expir}$ = End-expiratory pressure	(see C_{EFF}) 35-50 ml/cm H_2O
Airway resistance	Directly proportional to driving pressure and inversely proportional to r^4 (laminar flow) or r^5 (tubulent flow)	$R_{aw} = \frac{P_{peak} - P_{static}}{V}$	R_{aw} = Airway resistance P_{peak} = Peak airway pressure P_{static} = Static pressure required to overcome flow resistance V = Flow	2-3 cmH_2O/L/sec in the older child and adult; 25-30 cm H_2O/L/sec in the infant

3. The primary site of airway resistance (R_{AW}) is the upper airway (60% from nose and mouth to trachea) and large central bronchi (another 30%), with only 10% of R_{AW} in small-diameter airways. Since babies are obligate nose breathers, any additional imposed upper airway resistance (e.g., by nasogastric tube, macroglossia, adenotonsillar hypertrophy, laryngeal edema, cricoid edema, tracheal stenosis, or webs) may severely limit air flow. Similarly small-diameter endotracheal tubes (ETTs) impose considerable resistance to flow.
4. As gas flows through tubes (i.e., airway passages), a pressure difference (driving pressure) is created between the two ends of the tube, which is dependent on the rate and pattern of flow.
   a. At low flow rates through straight, unbranched tubes, *laminar flow* predominates, producing a cone front of flowing gas with the highest velocity at the center of the tube and the lowest velocity at the periphery because of friction. Resistance to laminar flow is inversely proportional to tube radius to the fourth power ($1/r^4$) and depends on gas viscosity, not density. The relationship is described by Poiseuille's law, as follows:

$$R = \frac{8ln}{\pi r^4}$$

   where
   R = Resistance
   l = Length of the tube
   n = Viscosity
   π = pi
   r = Radius of the tube
   b. *Reynold's number* is a nondimensional quantity that predicts the nature of gas flow in long, straight unbranched tubes. It is derived from the following equation:

$$Re\# = \frac{2r \times v \times d}{n}$$

   where
   Re# = Reynold's number
   r = Tube radius
   v = Linear velocity of gas
   d = Gas density
   n = Gas viscosity

   When Reynold's number is less than 1,000, flow is laminar. When Reynold's number is greater than 1,500 to 2,000, flow becomes turbulent.
   c. Effective alveolar ventilation is best served by preserving laminar flow and diminishing the ineffective gas exchange that occurs with turbulent eddies of flow. To maintain laminar flow, therefore, one

should choose low flow rates through ventilator circuits, gas mixtures with low density to viscosity ratios (e.g., helium-O_2), and ETTs of the largest possible diameter and shortest possible length.

d. In contrast, *turbulent flow* predominates with:
   - High flow rates (greater than critical velocity)
   - Flow through constrictions and changing tube diameters
   - Flow that changes direction at angled turns or branch points

   Therefore, to diminish turbulence curved or straight rather than angled circuit connectors are chosen. Turbulent flow is inversely proportional to tube radius to the fifth power ($1/r^5$) and depends on gas density, not viscosity.

e. *Orifice flow* predominates when there is high flow through a very narrow constriction (e.g., severe tracheal stenosis). It is directly proportional to the tube radius squared (r^2) and inversely proportional to the square root of driving pressure over gas density. Therefore, the less dense the gas, the more flow will cross the orifice. Again, helium-O_2 mixtures may be beneficial in improving pulmonary mechanics and gas exchange in cases of severe intrinsic or extrinsic tracheal or bronchial narrowing.

OXYGEN THERAPY

Indications

O_2 therapy (increased F_IO_2) is indicated in the following situations:

- In the presence of arterial hypoxemia in room air ($PaO_2 \leq 70$ mm Hg or $SaO_2 \leq 93\%$).
- As therapy for smoke inhalation and carbon monoxide intoxication
- To accelerate resorption of intrapleural air from pneumothorax
- During emergence and recovery from general anesthesia
- During conscious sedation (e.g., diagnostic and radiologic procedures, regional anesthesia)
- To decrease pulmonary vascular resistance and improve pulmonary blood flow in the presence of a right-to-left intracardiac shunt

Limitations of Oxygen Therapy

1. In the presence of an *intrapulmonary right-to-left shunt* in excess of 20% to 30%, increasing F_IO_2 will not improve oxygenation. This situation occurs when there are large areas of very low $\dot{V}/\dot{Q}$ with inadequate ventilation to match pulmonary capillary blood flow (Fig. 9-3, Isoshunt chart).
2. Increased F_IO_2 does not improve oxygenation in fixed *extrapulmonary right-to-left shunts*, such as tetralogy of Fallot, Eisenmenger's syndrome, truncus arteriosus, pulmonary atresia, tricuspid atresia, and transposition of the great vessels. However, increasing F_IO_2 may improve oxygenation in a fixed extrapulmonary shunt by its ability to dilate the pulmonary vasculature, which increases pulmonary blood flow.
3. The occurrence of pulmonary *oxygen toxicity* or retinopathy of prematurity may counteract advantages of increasing the delivered oxygen concentration.
4. The onset of alveolar nitrogen washout and *resorption atelectasis* in

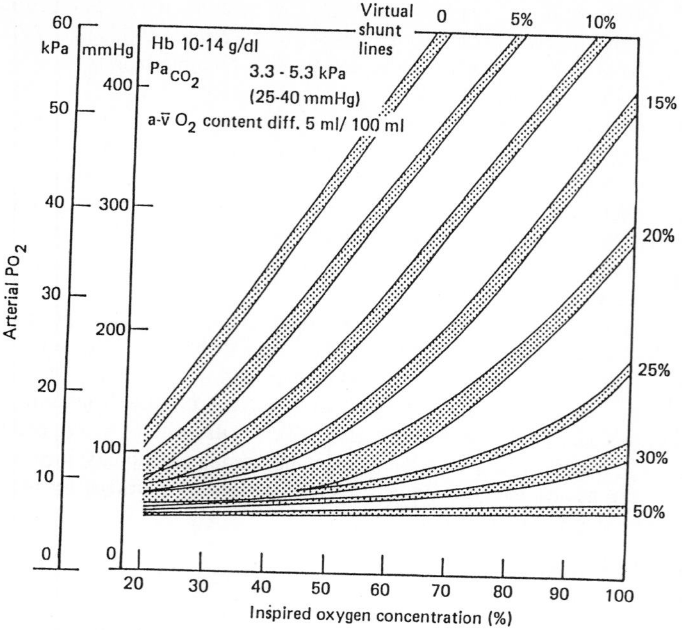

Fig. 9-3. Iso-shunt chart. The iso-shunt chart describes the theoretical relationship between PaO_2 and inspired oxygen concentration at different levels of virtual shunt (arterial-mixed venous oxygen content difference equals 5 ml/100 ml). The shaded lines are limited by the following parameters: hemoglobin 10–14 g/dl and $PaCO_2$ 25–40 mm Hg. This diagram is useful for adusting the F_IO_2 in patients requiring oxygen therapy. If the F_IO_2 and PaO_2 are known, the percent of shunt can be derived from the chart. When the percent of shunt is known, the F_IO_2 may be changed to achieve a desired PaO_2. A decrease in shunt usually indicates patient improvement. Note the minimal effect of F_IO_2 on PaO_2 in the presence of a 50% shunt. (Reproduced from Benatar SR, Hewlett AM, and Nunn JF: The use of iso-shunt lines for control of oxygen therapy, Br J Anaesth 45:711, 1973. With permission.)

patients with hyperoxia may increase intrapulmonary shunt by converting areas of low $\dot{V}/\dot{Q}$ to $\dot{V}/\dot{Q} = 0$.

Types of Oxygen Therapy

The type of oxygen delivery system selected for the unintubated patient is dependent on the age, size, and degree of cooperation of the patient and the goals of therapy (Table 9-3, Modes of oxygen therapy).

Oxygen Therapy During Patient Transport

Oxygen Source

1. A green "E" cylinder contains compressed oxygen gas and is fitted with a gas regulator, serving both as a pressure-reducing valve and a flowmeter.
2. When filled, the "E" cylinder weighs approximately 7 kg and contains 625 L of oxygen pressurized to 2200 PSI.

3. Its duration of use depends on two factors:
   a. The gas capacity of the cylinder (measured indirectly by cylinder pressure)
   b. The rate of gas flow delivered
4. Approximate usable duration can be calculated by the following formula:

$$\text{Duration of flow (min)} = \frac{\text{Cylinder pressure (PSI)} \times 0.28}{\text{Flow rate (L/min)}}$$

For example, following are calculated durations of flow for two flow rates and three cylinder pressures:

	Cylinder pressure		
Flow rate	**2200 PSI (full)**	**1200 PSI (½ full)**	**600 PSI (¼ full)**
10 L/min	61 min	33 min	16 min
6 L/min	102 min	56 min	28 min

Delivery Systems

1. Any of the following can be used for oxygen delivery: nasal cannulae, oxygen hood, any of the previously discussed mask systems, or a positive-pressure delivery system connected to a mask, ETT, or tracheostomy tube.
2. An Ambu bag with nonrebreathing valve, or a Jackson-Rees modification of the Ayre's T-piece are useful for delivery of positive pressure. Their important features include the following:
   - Ability to use the system with both spontaneous or controlled ventilation. Some Ambu bags contain valves that only allow inspiration of room air, not O_2, during spontaneous ventilation.
   - High fresh gas flows (either 8 to 10 L/min or 2 times minute ventilation) are required to avoid CO_2 rebreathing and ensure delivery of F_iO_2 greater than 90%.
   - Pressure-limiting relief valves are needed to minimize the risk of barotrauma or overdistension.
   - The Ambu system may be fitted with a PEEP valve as well.

Emergency Equipment

1. Critically ill patients requiring oxygen therapy are vulnerable to airway and respiratory emergencies during transport from the operating room, intensive care unit, recovery room, or to remote hospital locations.
2. Extra equipment to manage a resuscitation includes the following:
   - Appropriately sized masks, oral and nasal airways, ETTs with stylets, and tracheostomy tubes
   - Laryngoscope with appropriate blades and functioning light systems
   - Positive-pressure delivery system (Ambu resuscitator or Jackson-Rees)
   - Full oxygen cylinder

TABLE 9-3. Modes of oxygen therapy

Mode	Apparatus	Inspiratory reservoir	Ambient air entrainment	Re-breathing	Valves
Nasal cannulae	Nasal prongs	Yes (anatomic naso- and oro-pharynx)	Possible	No	No
Oxygen hood	Plastic hood, which covers the head and neck	Yes (mixing of gases within the hood)	No	Yes	No
Simple mask	Mask with exhalation side-ports	No	Yes (through sideports)	No	No
Partial re-breathing mask	Mask with exhalation side-ports and a reservoir bag	Yes (bag)	Yes (through side-ports)	Yes	Yes
Venturi, or entrainment, mask	Mask fitted with O_2 jet nozzle and entrainment ports	No	Yes (oxygen jet velocity is transferred to entrained air)	No	No

O_2 flow delivery rate (set on flow meter)	Delivered F_IO_2*	Comments	Disadvantages
2-6 L/min	Variable: .27-.39 (usually increases F_IO_2 by 0.03 for each L/min of flow)	• Ensure proper fit and positioning of prongs	• Inability to measure F_IO_2 • Nasal irritation and drying
6-8 L/min	Preblended range of 0.28-0.60	• Must provide adequate fresh gas flow to ensure mixing of delivered gases and flushing of exhaled gases	• O_2 gradients can form from the top to the bottom of the hood • Cold, humidified gases can contribute to thermal stress in small infants
6-10 L/min	Variable: 0.35-0.55	• Limited concentration of delivered oxygen	• Delivered F_IO_2 varies with O_2 delivery, patient's inspiratory time, and peak inspiratory flow rate.
8-15 L/min	Variable: 0.60-0.80	• Tight fit of mask is essential • Delivered flow must exceed peak inspiratory flow so reservoir doesn't collapse on inspiration	• Requires high gas flows to maintain reservoir
8-15 L/min	Variable: 0.24-0.60 (depends on jet velocity and size of entrainment ports)	• Delivered flow must exceed peak inspiratory flow to ensure accurate F_IO_2 delivery	• If fresh gas flow fails, total rebreathing may occur (some are fitted with either nonvalved perforations or a valve to allow ambient air to enter)

*For all the above modes, desired F_IO_2 is delivered only if delivered fresh gas flow exceeds the patient's peak inspiratory flow rate (typically $\geq$6 L/min for an infant and from 20 to 60 L/min in the adult).

- Resuscitation drugs (atropine, epinephrine, succinylcholine) and IV flush syringes
- Stethoscope to assess breath sounds
- Transport monitor with a mobile, battery-powered pulse oximeter and ECG capacity. Portable capnography is also available.

MECHANICAL VENTILATION

Positive-pressure mechanical ventilation is an important technique in the management of surgical and critically ill pediatric patients. As technical advances increase, the indications for mechanical ventilation in infants and children also increase (see box on p. 171 for indications for mechanical ventilation). An understanding of pulmonary pathophysiology, basic pulmonary mechanics, and the specific technical features of pediatric mechanical ventilators is necessary for the safe and proper application of positive-pressure ventilation.

Classification of Pediatric Ventilators

Several physical characteristics define and classify positive-pressure ventilators. These include the following. (See also Table 9-4.)

1. Trigger for initiation of inspiration (cycling)
   a. The patient's spontaneous inspiratory effort ("assistor")
   b. A preset time interval ("controller")
   c. A combination ("assistor-controller")
2. Signal for end of inspiration (changeover to expiratory phase)
   a. Time-limited: inspiration ends after a preset time interval.
   b. Pressure-limited: inspiration ends when a preset airway pressure is reached.
   c. Volume-limited: inspiration ends when a preset circuit volume is delivered.
3. Inspiratory flow generator pattern
   a. Constant (or square wave): inspiratory flow remains constant during inspiration. 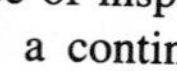
   b. Nonconstant:
      i. Decelerating flow is highest at the start of inspiration and then steadily decreases. 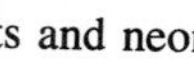
      ii. A sine wave pattern shows a flow that increases until mid-inspiration and then decreases. 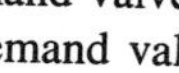
4. IMV circuitry (source of inspired gas for spontaneous breaths)
   a. Continuous flow: a continuous flow of fresh gas at the airway opening serves as an inspiratory reservoir for spontaneous breaths. The patient does not exert effort to open an inspiratory valve, so it is preferred for infants and neonates.
   b. Noncontinuous flow inhalation demand valve: spontaneous inspiratory efforts open the reservoir demand valve, which results in increased work of breathing.
5. Expiratory phase
   a. Retardation: the expiratory valve is gradually depressurized to simulate pursed-lip breathing (grunting) and thereby prevent airway collapse.

INDICATIONS FOR POSITIVE-PRESSURE MECHANICAL VENTILATION AND RESPIRATORY SUPPORT OF THE PEDIATRIC PATIENT

1. **Acute respiratory failure**
   a. Inadequate ventilation
      - Apnea
      - Hypopnea
      - $V_D/V_T > 0.6$
      - VC < 15 ml/kg
      - Rising $PaCO_2$ or $PaCO_2 > 50$ mm Hg (acutely)

   b. Inadequate oxygenation
      - $PaO_2 < 70$ mm Hg or $SaO_2 < 93\%$ with $F_IO_2 \geq 0.6$
      - $A - a\ DO_2$ gradient > 300 mm Hg with $F_IO_2 = 1$
      - $Q_s/Q_T > 15 - 20\%$
2. **To secure the airway**
   a. Neurologic dysfunction (obtundation, coma, high spinal cord injury, intractable seizures)
   b. Upper GI bleed/aspiration risk
   c. Toxic or foreign body ingestion
   d. Upper airway obstruction (e.g. croup, epiglottitis, laryngeal papillomas or webs, vascular ring)
   e. Airway edema, trauma, or burn
3. **To control ventilation**
   a. Elevated ICP (e.g., hydrocephalus, intracranial tumor, closed head injury, Reye's syndrome)
   b. Neuromuscular disease (e.g., spinal cord injury, phrenic nerve injury, Werdnig-Hoffman, muscular dystrophy, myasthenia gravis, Guillain-Barré)
   c. Acute reactive airways disease or bronchospasm (e.g., asthma, bronchiolitis)
   d. Consolidative processes (e.g., pneumothorax, atelectasis, hemorrhage, contusion, near-drowning)
   e. Acute postoperative state
   f. Restrictive lung disease due to abdominal distention, obesity, kyphoscoliosis, flail chest, pleural disease, or tumor
4. **To decrease the work of breathing**
   a. Sepsis
   b. Metabolic acidosis (e.g., diabetic ketoacidosis, acute renal failure)
   c. Chronic pulmonary disease (e.g., bronchopulmonary dysplasia, cystic fibrosis)
   d. Congestive heart failure, pulmonary edema
   e. Acute reactive airway disease
   f. Shock/circulatory failure

b. PEEP: a preset positive-end expiratory pressure is applied, most commonly by a threshold-resistor type of expiratory valve. PEEP can increase FRC and lung volumes, improve compliance, recruit atelectatic alveoli, improve $\dot{V}/\dot{Q}$ matching, and allow a decrease in F_IO_2 while maintaining adequate oxygenation.

TABLE 9-4. Pediatric ventilators: technical features

	Age Group		
	Neonate 0.5-5.0 kg	**Infant 3.5-10 kg**	**Infant or Child 10-70 kg**
How driven	Pneumatic/Electrical	Electrical	Electrical/Pneumatic
Inspiratory factors:			
Cycling	Time	Time	Time
Limit	Time or pressure	Volume or pressure	Volume or pressure
Flow generator pattern	Constant	Constant	Constant or decelerating or sine wave
Pressure plateau ("pause")	Yes, if pressure limited	Yes, 0-2.0 sec	Yes, variable duration
Flow rate	8-12 L/min	75-125 ml/sec	10-30 L/min
Inspiratory time setting	0.4-0.7 sec	0.7-1.0 sec	0.7-1.0 sec
I:E ratio	4:1 → 1:10	4:1 → 1:6	4:1 → 1:6
IMV modes	IMV only	IMV and SIMV	IMV and SIMV
IMV circuitry	Continuous flow	Demand valve	Demand valve
Circuit compressible volume	1 ml/cm H_2O	0.3-0.5 ml/cm H_2O	3-4 ml/cm H_2O
PEEP/CPAP range	0-20 cm H_2O	0-25 cm H_2O	0-50 cm H_2O
Pressure support mode	No	No	Yes (Servo 900C only) 5-15 cm H_2O
Tidal volume	Not preset	12-15 ml/kg Max = 150 ml	12-15 ml/kg
Rate (breaths/min)	25-40	15-40	8-20
Examples	Baby Bird Bear Cub Sechrist BP200	Bear LS104-150 Infrasonics Infant Star	Bear 2 or 5 Puritan Bennett 7200A Siemens Servo 900C

ADVANTAGES AND DISADVANTAGES OF COMMONLY USED VENTILATORS

Pressure limited

Advantages

- Preset peak inspiratory pressure prevents excessive inflating pressures
- Decreased risk of barotrauma
- Provides static inspiratory pressure plateau, which helps $\dot{V}/\dot{Q}$ matching and intrapulmonary shunting in diseases of decreased compliance and low FRC (neonatal RDS)

Disadvantages

- Delivered tidal volume is variable, depending on inspiratory flow, inspiratory time, circuit, and patient compliance
- Changes in lung compliance and airway resistance are difficult to detect because the peak inflating pressure is constant

Volume limited

Advantages

- A constant preset tidal volume is delivered to the circuit
- Changes in the patient's pulmonary mechanics (compliance, airway resistance) are suggested by changes in inflating pressures
- Better suited to ventilating patients with severe pulmonary pathology

Disadvantages

- Delivered tidal volume to the patient can vary with extremes of circuit compliance and peak inspiratory pressure (also referred to as "lost" compressible volume)
- High peak inflating pressures may be reached to deliver preset V_T
- Increased risk of barotrauma
- Delivered tidal volumes less than 100 ml are difficult to ensure even with sophisticated circuitry

Specific Advantages and Disadvantages of Different Ventilators

The most commonly used pediatric positive-pressure ventilators are the constant-flow generator, time cycled, and assistor-controller devices that are either volume or pressure limited. The relative advantages and disadvantages of these ventilators are compared in the accompanying box.

Modes of Mechanical Ventilation

1. The most common modes of mechanical ventilation are asynchronous controlled intermittent mandatory ventilation (IMV), in which positive-pressure breaths are delivered at a preset time interval, and synchronous assisted IMV (SIMV), in which the patient's spontaneous inspiratory effort triggers an assisted breath. If there is no spontaneous effort within a preset time interval, then a positive pressure breath is delivered. SIMV offers the following advantages:
   - Diminishing ventilator-patient asynchrony ("bucking" and "respiratory stacking" of spontaneous and mechanical breaths)

- Diminishing peak intrathoracic and airway pressures during positive-pressure ventilation, potentially minimizing hemodynamic embarrassment caused by decreased systemic venous return, decreased cardiac output, and left ventricular dysfunction
- Improving $\dot{V}/\dot{Q}$ matching, as spontaneous breaths are better distributed to dependent lung regions with higher perfusion
- Decreasing the work of breathing, while preserving spontaneous inspiratory efforts, particularly useful during weaning from mechanical ventilatory support

2. Inspiratory pressure support is another mode of ventilation increasingly in use. Primarily used in weaning from mechanical support, this method applies 5 to 15 cm H_2O of inspiratory plateau pressure "assistance" with each spontaneous patient breath, for the duration of the patient inspiratory flow. The patient maintains control over respiratory frequency, inspiratory time, and ultimately delivered V_T. However, pressure assistance increases both inspiratory flow and V_T, thereby decreasing the respiratory rate required to maintain a given alveolar ventilation. The patient shifts to a slower frequency, larger tidal-volume pattern. Pressure support also acts to decrease the work of breathing done by ventilatory muscles and that associated with breathing through an endotracheal tube.
3. Continuous positive airway pressure, or CPAP, refers to the application of positive airway pressure throughout the ventilatory cycle in spontaneously breathing patients (i.e., no positive pressure mechanical breaths are delivered). CPAP is also primarily used for weaning. Physiologically, CPAP, like PEEP, maintains intrathoracic airway patency and lung volumes, preserves or improves FRC, recruits atelectatic alveoli, improves $\dot{V}/\dot{Q}$ matching, and diminishes intrapulmonary shunting. CPAP weaning through small-diameter, high-resistance endotracheal tubes can substantially increase the work of breathing and precipitate ventilatory muscle fatigue and respiratory failure. CPAP weaning in pediatric patients should therefore include between 4 and 6 IMV positive-pressure breaths per minute.

Initiating Mechanical Ventilation

Selection of ventilators and operational variables may be initiated in the immediate postoperative period by the anesthesiologist and intensive care team, based on the age and size of the patient, the underlying disease and surgical procedure, and therapeutic goals (see box on p. 175 for procedures to initiate ventilation).

Complications of Mechanical Ventilation

PEEP/CPAP

PEEP and CPAP are critical modalities for maintaining alveolar patency and FRC while diminishing atelectasis and shunt. However, their use can be limited by multisystem complications, as described in the box on p. 176.

Barotrauma

Barotrauma caused by positive pressure ventilation (see box on p. 177) can result in pneumothorax, pneumomediastinum, pneumopericardium, and pul-

PROCEDURES FOR INITIATING POSITIVE PRESSURE MECHANICAL VENTILATION

1. Select ventilator based on:
   - Patient/disease characteristics
   - Therapeutic goals
   - Specific technical features (see Table 9-5)
2. Ensure proper set-up of machine
   - Correct wall-source connections for gases
   - Cycling and flow rates
   - Humidification and warming of gases
   - Alarms activated (apnea, disconnect, low V_T, low pressure)
   - Oxygen analyzer in circuit
3. Choose mode
   - Volume or pressure limited
   - IMV or SIMV
   - CPAP with spontaneous ventilation
   - Inspiratory pressure support
4. Choose inspiratory parameters
   - Peak inspiratory pressure
   - Inspiratory time
   - Preset V_T (12-15 ml/kg)
   - I:E ratio (typically 1:2) (for obstructive diseases choose low I:E of 1:3 or 1:4 to allow prolonged expiratory time)
   - Inspiratory flow generator pattern
5. Choose frequency (bpm)
   - Use age-specific norms
6. Choose F_IO_2
   - Aim for <0.50 to avoid O_2 toxicity
7. Select end-expiratory distending pressure
   - CPAP (usually 3-5 cm H_2O)
   - PEEP (usually 3-5 cm H_2O)
8. Assess adequacy of ventilation and oxygenation
   - Color and perfusion
   - Chest excursion
   - Breath sounds
   - ABG for PaO_2 ($\geq$70 mm Hg) and $PaCO_2$ (35-45 mm Hg)
   - Pulse oximetry
   - Capnography/capnometry for E_TCO_2
   - Hemodynamics (esp. with PEEP $\geq$10 cmH_2O)
9. Consider sedatives and muscle relaxants
   - Narcotics
   - Benzodiazepines
   - Intermediate or long-acting nondepolarizing muscle relaxants
10. Ensure good pulmonary toilet
    - ETT suction
    - Change ventilator circuits at 24°-48°
    - Chest physiotherapy
    - Bronchodilator/nebulizer therapy
11. Maintain optimal matching of O_2 delivery to consumption
    - Sedation/muscle relaxation
    - Fever control
    - Nutritional support (enteral or parenteral feeding)
    - Correct anemia to maximize O_2 content
    - Elevate head of bed 30-45° to improve $\dot{V}/\dot{Q}$

COMPLICATIONS OF PEEP/CPAP

Hemodynamic

↓ Cardiac output
↓ Venous return
↑ Right ventricular afterload
↑ Pulmonary vascular resistance
↓ Myocardial blood flow

Neurologic

↓ Cerebral perfusion pressure
↑ Intracranial pressure

Renal

↓ Renal blood flow
Hyponatremia
Syndrome of inappropriate ADH secretion
↓ Free water clearance
↓ Creatinine clearance

Splanchnic

↓ Hepatic blood flow
↓ Portal venous blood flow
↓ Mesenteric blood flow

Pulmonary

↑ Barotrauma
- Pneumothorax
- Pneumomediastinum
- Pneumopericardium
- Subcutaneous emphysema

↑ Physiologic dead space (V_D)

monary interstitial emphysema. The occurrence of any of these complications in the infant or the older child with marginal reserve may result in immediate and profound decompensation.

Oxygen Toxicity

Pulmonary effects

1. Pulmonary damage from prolonged hyperoxia is caused by O_2 free radicals, usually in the presence of an F_IO_2 greater than 60% for more than 24 hours.
2. Clinical manifestations include tracheitis, hyaline membrane formation, pleural effusions, severe respiratory distress, chronic pulmonary fibrosis, and hypertension.
3. Young age, chemotherapeutic agents, radiation therapy, and a hypermetabolic state may worsen oxygen toxicity.

MECHANISMS OF BAROTRAUMA WITH POSITIVE PRESSURE VENTILATION

Factors	Mechanism	Result
• Long inspiratory times • High peak inflating pressures • Inspiratory "pause" • CPAP/PEEP • Excessive V_T	Overdistension	Barotrauma
• Decreased lung volume (e.g., consolidation, atelectasis, vascular engorgement) • Increased alveolar surface tension (e.g., neonatal RDS) • Increased elastic recoil (e.g., pulmonary fibrosis) • Chest wall restriction (e.g., kyphoscoliosis, burn or scar contractures, collagen-vascular disease)	Decreased compliance	
• ETT plugging or kinking • Small ETT • Reactive airway disease or bronchospasm • Short expiratory time (air trapping) • Ventilator-patient asynchrony	High airway or circuit resistance	
• Focal lung disease (areas of low compliance and high resistance) • Main-stem bronchus intubation	Unequal distribution of ventilation	

Retinopathy of prematurity (ROP, retrolental fibroplasia)

1. ROP probably occurs as a result of hyperoxia-induced responses in the retinal vascular bed.
2. Low birth weight (less than 1,000 g), extreme prematurity, and prolonged duration of supplementary oxygen therapy are important factors that correlate with the development of ROP. ROP may also occur in full-term infants not receiving oxygen.
3. An F_IO_2 greater than 50% should be avoided while maintaining a PaO_2 between 60 and 100 mm Hg until the infant is 44 weeks postconceptual age.

Negative Pressure Pulmonary Edema

1. Negative pressure or postobstructive pulmonary edema results from the large transpulmonary gradients that develop as the patient attempts to inspire against a closed glottis.

2. Typically, it develops soon after extubation as a result of laryngospasm, airway obstruction, or insufficient reversal of muscle relaxants.
3. With reintubation and positive pressure ventilation, symptoms usually resolve within a few hours.

Other Complications

Numerous other complications of mechanical ventilation exist, including atelectasis, infection, aspiration, ventilator asynchrony, subglottic stenosis, tracheomalacia, and inability to wean (Table 9-5, Complications of mechanical ventilation). Treatment of these complications usually prolongs the course of mechanical ventilation, making prevention of prime importance.

High-Frequency Ventilation (HFV)

Definition

HFV consists of low tidal volume (often less than anatomic dead space) and high-frequency ventilation (60 to 150 breaths per minute), using low circuit volume and noncompliant circuit tubing. Flow generators are fitted with either valved flow-interruption devices or high-frequency oscillators. Most clinical experience is with high-frequency flow interrupters (HFFI) and high-frequency jet ventilators (HFJV) (see box on p. 180 for characteristics of high-frequency ventilation). At present, high-frequency oscillation (HFO) is essentially an investigative technique.

Goals

High-frequency ventilation provides normal gas exchange for oxygen and carbon dioxide while potentially minimizing $\dot{V}/\dot{Q}$ mismatching, barotrauma, and adverse hemodynamic consequences of positive pressure ventilation.

Applications

- Surgery:
  Laser and bronchoscopic airway procedures
  Cardiac and microneurosurgical procedures
- Bronchopleural fistula and air leak syndromes
- Pulmonary interstitial emphysema
- Adult respiratory distress syndrome
- As a weaning technique for patients who have failed more conventional procedures
- CPR (particularly with transtracheal HFJV)
- Pericardial tamponade

Physiology

Theoretical mechanisms of gas exchange in high-frequency ventilation include the following:

- *Augmented dispersion*—a combination of turbulent mixing, convective bulk flow (in larger proximal airways), and enhanced diffusion (especially radial diffusion in smaller airways)
- *Interregional gas mixing*
- *Axial dispersion* (especially in very small distal airways)

Gas flow and exchange appear to be less dependent on mechanical factors of airway resistance and compliance during HFV than during conventional

TABLE 9-5. Complications of mechanical ventilation

Complication	Prevention	Treatment
Barotrauma	• Avoid excessive inspiratory times, pressure, and volume	• May require thoracostomy (chest tube placement)
Oxygen toxicity	• Prevent hyperoxia	• Support ventilation
Atelectasis or collapse	• Ensure correct tube positioning to avoid endobronchial intubation • Ensure adequacy of tidal volumes, use continuous distending pressure, and provide intermittent "sigh" or manual ventilation	• Vigilant airway suction, pulmonary toilet, humidification and bronchodilator therapy • Consider interventional bronchoscopy
Infection	• Vigilant ETT and tracheostomy care • Frequent changing of ventilator circuits and humidification systems (every 24-48 hr)	• Treat with appropriate antibiotics and chest physiotherapy
Aspiration	• Use high-volume, low-pressure cuffed ETT if possible (patient >6-8 yr) • NG drainage, H_2 blockers, and antacids • Elevate head of bed 30 degrees	• Treat with appropriate antibiotics and chest physiotherapy
Ventilator-patient asynchrony	• Use SIMV mode when possible	• Alternatively, use sedation or muscle relaxants
Subglottic stenosis or tracheomalacia	More likely to occur in patients with: • Prematurity • Tight ETT fit with small air leak • Cuffed ETT • Excessive head and neck movement while intubated • Prolonged intubation	• May ultimately require tracheostomy
Failure to wean	• Correct underlying pulmonary pathology (intra- and extrathoracic) as much as possible • Minimize use of depressant drugs (sedatives, narcotics, muscle relaxants) • Fever control • Metabolic homeostasis (thyroid, pituitary-adrenocortical axis, etc.)	• Provide adequate nutritional support to meet metabolic needs for increased work of breathing • Correct anemia

TECHNICAL CHARACTERISTICS OF HIGH-FREQUENCY VENTILATION: HFFI AND HFJV

1. Flow generator: high-pressure air-oxygen mixture
2. Delivery system: valved flow interrupter (either solenoid, fluidic, or motorized rotating interrupter)
3. Adapter: continuous flow circuit plus jet cannula *or* specialized ETT*
4. Expiratory phase: passive (>100 bpm → gas trapping)
5. Frequency: HFFI = 60-120 bpm
   HFJV = 60-300 bpm
6. Waveform: sinusoidal
7. Regulation of V_T: relative I:time *and* inspiratory driving pressure (range 20-50 PSI *or* 1,400-3,500 cm H_2O)

*Gas accelerates through the jet and entrains fresh gas from the continuous flow circuit by Bernoulli's effect.

ventilation. At lower ranges of HFV it appears that convective flow is most important, while augmented dispersive exchange predominates at higher ranges. At rates over 100 breaths per minute, CO_2 retention becomes a limiting phenomenon, probably because of air trapping (insufficient expiratory time), increased V_D/V_T, and decreased insufflating or tidal volumes at higher frequencies. Maximal oxygenation and diminished intrapulmonary shunting are favored by increases in mean airway pressures and lung volume.

Complications

- To ensure adequate ventilation, close observation of the patient's clinical status, serial ABGs, and CXRs is mandatory, since neither airway pressures nor distending volumes can be easily measured.
- Auto-PEEP occurs at frequencies greater than 100 to 120 beats per minute, causing increased end-expiratory lung volume because passive exhalation to FRC doesn't occur at high frequencies.
- Barotrauma remains a potential complication, particularly with poorly compliant lungs.
- Exhaled gases must be properly vented and airway or circuit obstructions diligently avoided to prevent over-distention and/or rupture.
- Inadequate minute ventilation and alveolar distension may lead to a decrease in surfactant production; "sighs" should be incorporated if possible.
- Large left-to-right shunts (e.g., PDA) persist during HFV, even at the same mean airway pressure as with conventional, phasic positive pressure ventilation.
- HFV attenuates hypoxic pulmonary vasoconstriction, probably by increasing release of prostacyclin (PGI_2), which may worsen intrapulmonary shunt.
- HFV does *not* seem to differ significantly from conventional ventilation with respect to cardiovascular and hemodynamic effects of positive pressure or PEEP. It appears that mean pressure changes are most important in producing these effects, regardless of the mode of ventilation.

TABLE 9-6. Techniques of extracorporeal membrane oxygenation

Methods and variables	Cannulation sites: Veno-arterial V: internal jugular vein to right atrium A: right common carotid retrograde to aortic arch	Cannulation sites: Veno-venous V: internal jugular vein to right atrium V: right femoral vein
Circuit perfusion rates	Low	High
Oxygenator	Membrane	Membrane
Assisted systemic circulation	Yes (partial CPB)	No
Pulmonary circulation	Decreased blood flow	Full blood flow
Pulmonary artery pressure	Decreased	Decreased or no change
Pulmonary artery mixed venous O_2	No change	Increased
PaO_2	Higher	Lower
Mechanical ventilation	Continued, with lower F_IO_2 and airway pressures	Continued, with lower F_IO_2 and airway pressures
Systemic heparinization	Yes	Yes
Duration of therapy	Hours to weeks	Hours to weeks

Extracorporeal Membrane Oxygenation (ECMO)

See Table 9-6 above.

Indications

Severe neonatal respiratory failure secondary to any of the following:
- RDS/hyaline membrane disease
- Meconium aspiration syndrome
- Congenital diaphragmatic hernia
- Persistent fetal circulation (PFC)
- Severe hypoxic pulmonary vasoconstriction

Goals

1. To allow the lungs to recover from ongoing hyperoxia exposure (oxygen toxicity) and barotrauma
2. To maintain normal gas exchange for oxygen and carbon dioxide
3. To wean eventually from ECMO and return to conventional mechanical ventilatory support

Complications

- Ischemia at cannulation sites
- Permanent ligation of the common carotid artery with veno-arterial ECMO and permanent ligation of the femoral vein with veno-venous ECMO
- Hemorrhage (particularly intraventricular)
- Heparin-induced thrombocytopenia
- Sepsis
- Embolic events
- Persistent hypoxemia/acidosis
- Death

Discontinuation of Mechanical Ventilatory Support (Weaning to Extubation)

Extubation in the Operating Room

1. Discontinuation of anesthetic gases
2. Maintenance of normothermia. The infant or child should have a core temperature greater than 36° C before attempting tracheal extubation.
3. Reversal of neuromuscular blockade. Adequate train-of-four and tetanus measured peripherally may not assure sufficient intercostal and diaphragmatic strength to support respiration. Clinical assessment is required.
4. Onset of spontaneous respiration. Often children exhibit irregular respiratory patterns on emergence. Extubation should not be attempted before the return of regular respiration.
5. Return of consciousness. Purposeful movement of arms and legs and eye-opening will help to assess the level of consciousness.

Extubation in the ICU

Tracheal extubation in the ICU setting usually occurs in patients who have required prolonged mechanical ventilation (more than 24 hours). Guidelines to assess adequacy of ventilatory reserve include the following:

- Normal pH with satisfactory PaO_2 and $PaCO_2$ by arterial blood gas
- F_IO_2 requirements less than 40%
- CPAP or PEEP less than 5 cm H_2O
- Negative inspiratory force (NIF) equal to −20 to −30 cm H_2O
- Dead space (V_D/V_T) less than 0.6
- Vital capacity greater than 15 ml/kg
- Clear chest radiograph
- Adequate level of consciousness
- Complete resolution or reversal of neuromuscular blockade
- Presence of a leak (of less than 25 cm H_2O) around the endotracheal tube

Before extubation of the trachea, all equipment for airway support or possible reintubation should be assembled. This will include the following:

- Suction with appropriate size flexible catheters and Yankauer
- Oxygen supply with oxygen hood, masks, or nasal cannulae and humidifying system
- Circuit with bag, mask, and relief valve in case positive pressure ventilation is required
- Nasal and oral airways

- Appropriate monitoring: ECG, pulse oximetry, and blood pressure
- IV access
- Equipment for reintubation, including appropriate size laryngoscopes and endotracheal tubes
- Drugs for reintubation: atropine, thiopental, succinylcholine

THE EFFECTS OF ANESTHESIA ON PULMONARY PHYSIOLOGY

The Normal Infant and Child

1. All general anesthetics depress respiration by decreasing FRC and vital capacity, impairing normal mechanisms for pulmonary toilet, decreasing function of respiratory musculature, and by central depression of ventilatory drive (Table 9-7).

TABLE 9-7. Effects of anesthesia and surgery on respiration

Respiratory variable	Effects of anesthesia
Lung volumes and mechanics of breathing	
↓ VC	• Essentially a restrictive pattern with diminished lung volumes. • 60%-70% with thoracic and high-abdominal procedures. • 50%-60% with subcostal and mid-abdominal procedures. • 25%-30% with lower abdominal procedures.
↓ FRC	• Decreases 25%-30% with general anesthesia and in the supine position. • Persists up to 5-7 days postoperatively.
↓ V_T	• Decreases 20% with inhalation anesthesia.
↑ V_D/V_T ratio	• 0.3 awake. • 0.5 anesthetized with an ETT. • 0.7 anesthetized with a mask.
↑ RR	• Increases 25% with inhalation anesthesia. • Hyperventilation postoperatively reflects a compensatory response for the decreased FRC. • May also be associated with pain.
↑ $\dot{V}/\dot{Q}$ mismatching	• Secondary to alveolar hypoventilation and increased closing capacity. • Absent "sigh." • Increased airway resistance leads to loss of lung volume.
Pulmonary toilet	• A decrease in cough, mucociliary transport, and "sigh" occur because of pain, splinting, inhalation anesthetics, narcotics, mechanical ventilation, and immobilization.

Continued.

TABLE 9-7. Effects of anesthesia and surgery on respiration—cont'd

Respiratory variable	Effects of anesthesia
Inspiratory muscle tone	• Impaired diaphragmatic function is thought to be centrally mediated by increased descending inhibitory input. • Decreased genioglossus and pharyngeal/laryngeal abductor motor tone contributes to upper airway obstruction (relieved with nasal and oropharyngeal airways). The genioglossus is most sensitive as depth of anesthesia increases, followed by the intercostal muscles, and finally by the diaphragm.
Respiratory depression and CO_2/O_2 ventilation response curves	• All inhalation anesthetics produce respiratory depression in a dose-related fashion, mostly by decreasing tidal volume. Minute ventilation is preserved by increasing respiratory rate. • All inhalation anesthetics depress hypoxic ventilatory drive, even at low concentrations. The normal augmentation of ventilation produced in the awake patient by the combination of increased $PaCO_2$ and decreased PaO_2 is *not* seen in the anesthetized patient. • All inhalation anesthetics depress the ventilatory response to CO_2 in a dose-dependent manner. The $PaCO_2$ is expected to be approximately 50-55 mm Hg at surgical planes of anesthesia in spontaneously breathing patients. At 1 MAC, $PaCO_2$ is highest with enflurane, and is followed in descending order by isoflurane, halothane, and nitrous oxide. The stimulus of surgery causes a partial reversal of this effect. • Respiratory depression produced by the inhalation anesthetics is potentiated by systemic narcotics and sedative/hypnotic drugs.

2. The neonate is particularly susceptible to respiratory depression because of increased O_2 requirements (higher metabolic rate) and decreased reserve (FRC) (see box on p. 185 for neonatal characteristics that increase anesthetic risk). Although the FRC approaches adult levels within hours to days, the persistently high closing capacity increases the likelihood of alveolar collapse and intrapulmonary shunt.
3. The oxyhemoglobin dissociation curve for neonates is shifted to the left. This shift represents the increased affinity for oxygen of fetal hemoglobin (HbF), indicated by a P_{50} of 19 as compared to a P_{50} of 27 for adult hemoglobin (P_{50} = PO_2 of whole blood at 50% saturation). A relatively low concentration of 2,3-DPG in fetal hemoglobin is responsible for the increased oxygen affinity. In contrast, children between the ages of 3 months and 10 years have a P_{50} of approximately 30, which is probably related to accelerated growth and development.
   As a result of the leftward shift of the curve, neonates require a higher hemoglobin level to maintain adequate O_2 delivery to the tissue. Alkalosis,

NEONATAL RESPIRATORY CHARACTERISTICS THAT INCREASE ANESTHETIC RISK

- Decreased FRC until about 24 hours old; after which FRC approaches normal infant/adult levels.
- Closing volume and closing capacity encroach upon FRC and tidal breathing.
- Chest wall compliance is high, secondary to poorly developed musculature and nonossified ribs, and lung compliance is low, contributing to increased work of breathing to maintain lung volume and airway caliber.
- $\dot{V}O_2$ is twice that of the adult and increases with hypothermia.
- Increased CO_2 production is a result of a high metabolic rate.
- Increased respiratory rate is required to maintain alveolar minute ventilation, which increases susceptibility to fatigue.
- Work of breathing increases because of high-resistance, small caliber airways.
- Reduced Type I sustained-twitch muscle fibers in the diaphragm increases susceptibility to fatigue.
- Immature central nervous system predisposes to periodic breathing and apnea.
- Residual left-to-right shunt (through the patent ductus) worsens intrapulmonary shunt.

hypocarbia, and hypothermia will also cause a leftward shift of the curve (Fig. 9-4).

Anesthetic Implications of Pulmonary Diseases in Children

Upper Respiratory Infections

Differential diagnosis (see box on p. 186). One of the more confusing and common issues presented to the pediatric anesthesiologist is the child with symptoms consistent with an upper respiratory infection (URI), especially since the average child will have six viral respiratory infections per year (approximately one every 2 months).

It is important to distinguish between an upper respiratory illness and an allergic response. Many children have seasonal allergies, and a thorough history must be obtained from the parents to determine whether the child's rhinorrhea, cough, and infected mucosa are a chronic problem or represent an acute change.

Children with rhinorrhea that is not of infectious origin have a smaller incidence of anesthetic complications (i.e., coughing, hypoxia, laryngospasm, apnea, bronchospasm) than children whose rhinorrhea is infectious in nature. Asthma, sinusitis, cystic fibrosis, or a history of prematurity requiring intubation may be exacerbated by an acute URI, increasing anesthetic risk.

Children who seem to "always have a cold." Some conditions produce symptoms of recurrent and chronic URI. These conditions include the following:

- Recurrent tonsillitis

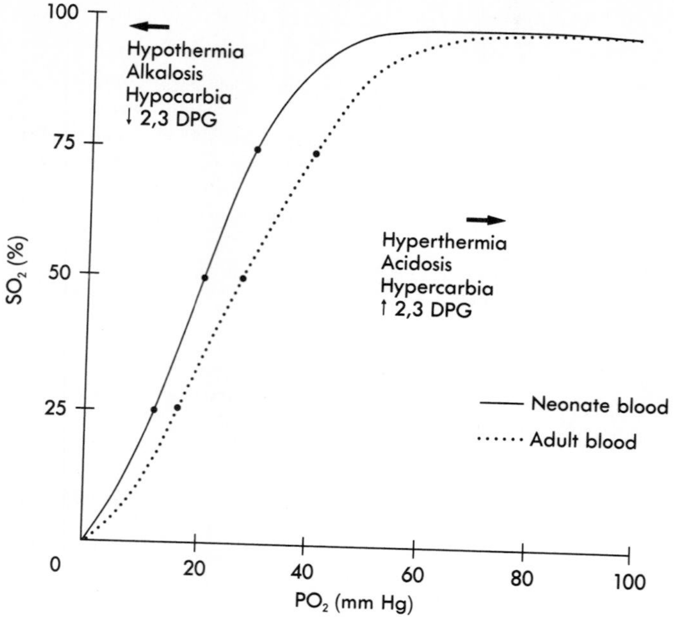

Fig. 9-4. Oxyhemoglobin curve. The oxyhemoglobin dissociation curve for fetal hemoglobin is shifted leftward (P_{50} = 19) compared to adult hemoglobin (P_{50} = 27), indicating an increased affinity of hemoglobin for oxygen. Alkalosis, hypocarbia, and hypothermia will also result in a leftward shift. Conversely, acidosis, hypercarbia, and hyperthermia shift the curve to the right, increasing the unloading of oxygen at the tissue level.

DIFFERENTIAL DIAGNOSIS OF THE "RUNNY NOSE"

Allergies
Crying child
Foreign body
Infection
- Viral infections
  - Adenovirus
  - Respiratory syncytial virus
  - Parainfluenza
- Viral exanthems
  - Varicella
  - Rubeola
- Bacterial
  - Epiglottitis
  - Retropharyngeal abscess
  - Streptococcal pharyngitis

Spinal fluid leak
Change in ambient temperature or humidity

- Recurrent otitis
- Cleft palate
- Chronic sinusitis
- Highly allergic child

The child will often persist with symptoms until the necessary operation is performed (e.g., tonsillectomy, myringotomy).

Risk of general anesthesia in the child with a URI

1. General anesthesia (GA) may precipitate bronchospasm, cough, laryngospasm, and/or apnea.
2. If this airway irritability causes acute obstruction, then hypoxia and negative pressure pulmonary edema may result.
3. Laryngospasm may be relieved by positive pressure ventilation, which adds to the risks of stomach distention and aspiration.
4. Postoperatively, pneumonia and atelectasis can prolong recovery.

Anesthesia for nonelective surgery in children with URIs

The following techniques can be used to minimize the risks of GA in children with upper respiratory infections.

1. Preoperatively, the patient should receive an anticholinergic agent (atropine or glycopyrrolate) to dry secretions and block vagal tone. Laryngospasm and bronchospasm are mediated by the vagus nerve and may precipitate bradycardia.
2. Inhalation inductions with halothane result in less airway irritability than those with enflurane or isoflurane. Intravenous or rectal inductions may also be well tolerated.
3. Anesthesia is maintained using humidified gases delivered at low flows to prevent inspissation of secretions.
4. It may be useful to avoid narcotics until airway reflexes are regained and spontaneous ventilation is resumed in young children who may be at increased risk for apnea.

Asthma

Asthma is a disease of the respiratory tree that is manifested by various symptoms from chronic cough to wheezing to respiratory failure. Most children with asthma show symptoms within the first 5 years of life. Bronchospasm may result from dysfunction of the autonomic nervous system's control mechanism or mast cell degranulation. Children develop respiratory compromise as a result of ventilation-perfusion mismatching, atelectasis, and air trapping, all of which further compromise gas exchange. Long-term effects of severe asthma can include pulmonary hypertension and resultant right ventricular hypertrophy and cor pulmonale. In children with status asthmaticus, the degree and severity of symptoms can be computed from the clinical asthma evaluation score (Table 9-8).

1. The preoperative evaluation of the asthmatic child (see box on p. 188) will help to determine the appropriate method of anesthetic management.

   The symptomatic patient scheduled for elective surgery should be delayed until symptoms resolve.
2. The asymptomatic patient should be anesthetized using induction techniques that minimize airway irritability (Table 9-9).

TABLE 9-8. Clinical asthma evaluation score (impending respiratory failure ≥5; existing respiratory failure ≥7 + PaO_2 ≥65 mm Hg)

Variables	0	1	2
PaO_2	70-100 in air	≤70 in air	≤70 in 40% O_2
Cyanosis	None	In air	In 40% O_2
Inspiratory breath sounds	Normal	Unequal	Decreased to absent
Accessory muscles used	None	Moderate	Maximal
Expiratory wheezing	None	Moderate	Marked
Cerebral function	Normal	Depressed or agitated	Coma

Reprinted from Wood DW, Downes JJ, and Lecks HI: A clinical scoring system for the diagnosis of respiratory failure, Am J Dis Child 123:227, 1972. With permission.

PREOPERATIVE EVALUATION OF THE ASTHMATIC CHILD

History

- Age at onset
- Nature and severity of symptoms
- Triggering events
- Management of acute episodes
- Hospital visits (i.e., clinic, emergency room, ward, ICU)
- Aggressive therapy (e.g., intubation or mechanical ventilation, isoproterenol infusions)
- Medication regimen

Physical examination

- Vital signs
- Use of accessory muscles
- Wheezing
- Cough
- Nature and symmetry of breath sounds
- Cyanosis
- Altered mental status (i.e., CNS depression from hypercarbia/hyperoxia)
- Hydration status

Laboratory data (as indicated)

- CBC with differential
- CXR if acute event is atypical or associated with fever
- Arterial blood gas
- ECG if signs and symptoms of right ventricular hypertrophy
- Spirometry (FEV_1, FVC) in compliant patients

TABLE 9-9. Effects of induction agents on the asthmatic patient

Technique or drug	Advantages	Disadvantages
Intravenous		
Thiopental	Rapid onset; blunts reflexes	Histamine release may precipitate bronchospasm
Ketamine	Bronchodilation	Increased secretions and airway irritability
Inhalation		
Halothane	Bronchodilation	May precipitate dysrhythmias when used with theophylline
Enflurane	Bronchodilation	Respiratory depression; elevated $PaCO_2$ with spontaneous ventilation
Isoflurane	Bronchodilation	Increased incidence of breath-holding and laryngospasm

The following should be considered preinduction:

- Premedication
- Preoperative bronchodilators
- Stress steroid coverage if the patient has required steroid therapy within the past 6 months
- Anticholinergics to decrease secretions and prevent reflex bradycardia

3. Regional techniques avoid airway manipulation but may prevent effective cough by decreasing vital capacity if thoracic muscles are blocked. General anesthesia is advantageous for controlling ventilation but may increase airway irritability, particularly with intubation.
4. Wheezing can occur at any time during the operation, even in the asymptomatic patient (see Table 9-10 for differential diagnoses of intraoperative wheezing).

TABLE 9-10. Differential diagnosis of intraoperative wheezing

Cause	Treatment
Light anesthesia	Deepen anesthesia
Obstructed tube	Suction
Pneumothorax	Aspirate air and insert chest tube
Mainstem intubation or tube positioned at carina	Reposition endotracheal tube
Aspiration	Consider antibiotics or inhaled bronchodilators
Bronchospasm	Consider IV theophylline or IV steroids

5. Intraoperatively, all gases should be humidified to prevent inspiration of dried secretions.
6. Suction of the trachea should only be performed while the patient is deeply anesthetized.
7. Mechanical ventilation should be instituted with low inflating pressures and prolonged expiratory time.
8. Deep extubation of the trachea avoids the risks of bronchospasm from coughing on the endotracheal tube during emergence but adds the risk of aspiration.
9. Humidified oxygen should be administered during recovery from anesthesia along with nebulized or intravenous bronchodilators, if needed.
10. Aggressive pain management increases the likelihood of adequate pulmonary toilet postoperatively.

It is occasionally necessary to anesthetize the acutely symptomatic asthmatic child for emergency surgery (see box).

ANESTHETIC TECHNIQUES FOR THE CHILD WITH SYMPTOMATIC ASTHMA

- Preoperative therapy with inhaled and intravenous bronchodilators and steroids (Table 9-11) may be continued intraoperatively.
- Preoperative laboratory studies include CBC, CXR, bedside pulmonary function tests, arterial blood gas, and theophylline levels.
- Premedication is usually avoided to prevent further respiratory depression.
- Regional anesthesia, if appropriate for patient age and level of cooperation, will avoid intubation. However, loss of accessory muscles of respiration can diminish vital capacity.
- Atropine may help to dry secretions and prevent reflex bradycardia but may also cause inspissated mucus that will exacerbate wheezing.
- Intravenous lidocaine or fentanyl preintubation helps to decrease airway reactivity.
- Agents that release histamine are avoided if possible (thiopental, succinylcholine, d-tubocurare).
- Intraoperative management includes inhalation agents for bronchodilatory effect, humidified gases, aggressive hydration, and mechanical ventilation with long expiratory times and low inflation pressures.
- Deep extubation is usually not useful in emergency situations because of aspiration risks. Intravenous lidocaine may attenuate airway reactivity on emergence. Severely symptomatic patients may require prolonged intubation and ICU admission.

Respiratory Distress Syndrome

Respiratory distress syndrome (RDS) has become a major medical problem in the field of neonatology. Children with RDS are generally born prematurely and require mechanical ventilation within the first 12 hours of life. Approximately 1% of all live births and 10% to 15% of all premature births are associated with RDS, the incidence being inversely related to the ges-

TABLE 9-11. Pharmacologic therapy for asthma

Classification	Drug (brand name)	Preparation*	Dose/route
Methylxanthines	Aminophylline	As per commercial preparation	IV: 6 mg/kg loading dose over 30 min in the absence of any level in blood. Begin infusion at 1 mg/kg/hr. Check level. Optimal level = 10-20 μg/dl. Adjust infusion accordingly.
Adrenergic agents	Epinephrine	1:1000 = 1 mg/ml	SC: 0.01 ml/kg/dose every 20 min × 3, as needed. *Max:* 0.4 ml.
	Terbutaline (Brethine, Bricanyl)	.05% = 0.5 mg/ml	SC: 0.01 mg/kg/dose every 20 min × 3, as needed. *Max:* 0.25 mg.
		1% solution = 10 mg/ml	Inhaled: 0.03 ml/kg in 1-2 ml of NS every 4 hr, as needed. *Max:* 1 ml.
	Metaproterenol (Alupent)	0.1% solution = 1 mg/ml	SC: 0.01 ml/kg every 20 min × 3, as needed.
		5% solution = 50 mg/ml	Inhaled: 0.005-0.01 ml/kg in 1-2 ml every 4 hr, as needed. *Max:* 0.4 ml.
	Albuterol (Ventolin, Proventil)	0.1% solution = 1.0 mg/ml	IV: 0.2-2 μg/kg/min
		0.5% solution = 5 mg/ml	Inhaled: 0.01-0.03 ml/kg in 1-2 ml NS every 4 hr, as needed. *Max:* 1 ml.
	Isoproterenol (Isuprel)	0.02% solution = 0.2 mg/ml	IV: 0.02-0.2 μg/kg/min
		0.5% solution = 5 mg/ml	Inhaled: 0.01-0.02 ml/kg in 1-2 ml NS every 2-6 hr, as needed. *Max:* 0.5 ml.

*Note: 1% = 10 mg/ml, 2% = 20 mg/ml, etc.

Continued.

TABLE 9-11. Pharmacologic therapy for asthma—cont'd

Classification	Drug (brand name)	Preparation*	Dose/route
	Isoethrane (Bronkosol)	1% solution = 10 mg/ml	Inhaled: 0.01 ml/kg in 1-2 ml NS every 2-6 hr, as needed. *Max:* 0.5 ml.
Steroids	Hydrocortisone	As per commercial preparation	IV: 5-7 mg/kg load followed by 5 mg/kg/dose every 6 hr.
	Methylprednisolone	As per commercial preparation	IV: 1 mg/kg load followed by 0.8 mg/kg every 4-6 hr.
Anticholinergics	Atropine	As per commercial preparation	Inhaled: 0.03-0.05 mg/kg nebulized.

*Note: 1% = 10 mg/ml, 2% = 20 mg/ml, etc.
Adapted from Chantarojanasiri T, Nichols DF, and Rogers MC: Status asthmaticus. In Rogers MC, editor: Handbook of pediatric intensive care, Baltimore, 1989, Williams & Wilkins.

tational age. RDS is a result of a deficiency in the formation of pulmonary surfactant, which is produced by the Type II pneumocytes.

Anesthetic considerations in the patient with RDS include the following:

- Preoperative assessment of umbilical artery line function and location
- Close monitoring of oxygen saturation and arterial blood gases to avoid both hypoxemia and O_2 toxicity
- Avoidance of hypocarbia by adequate ventilation
- Prevention of atelectasis by providing adequate tidal volumes
- Provision of end-expiratory pressure as needed for oxygenation
- Prevention of metabolic acidosis
- Evaluation of potential intracardiac shunting through a patent foramen ovale or ductus arteriosus
- Monitoring for pneumothorax
- Maintenance of a patent airway by suction of the endotracheal tube
- Postoperative apnea monitoring

Bronchopulmonary Dysplasia

Bronchopulmonary dysplasia (BPD) is a form of chronic pulmonary disease seen in children after a prolonged period of respiratory compromise, which has its onset in the neonatal period. Most often these children are born prematurely and have a prolonged requirement for supplemental oxygen as well as a significant period of mechanical ventilation to support gas exchange.

1. Anesthetic considerations for the child with BPD include the following:
   - Optimal nutrition status preoperatively
   - Continuation of chronic medication throughout the pre- and postoperative periods
   - High minute ventilation
   - Requirement for bronchodilators (nebulized and/or intravenous)
   - Diuretic requirement to reduce edema
   - Maintenance of acid-base balance
   - Adequate sedation and possibly tracheostomy if requirements for mechanical ventilation are prolonged
2. Anticipated postoperative complications include the following:
   - Pneumothorax from high inflating pressures
   - Bronchospasm upon placement of the endotracheal tube
   - Postoperative atelectasis and/or infection
   - Congestive heart failure as a result of possible right ventricular hypertrophy, cor pulmonale, and/or myocardial dysfunction
   - Complications involving other medical problems that occur in children who are prone to bronchopulmonary dysplasia (intracranial bleeding, retinopathy of prematurity, poor musculoskeletal development)
3. The goals of the anesthesiologist should be to:
   - Maintain adequate oxygenation to meet the demands of all tissues (PO_2 between 50 and 70 mm Hg)
   - Avoid triggers that increase pulmonary hypertension (acidosis, hypercarbia, hypothermia)
   - Maintain peak inflating pressures at the lowest acceptable level
   - Restrict fluid administration
   - Prevent bronchospasm by use of prophylactic bronchodilators

Cystic Fibrosis (CF)

CF is a congenital disease of autosomal recessive inheritance that results in pulmonary and hepatobiliary problems. Elevated sodium and chloride levels in the sweat are notable and often diagnostic. Given the obstruction in the respiratory tract, children and adolescents with this disease often develop bronchitis and bronchiolitis, with significant damage to the airway and ultimately cystic changes in the pulmonary parenchyma. Hyperinflation of lung fields is common.

1. Complications of cystic fibrosis include pneumonia, lung abscesses, pneumothoraces, pneumomediastinum, right ventricular hypertrophy, and atelectasis. As a result, these children often have $\dot{V}/\dot{Q}$ mismatching and hypoxemia. Bacterial and viral opportunistic infections are common.
2. Associated gastrointestinal findings in patients with cystic fibrosis include the following:
   - Rectal prolapse
   - Meconium ileus
   - Cholelithiasis, causing obstructive jaundice

- Portal hypertension and esophageal varices
- Malabsorption

3. The following operations are often required by children with CF:
   - Nasal polypectomy
   - Pleurodesis for recurrent pneumothorax
   - Alleviation of intestinal obstructions

Anesthetic management for patients with cystic fibrosis is as follows:

Preoperative

- All medications are continued (for pancreatic insufficiency, right ventricular hypertrophy).
- Pulmonary function is maximized by chest physiotherapy.
- Laboratory data are obtained including electrolytes, arterial blood gases, and pulmonary function tests.

Intraoperative

- Nitrous oxide is avoided if cystic lesions are present by x-ray.
- Narcotics should be titrated to effect to prevent further respiratory depression.
- Lower pressure settings are used for mechanical ventilation to avoid pneumothorax.
- Aggressive hydration helps to prevent inspissation of mucus. Frequent endotracheal suction of mucous plugs is required.
- Regional techniques avoid the need for intubation but may cause decompensation if accessory muscles of respiration are blocked. Many children with CF must also sit up to spontaneously ventilate, which may make the use of regional techniques for certain operative procedures less favorable.

Postoperative

- Prolonged mechanical ventilation is often required.
- Regional pain management techniques and neuraxis opioids allow for vigorous chest physiotherapy and earlier extubation.
- All medications should be resumed as soon as possible.

Apnea of Prematurity

Apnea is defined as the absence of breathing for 20 seconds or longer or with associated signs of cyanosis and/or bradycardia. Central apnea (absence of respiratory effort) is often associated with prematurity. Obstructive apnea may be due to adenotonsillar hypertrophy, micrognathia, macroglossia, or obesity and is more common in older children (see Chapter 8).

1. Immature physiology and specific perinatal events have a high association with the development of apnea. In premature infants apnea may result from the following:
   - CNS immaturity
   - A diminished response to increased $PaCO_2$ and decreased PaO_2
   - A reflex response to airway stimulation
   - A history of patent ductus arteriosus
   - Medications (PGE_1, narcotics)
   - Sepsis
   - Respiratory distress syndrome
   - Hypothermia, fever

- Gastroesophageal reflux
- General anesthesia

2. Anesthetic management of infants with a history of apnea includes the following:
   - Optimization of the preoperative medical condition
   - Careful titration of intra- and postoperative narcotics
   - Postoperative hospitalization for at least 24 hours (or 12 hours after an apneic event) for all term infants less than 44 weeks of gestational age and all preterm infants less than 60 weeks of gestational age
   - Continuous cardiorespiratory monitoring and oximetry in the postoperative period
   - Theophylline or caffeine are frequently used as central stimulants to diminish apneic episodes.

BIBLIOGRAPHY

Barker SJ and Tremper KK: Physics applied to anesthesia. In Barash PG, Cullen BF, and Stoelting RK, editors: Clinical anesthesia, Philadelphia, 1989, JB Lippincott Co.

Berry FA: Anesthesia for the child with a difficult airway. In Berry FA, editor: Anesthetic management of difficult and routine pediatric patients, New York, 1986, Churchill Livingstone.

Berry FA: The child with a runny nose. In Berry FA, editor: Anesthetic management of difficult and routine pediatric patients, New York, 1986, Churchill Livingstone.

Bikhazi GB and Davis PJ: Anesthesia for neonates and premature infants. In Motoyama EK and Davis PJ, editors: Smith's Anesthesia for infants and children, ed 5, St Louis, 1990, The CV Mosby Co.

Chantarojanasiri T, Nichols DG, and Rogers MC: Lower airway disease: broncholitis and asthma. In Rogers M: Textbook of pediatric intensive care, Baltimore, 1987, Williams & Wilkins.

Cote CJ and Todres ID: The pediatric airway. In Ryan JF and others, editors: A practice of anesthesia for infants and children, Orlando, 1986, Grune & Stratton.

Gibney N: Respiratory intensive care. In Lebowitz PW, Newberg LA, and Gillette MT, editors: Clinical anesthesia procedures of the Massachusetts General Hospital, ed 2, Boston, 1982, Little, Brown & Co.

Gioia FR, Stephenson RL, and Alterwitz SA: Principles of respiratory support. In Rogers MC, editor: Textbook of pediatric intensive care, vol 1, Baltimore, 1987, Williams & Wilkins.

Gregory GA: Anesthesia for premature infants. In Gregory GA, editor: Pediatric anesthesia, ed 2, New York, 1989, Churchill Livingstone.

Harrison RA: Respiratory function and anesthesia. In Barash PG, Cullen BF, and Stoelting RK, editors: Clinical anesthesia, Philadelphia, 1989, JB Lippincott Co.

Kirby RR, Smith RA, and Desautels DA, editors: Mechanical ventilation, New York, 1985, Churchill Livingstone.

Klein J: Normobaric pulmonary oxygen toxicity, Anesth Analg 70:195-207, 1990.

Motoyama EK: Respiratory physiology in infants and children. In Motoyama EK and Davis PJ, editors: Smith's Anesthesia for infants and children, ed 5, St Louis, 1990, The CV Mosby Co.

Nugent J, Matthews BJ, and Goldsmith JP: Pulmonary care. In Goldsmith and Karotkin E, editors: Assisted ventilation in the neonate, ed 2, Philadelphia, 1988, WB Saunders Co.

Nunn JF: Applied respiratory physiology, ed 3, London, 1987, Butterworths Co.

O'Rourke PP and Crone RK: The respiratory system. In Gregory GA, editor: Pediatric anesthesia, ed 2, New York, 1989, Churchill Livingstone.
Thompson AE and Cook DR: Respiratory care. In Cook DR and Marcy JH, editors: Neonatal anesthesia, Pasadena, 1988, Appleton Davies, Inc.
Todres ID: Diseases of the respiratory system. In Katz J and Steward DJ, editors: Anesthesia and uncommon pediatric disorders, Philadelphia, 1987, WB Saunders Co.
Willson DF: The child with asthma. In Berry FA, editor: Anesthetic management of difficult and routine pediatric patients, New York, 1986, Churchill Livingstone.

10

ANESTHESIA FOR GASTROINTESTINAL DISORDERS

Edward Weingarden

Jack Sprat could eat no fat
  His wife could eat no lean;
And so between them both, you see
  They licked the platter clean.
ANON

NORMAL PATTERNS OF GASTROINTESTINAL FUNCTION IN THE NEWBORN

Swallowing

The fetus is able to swallow by 11 weeks in utero; esophageal peristalsis also begins at this time. It is not until the seventh month of age that the infant can coordinate the movement of food from the front of the tongue to the pharynx. Withholding solid foods because of illness beyond seven months of age leads to the infant having difficulty accepting solid foods.

Gastric Emptying

The gastric emptying time for a healthy full-term infant varies from 1.5 to 25 hours. Gastric emptying is slow in the first 12 hours of life and "full stomach" precautions prevail for any anesthetic conducted in a neonate during this period of time. Pathologic conditions including cardiovascular disease, respiratory distress, and gastroesophageal reflux are also associated with delayed gastric emptying.

Intestinal Motility

Intestinal motility is disorganized in the preterm infant (<34 weeks gestation). After 34 weeks gestation a more cyclical pattern of smooth muscle activity develops with corresponding neurologic development. It is not until the end of the first year of life that a normal adult pattern of gastrointestinal motility is present.

Gastroesophageal Reflux (GER)

Passive gastroesophageal reflux is a common condition in a newborn infant. As many as 40% of infants will regurgitate or "spit up" gastric contents. This results from an immature sphincter, absent or disorganized peristaltic waves, and a lower pressure in the esophagus than in the stomach. Adequate NPO times and safe principles of airway management are essential in even the healthiest neonates.

COMMON GASTROINTESTINAL DISORDERS

Common GI disorders may be symptoms representative of more severe underlying pathology or entities within themselves.

Gastroesophageal Reflux

Normal passive GER will either improve or resolve in 70% of all children by 18 months of age. Conditions such as apnea and bradycardia in the preterm infant are associated closely with GE reflux. Persistent vomiting, failure to thrive, and chronic respiratory infections also are associated with chronic reflux. Medical therapy for reflux includes administration of antacids, H_2 antagonists, bethanechol (to increase lower esophageal sphincter tone), and metoclopramide.

1. Surgical correction of GER is seldom indicated unless the reflux causes recurrent aspiration pneumonia or malnutrition with failure to thrive, severe esophagitis or stricture, or Barrett's esophagus. Problems that commonly result in reflux include hiatal hernia, achalasia of the esophagus, or tracheoesophageal fistula repair.
2. Preoperative medical management should aim to resolve any respiratory infections, maintain adequate fluid and electrolyte balance, and treat acidic reflux with H_2 antagonists and bethanechol or metoclopramide (Table 10-1).
3. A child with severe reflux should be treated as having a "full stomach"

TABLE 10-1. Drug therapy for GI problems

Medication	Dose	Action	Time course
Cimetidine	7.5 mg/kg PO/ IV	Reduces gastric acid secretion	1-3 hr before induction
Metoclopramide	0.1-.2 mg/kg IV	Improves gastric emptying	30 min before induction
Glycopyrrolate	10 μg/kg IV or IM	Antisialologue; vagolytic	30 min before induction
Atropine	10-20 μg/kg IV or IM	Antisialologue; vagolytic	15-30 min before induction
Droperidol	50-75 μg/kg IV or IM	Antiemetic	Before emergence from anesthesia

RAPID SEQUENCE INDUCTION IN AN INFANT

1. Secure IV access is established.
2. Monitors including ECG, precordial stethoscope, oximeter, and BP cuff should be placed, and baseline values obtained before proceeding.
3. A small towel placed under the child's neck and shoulders may help to accommodate the relatively large occiput of the infant.
4. The stomach should be emptied with an orogastric suction tube, especially in pyloric stenosis or duodenal atresia.
5. Administration of atropine (0.01 to 0.02 mg/kg IV) before gastric decompression will decrease vagal tone.
6. Oxygen should be administered with a face mask.
7. Thiopental (4 to 6 mg/kg) or ketamine (1 to 2 mg/kg) and succinylcholine (2 mg/kg) are given intravenously by bolus. Firm but gentle cricoid pressure should be applied before laryngoscopy and orotracheal intubation. Correct placement of the endotracheal tube should be confirmed by auscultation and presence of CO_2 by capnography before releasing cricoid pressure.

and either a rapid-sequence induction (see the box above) or awake intubation (see the box on p. 200) should be performed.

4. An inhalation induction may be appropriate in the child whose symptoms are well controlled.
5. A Nissen fundoplication (see Table 10-5 for common surgical procedures) is the most common operative procedure for correction of GER. The surgeon may approach the operative site through either a high midline abdominal or thoracic incision. A gastrostomy tube usually is placed. The patient will require prolonged postoperative ventilation depending on age, weight, site of incision, preoperative pulmonary status, and anticipated postoperative analgesic needs.

Nausea and Vomiting

The causes of nausea and vomiting are numerous. Because young infants have high caloric and fluid requirements, they can rapidly develop dehydration, starvation ketosis, and hypochloremic/hypokalemic metabolic alkalosis with persistent vomiting. An assessment of the degree of dehydration and adequate fluid and electrolyte therapy are necessary. Although reflux and regurgitation may be normal in newborn infants, vomiting often heralds significant disease and probably indicates radiographic examination.

Diarrhea

Diarrhea is a major cause of infant mortality. Common etiologies include infection, inborn errors of metabolism, food allergy, carbohydrate intolerance, and inflammatory bowel disease. Factors that contribute to the increased morbidity and mortality from diarrhea in children include the large intestinal surface/body weight ratio and the large extracellular fluid compartment, which makes them particularly susceptible to dehydration. Evaluation of a child with diarrhea includes the assessment of fluid and electrolyte imbalances and proper replacement therapy (Table 10-2).

AWAKE INTUBATION IN A NEONATE

1. Indications for awake intubation include:
   a. Avoiding hemodynamic alterations from drugs commonly used for rapid-sequence induction (hemodynamic instability from GI bleeding, septic shock, necrotizing enterocolitis, or congenital heart disease).
   b. Insufficient respiratory reserve to tolerate any sustained period of apnea (respiratory distress syndrome).
   c. Questionable airway for bag-mask ventilation.
   d. Bowel obstruction or full-stomach considerations.
   e. Severe GE reflux.
2. Airway support equipment should be present and ready to be used including: suction, O_2 delivery system, masks, oral airways, checked circuit, and ventilator.
3. Resuscitative drugs should include atropine, epinephrine 1:10,000, sodium bicarbonate 0.5 mEq/ml, and calcium chloride.
4. Routine monitors should be placed (ECG, precordial stethoscope, blood pressure, oximeter) and baseline values obtained.
5. Atropine 0.02 mg/kg IM or IV should be given.
6. An orogastric tube should be placed to decompress the stomach and then removed.
7. A rolled towel can be placed below the infant's neck/shoulders to accommodate the large occiput and help stabilize the head.
8. Oxygen should be insufflated in the vicinity of the infant's airway or with an oxygenating laryngoscope.
9. Three different sizes of endotracheal tubes (ID equaling 2.5, 3.0, and 3.5 mm) with stylets should be opened and ready to use.
10. An assistant should restrain the infant while laryngoscopy and tracheal intubation is performed.
11. The thumb and index finger of the left hand can hold the pediatric laryngoscope at the junction of blade and handle. This technique leaves the hand free to cup the chin for stabilizing a wiggling infant. The fifth finger is used for cricoid pressure.
12. Passing the blade from the right corner of the mouth toward the left in an oblique fashion helps to fix the tongue.
13. The endotracheal tube should be held in the right hand before beginning laryngoscopy so that one's eyes are not diverted to locate the tube once the larynx is identified.
14. The vocal cords often close with stimulation during awake laryngoscopy. The endotracheal tube should be placed on the closed cords directly and advanced gently through the larynx when the cords first relax with inhalation.
15. The endotracheal tube should be held securely while the child is being anesthetized. Position of the tube should be confirmed before taping.

SEVERE GASTROINTESTINAL DISORDERS

Necrotizing Enterocolitis (NEC)

Necrotizing enterocolitis (see the box on p. 202 for features of NEC) is a disease process of premature infants characterized by varying degrees of bowel necrosis. It is the most common acquired gastrointestinal emergency in the intensive care nursery. The infant at greatest risk is less than 32 weeks

TABLE 10-2. Metabolic disturbances associated with diarrhea (See also dehydration in Chapter 6, Fluids and Electrolytes)

Metabolic disturbance	Etiology	Treatment
Metabolic acidosis	Bicarbonate loss in stool	If pH <7.29, give HCO_3 1 mEq/kg
Ketosis	Malabsorption; poor PO intake	Glucose-containing IV
Hypokalemia	Potassium loss in stool	K^+ 0.5 mEq/kg/hr IV after voiding twice
Hypoglycemia	Prolonged diarrhea	Glucose 0.5-1.0 g/kg
Hypocalcemia	Ca^{++} loss in stool	Calcium gluconate 100 mg/kg IV slowly
Hypernatremia	Severe fluid losses	IV therapy with D_5W

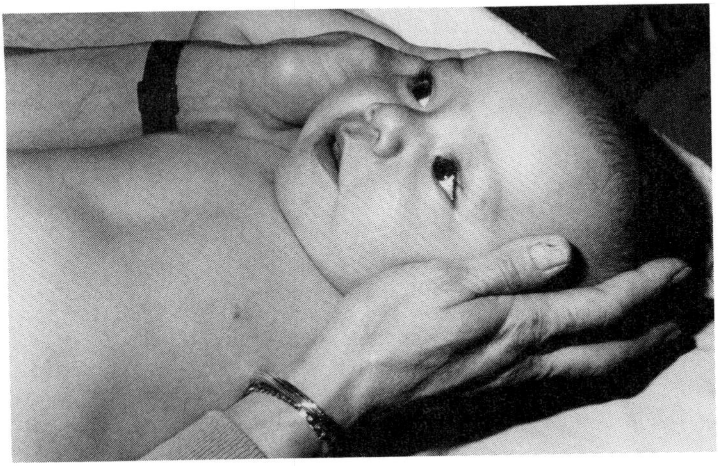

Fig. 10-1. During laryngoscopy, an assistant can restrain an awake infant by immobilizing the arms and trunk while holding the head securely in the neutral position.

gestational age and weighs less than 1500 grams, although the disease may occur in full-term infants. The exact cause remains an enigma and is probably multifactorial.

Anesthetic Management of NEC

Preoperative management. Only those infants failing medical therapy proceed to surgical intervention, so these infants by definition are critically ill and often moribund. Most infants are hypovolemic with a metabolic acidosis requiring colloid and crystalloid resuscitation. Coagulopathy and hypocalcemia also must be corrected. An arterial catheter allows direct blood pressure monitoring and frequent measurement of arterial blood gases, pH, hematocrit, coagulation parameters, and electrolytes to guide resuscitation

FEATURES OF NEC

Etiologies

Asphyxia, polycythemia, hyperosmolar feedings, umbilical artery catheterization, respiratory distress syndrome, exchange transfusions, congenital cardiac disease; an ischemic insult to the intestine is the final common pathway

Clinical features

Irritability and/or lethargy, abdominal distention, bloody mucus in stool, vomiting, high gastric residuals

Associated problems

Acidosis, hypothermia, apnea and bradycardia, thrombocytopenia, disseminated intravascular coagulation (DIC), septic/hypovolemic shock

Radiographic findings

Pneumotosis intestinalis (presence of air within the bowel wall); pneumoperitoneum

Medical management

Antibiotics, continuous nasogastric suction, discontinuation of enteral feedings for 10 to 14 days, IV fluids; medical therapy is successful in avoiding surgery in 85% of all cases

Surgical intervention

Indications for surgery include: intestinal perforation, mechanical obstruction, peritonitis, progressive acidosis, or failed medical therapy

efforts. The necessary blood and blood products should be ordered, especially if thrombocytopenia or coagulopathy are present.

Airway management. If the infant has not yet been intubated in the intensive-care unit the airway must be established by either a rapid-sequence induction or awake intubation. Although awake intubations may result in large increases in intracranial pressure and subsequent intracranial hemorrhage, most anesthesiologists believe this is the safest technique in the premature infant with an acute abdomen and marginal respiratory reserve.

Anesthetic agents. Appropriate anesthetic agents include narcotics and ketamine. Inhalation agents should be used judiciously because many infants with NEC requiring surgery are too critically ill to tolerate the depressant effects of these anesthetics. Nitrous oxide should be avoided because of bowel distention and the frequent presence of pneumotosis intestinalis. An air/oxygen mixture is used to maintain arterial oxygen tension between 50 and 70 mm Hg or SaO_2 around 90% by oximetry.

Intraoperative management. During the operation, attention must be paid to adequate fluid replacement, electrolyte deficiencies, acid-base balance, serum glucose, coagulation abnormalities, and hematocrit level. Dopamine may be needed for cardiovascular support.

Temperature maintenance. Hypothermia is a common problem in young infants with NEC. Normothermia is maintained with increased room temperature, radiant heat lamps, warming blankets, warmed and humidified gases, wrapping the extremities in clear plastic wrap, and covering the head. *Postoperative management.* The infant usually requires ventilatory assistance in the postoperative period and should be transported back to the intensive care unit in a warm isolette with ECG, oximetry, resuscitative drugs, and oxygen.

A prolonged ileus is expected and may necessitate placement of a central venous catheter for parenteral hyperalimentation.

Pyloric Stenosis

1. Congenital hypertrophy of the pyloric sphincter is most likely to present with persistent or projectile vomiting in the fourth to sixth week of life, commonly in male infants. An olive-sized mass is classically palpable in the pyloric region.
2. Dehydration and hypochloremic, hypokalemic metabolic alkalosis may develop if vomiting has been severe or prolonged. It must be emphasized that pyloric stenosis is first a medical emergency, requiring correction of fluid and electrolyte abnormalities, and then a surgically treatable condition (see Treatment of Dehydration in Chapter 6, Fluids and Electrolytes).
3. Preoperative management includes continuous nasogastric suction and intravenous replacement of fluids and electrolytes.
4. Before induction of general anesthesia, the stomach should be emptied with a 10 or 12 French suction catheter. Despite continuous low pressure nasogastric suction these infants will commonly have a large amount of fluid in their stomachs.
5. The airway is secured either by an awake intubation or rapid-sequence induction. The age, size, and overall medical condition of the child as well as the experience and expertise of the anesthesiologist will determine which method is more suitable.
6. Because pyloromyotomy is a relatively short procedure the newer short-acting muscle relaxants are useful in this setting.
7. Extubation of the trachea should follow when the child is wide awake and the stomach has been emptied.

Bowel Obstruction

1. Etiologies of bowel obstruction in children include: congenital bands, malrotation, intestinal atresia, volvulus, appendicitis, meconium inspissation, intussusception, Hirschsprung's disease, imperforate anus, meconium ileus and meconium peritonitis, and mucosal cysts and polyps (Tables 10-3 and 10-4).
2. Preoperative management consists of nasogastric suction and intravenous replacement of fluid and electrolytes.
3. A rapid-sequence induction or awake intubation is indicated.
4. Appropriate anesthetic agents include inhalation agents, narcotics, or ketamine. Nitrous oxide can be used judiciously once the abdomen is open. However, it may cause increased bowel distention and make the surgical closure of the abdomen more difficult in a small infant. An air/oxygen mixture is a better choice in the small infant and child.

TABLE 10-3. Bowel obstruction in neonates

Disorder	Signs and symptoms	Surgical management
Intestinal atresia		
• Duodenal atresia	Absence of abdominal distension because of proximal obstruction X-ray findings: double-bubble (air/fluid levels in stomach and proximal duodenum) Incidence of associated anomalies	Duodendenostomy
• Ileal and jejunal atresia	Abdominal distension Multiple loops of small bowel on x-ray; no air in colon	Duodenojejunostomy or ileal resection
Malrotation and volvulus	Duodenal obstruction because of anomalous peritoneal bands Volvulus of entire small bowel with early necrosis as superior mesenteric vessels twist with unfixed mesentery May present with distention and bloody stools	Exploration, Ladd procedure (see Table 10-5) to lyse bands and fix mesentery
Meconium ileus	Obstruction caused by unusually thick meconium Most often associated with cystic fibrosis	May resolve with hyperosmolar enemas of meglumine diatrizoate (Gastrograffin) Often requires bowel resection or colostomy
Meconium peritonitis	Caused by intrauterine intestinal rupture X-ray: spotty calcification in an area that does not contain loops of bowel	Exploration; correct cause of rupture
Hirschsprung's disease	Clinical symptoms range from constipation to severe colonic obstruction X-ray: narrowed distal segment of colon with proximal dilation Aganglionic section of bowel is usually segmental	Colostomy and biopsy Later, Swenson or Duhamel pull-through procedure (see Table 10-5)
Imperforate anus	Usually accompanied by fistula into bladder or vagina High incidence of associated renal or GI problems	May require colostomy Later, surgical reconstruction
Mucosal cysts	Obstruction by torsion or by compression from the mass Hemorrhage occurs in cysts lined with gastric mucosa	Resection of cyst or associated bowel

TABLE 10-4. Bowel obstruction in older children

Disorder	Signs and symptoms	Surgical management
Intussusception	Inversion of loop of bowel into the next one, usually at ileocecal valve Current jelly stools caused by blood and mucus secreted into bowel lumen Usually male, 5 to 9 months of age	Often can be reduced with barium enema Surgical intervention necessary for about 25% of patients
Appendicitis	Low-grade fever, mild leukocytosis Guarding and rebound on exam	Immediate operative intervention (mortality greatly increases if appendix ruptures) Rarely, a profoundly dehydrated child requires normalization of fluids and electrolytes preoperatively
Colonic polyps		
• Juvenile	Never malignant Rarely prolapse through rectum	Removal of polyps during sigmoidoscopy
• Multiple polypoid adenomatosis	Genetically determined All result in malignant conversion	Total proctocolectomy
Peutz-Jeghers	Hamartomatous bowel or stomach polyps; will occasionally bleed, causing anemia Pigment spots on skin and mucosa Not associated with malignancy	Treatment indicated if persistent bleeding

5. Stomach contents should continue to be aspirated via an orogastric or nasogastric tube after the airway is secured. This is an important maneuver before any surgical manipulation of the gut because regurgitation and leakage of stomach contents beyond an uncuffed endotracheal tube is an ever-present hazard.
6. The trachea should be extubated when the child is fully awake. The lateral position is advised for transport to the recovery room.

Gastrointestinal Bleeding

1. Gastrointestinal pathology that can lead to GI bleeding includes: intussusception, Meckel's diverticulum, polyps, hereditary telangiectasias, and inflammatory lesions (ulcerative colitis, peptic ulcer disease).
2. Melena is characteristic of upper GI bleeding, while bright red blood or bloody diarrhea is seen with lower GI bleeding. Currant jelly stools (bloody mucus) are present with intussusception.

TABLE 10-5. Eponym surgical procedures for GI disorders

Eponym	Diagnosis	Procedure	Comments
Swenson's procedure	Hirschsprung's disease	Resection of aganglionic intestine Eversion of rectal stump through anus Anastomosis of stump and normal colon Posterior sphincterotomy	Lengthy procedure Difficult pelvic dissection
Duhamel's procedure	Hirschsprung's disease	Aganglionic intestine resected to peritoneal reflection Rectum sutured closed Wide anastomosis of end of normal colon to posterior rectal wall	Eliminates much pelvic dissection Decreased blood and fluid losses Shorter procedure Preserves aganglionic rectum Sphincter mechanism is undisturbed
Soave, State, Soper, Ikeda, Martin	Hirschsprung's disease	Modifications of Duhamel	
Kasai (portoenterostomy)	Biliary atresia	Removal of extrahepatic bile ducts Bile drainage established by anastomosis of intestinal conduit to transected duct (usually, Roux-en-Y jejunostomy) Temporary exteriorization of conduit (decreases pressure and stasis, and allows monitoring of adequate function)	Cholangitis is a frequent complication (caused by stasis and contamination by enteric bacteria)

Ladd's procedure	Malrotation Division of Ladd's bands (peritoneal bands)	Reduction of volvulus (coils of intestine wrapped around root of unanchored mesentery) Resection of peritoneal bands Fixation of mesentery Appendectomy (cecum ends up in left lower quadrant; appendicitis in future may be misdiagnosed)	May need to be done emergently if obstructed Fluid, blood, and electrolyte losses may be severe, particularly if significant ischemia, or necrotic bowel
Nissen fundoplication	Gastroesophageal reflux	Wrapping gastric fundus around gastroesophageal junction May include gastrostomy	Assume "full stomach" precautions Patients often have a history of respiratory dysfunction from recurrent aspiration pneumonia Complications include inability to vomit and gas bloat syndrome
Thal-Ashcraft procedure	Gastroesophageal reflux	270-degree wrap of gastric fundus around gastroesophageal junction	Avoids complications of Nissen

3. Preoperative treatment consists of the establishment of an intravenous line that will be adequate for fluid resuscitation and the administration of blood products. A 22-gauge catheter is the smallest catheter appropriate for these purposes. Gastric decompression by continuous nasogastric suction or the passage of an orogastric catheter before the induction of anesthesia is indicated. Appropriate blood products should be ordered and available before bringing the child to the operating room.
4. "Full stomach" considerations apply; the airway is secured either by an awake intubation or rapid-sequence induction. Awake intubation can be performed in the lateral position to decrease the likelihood of aspiration.
5. The trachea is extubated when the child is fully awake and in the lateral position.

Inflammatory Bowel Disease

1. Inflammatory bowel disease (IBD) refers to colitis or ileitis of unknown etiology. The most common causes in developed countries are ulcerative colitis (UC) and Crohn's disease. The diagnosis is made on the basis of clinical, radiologic, colonoscopic, and pathologic findings.
2. Ulcerative colitis involves only the mucosa of the colon. It most commonly presents as bloody diarrhea. The two most important complications of UC are toxic megacolon and carcinoma. Extraintestinal involvement includes arthritis, uveitis, nephrolithiasis, growth retardation, and liver dysfunction.
3. Crohn's disease differs from UC in that there is transmural involvement of the bowel wall and involvement of the entire intestine. Common intestinal complications include the development of fistulas and bowel obstruction from fibrous adhesions. Extraintestinal complications include arthritis, skin lesions, uveitis, renal calculi, liver dysfunction, and cholelithiasis.
4. Patients with IBD are prone to develop the following problems: anemia, leukocytosis, hypoalbuminemia, hypokalemia, and hypomagnesemia.
5. Preoperative laboratory tests that will help to assess the severity of either disease include: leukocyte count and determination of hematocrit, albumin, and electrolyte levels.
6. Steroids and antibiotics commonly are used to treat IBD. Stress dose coverage may be required in the perioperative period. Hydrocortisone 4 to 8 mg/kg/day in three divided doses will cover surgical stress in a child. Similarly, any antibiotics should be continued through the operative period.
7. Patients with IBD frequently present to the operating room on an emergent basis for bowel obstruction or bleeding. All the same principles concerning airway management in the child with a full stomach apply.
8. It is not uncommon for the patient with IBD to be on total parenteral nutrition (TPN), administered either centrally or peripherally. (See p. 100 in Chapter 6, Fluids and Electrolytes.)

Biliary Atresia

1. Biliary atresia is the obliteration of the extrahepatic ducts by a progressive inflammatory process of unknown etiology. The disease is unique to infancy and is characterized by an inability to excrete bile and eventual biliary cirrhosis. Management and prognosis is determined by the type of atresia:
   a. Type I—atresia limited to common bile duct
   b. Type II—atresia limited to the hepatic duct
   c. Type III—atresia extends to the portahepatus

   In Types I and II, bile duct to bowel anastomosis may be possible. Type III is corrected by the Kasai procedure (see Table 10-5), which creates a conduit from a segment of jejunum to residual bile duct tissue at the portahepatus.
2. These infants are quite ill and generally debilitated. Associated problems include hyperbilirubinemia (conjugated type), increased liver enzymes (SGOT, SGPT, alkaline phosphatase), abnormal coagulation studies (prothrombin time, partial thromboplastin time, dysfunctional platelets, prolonged bleeding time), severe malnutrition (hypoalbuminemia), and anemia.
3. Preoperative management of the infant with biliary atresia includes paying careful attention to these associated problems and corrective therapy before starting surgical repair. The infant must be treated for any serious infections, be given transfusions until an acceptable level of hemoglobin/hematocrit is reached, and have had coagulopathies treated either with vitamin K or platelet/FFP transfusions. Often it is advisable to treat severe malnutrition with TPN.
4. Besides standard monitoring, placement of arterial and central venous catheters in the child undergoing the Kasai procedure is useful for close hemodynamic monitoring, frequent blood sampling, and infusion of inotropic or resuscitative drugs.
5. Postoperative complications include ascending cholangitis, portal hypertension, esophageal varices, and malabsorption.

BIBLIOGRAPHY

Kliegma RM and Fanaroff AA: Necrotizing enterocolitis, N Engl J Med 310:1093-1103, 1984.

Levy J: A practical approach to pediatric gastroenterology, Chicago, 1988, Year Book Medical Publishers, Inc.

Milla PJ and Muller DPR, editors: Harries' Paediatric Gastroenterology, ed 2, New York, 1988, Churchill Livingstone, Inc.

Rajn TNK and others: Intracranial pressure during intubation and anesthesia in infants, J Pediatr 96:860, 1980.

Steward DG: Diseases of the gastrointestinal system. In Katz J and Steward DG, editors: Anesthesia and uncommon pediatric diseases, Philadelphia, 1987, WB Saunders Co.

Welch KJ and others: Pediatric surgery, ed 4, Chicago, 1986, Year Book Medical Publishers, Inc.

Ziai M and Grand RJ: The abdomen & gastrointestinal tract. In Ziai M, editor: Pediatrics, Boston, 1984, Little Brown & Co.

11

ANESTHESIA FOR CHILDREN WITH CONGENITAL HEART DISEASE

Frederick C. Jacobson

Flesh will heal and pain will fade
As nature and time repair,
But when the heart is bruised and torn,
The scar—still lingers there
CLAIRE RICHCREEK THOMAS
POEMS THAT TOUCH THE HEART

The following is a list of abbreviations that are used in this chapter:

AS	Aortic stenosis
ASD	Atrial septal defect
AV	Aortic valve
CHD	Congenital heart disease
CHF	Congestive heart failure
CPB	Cardiopulmonary bypass
CVP	Central venous pressure
CXR	Chest x-ray
DPA	Dorsalis pedis artery
ECG	Electrocardiograph
EJ	External jugular vein
FTT	Failure to thrive
HR	Heart rate
HTN	Hypertension
ICS	Intercostal space
IJ	Internal jugular vein
IV	Intravenous
IVC	Inferior vena cava
LA	Left atrium

LLSB	Lower left sternal border
LV	Left ventricle
LVH	Left ventricular hypertrophy
MVO_2	Myocardial oxygen consumption
NG	Nasogastric
PA	Pulmonary atresia
PaO_2	Arterial oxygen tension
PAPVR	Partial anomalous pulmonary venous return
PCWP	Pulmonary capillary wedge pressure
PDA	Patent ductus arteriosus
PFO	Patent foramen ovale
PS	Pulmonic stenosis
PTA	Posterior tibial artery
PVO_2	Mixed venous oxygen tension
PVR	Pulmonary vascular resistance
RA	Right atrium
RBBB	Right bundle branch block
RV	Right ventricle
RVH	Right ventricular hypertrophy
RVOT	Right ventricular outflow tract
SaO_2	Oxygen saturation (%)
SCM	Sternocleidomastoid muscle
SEM	Systolic ejection murmur
SVC	Superior vena cava
SVR	Systemic vascular resistance
SVT	Supraventricular tachycardia
TA	Tricuspid atresia
TAPVR	Total anomalous pulmonary venous return
TOF	Tetralogy of Fallot
TOGA	Transposition of great arteries
TR	Tricuspid regurgitation
$\dot{V}O_2$	Oxygen consumption
VSD	Ventricular septal defect
WPW	Wolff-Parkinson-White syndrome

INCIDENCE AND ASSOCIATIONS

1. Congenital heart disease (CHD) occurs in approximately 6 to 8 births per 1,000.
2. The incidence is two to three times higher in premature births (excluding PDAs).
3. Of patients with CHD, 4% to 15% have genitourinary tract anomalies.
4. Siblings of an affected child are at higher risk for congenital heart disease.

DIAGNOSIS

A diagnosis of CHD can be confirmed by the following techniques:

- Physical examination for presence of murmur, rales (CHF), cyanosis, respiratory distress or tachypnea, failure to thrive, hypertension, or discrepancies in blood pressure in different extremities

- ECG for presence of chamber enlargement, conduction defects, or axis deviation
- Chest radiograph for size and shape of heart and for pulmonary vascularity
- Echocardiography to document presence of defect
- Cardiac catheterization to anatomically define size and location of defect and degree of stenosis or shunt

INTERPRETATION OF CARDIAC CATHETERIZATION DATA

The objective of cardiac catheterization is to obtain hemodynamic data about suspected cardiac anomalies by measuring pressures and oxygen saturations in each chamber and great vessel. Specific anatomic defects are ascertained by angiographic imaging using an organic iodide preparation for radiopaque contrast. The following types of data are obtained from cardiac catheterization. (See Table 11-2 for data commonly obtained at cardiac catheterization.)

Oxygen Saturations

- The mixed venous saturation obtained in the superior vena cava (SVC) gives the most reliable value in the presence of intracardiac shunts.
- Normally, a slight step-down in saturation occurs from the right atrium (RA) to the right ventricle (RV) because of the addition of coronary sinus blood.
- Low left atrium (LA), left ventricle (LV), or systemic arterial saturations are usually a result of right-to-left shunts.

Oxygen Content

The oxygen content is the amount of oxygen bound to hemoglobin plus the amount dissolved in blood. Oxygen content (CaO_2) is calculated by the following formula:

$$CaO_2 \text{ (ml } O_2/100 \text{ ml blood)} = (1.34 \times \text{hemoglobin} \times \text{saturation}) + (.0031 \times PaO_2)$$

Normal oxygen content is 15 to 20 ml O_2/100 ml blood.

Ratio of Pulmonary to Systemic Blood Flow (Q_p/Q_s)

The ratio of pulmonary to systemic blood flow (Q_p/Q_s) is used to quantitate intracardiac shunt in children. The magnitude of the shunt is usually calculated using the Fick equation (see box on next page). The oxygen saturation of blood in each vessel and chamber is measured during cardiac catheterization.

Pressures and Gradients

Pressures and gradients are obtained by percutaneous placement of catheters and transduction of pressure in chambers or central vessels or across valves. With very large shunts, pressure gradients can be measured in chambers or vessels in the absence of any actual valvular or obstructive lesions.

DETERMINATION OF Q_p/Q_s*

Equation

$$Q_p\ (L/min) = \frac{\dot{V}O_2}{SpvO_2 - SpaO_2}$$

$$Q_s\ (L/min) = \frac{VO_2}{SaO_2 - SmvO_2}$$

$$Q_p/Q_s = \frac{SaO_2 - SmvO_2}{SpvO_2 - SpaO_2}$$

Variables

$\dot{V}O_2$ = Oxygen consumption
$SpvO_2$ = Pulmonary venous oxygen saturation
$SpaO_2$ = Pulmonary artery oxygen saturation
SaO_2 = Systemic arterial oxygen saturation
$SmvO_2$ = Mixed venous oxygen saturation (SVC)

Interpretation	Physical findings
1-1.5: Minimal shunt	• Asymptomatic • Loud murmur • Normal ECG
1.5-3: Moderate shunt	• +/− symptomatic; CXR shows signs of CHF
3-5: Large shunt	• Very symptomatic: FTT, CHF, repeated respiratory infections, cyanosis • ECG shows biventricular enlargement • CXR reveals CHF and pulmonary congestion

*O_2 content may replace O_2 saturation: CaO_2, $CmvO_2$, $CpvO_2$, $CpaO_2$.

Vascular resistance can be calculated if pressure and flow (Q) are known (Table 11-1).

Valvular Area

The severity of stenotic valvular lesions can be determined by calculating the valvular area in conjunction with the pressure gradients across the affected valve. The equation for this is as follows:

$$A = \frac{Q}{K\sqrt{\Delta P}}$$

where

A = Valvular area (cm^2)
Q = Cardiac flow through the valve (ml/sec)
ΔP = Mean pressure gradient (mm Hg)
K = Constant specific for each valve (aorta, pulmonary: 44.5, mitral: 31.5)

TABLE 11-1. Calculation of resistance to cardiac flow

Equation	Variables	Normal values
$PVR = \frac{PAP - LAP}{Q_p}$	PVR = Pulmonary vascular resistance PAP = Mean pulmonary artery pressure LAP = Mean left atrial pressure (may use mean pulmonary capillary wedge pressure) Q_p = Pulmonary blood flow	• 1-3 Woods units (mm Hg/L/min/M^2) in older children and adults • 150-250 $\frac{\text{dynes} \times \text{sec}}{\text{cm}^5}$ (equation multiplied by 80) • Higher in the neonate until 2 months of age
$SVR = \frac{MAP - CVP}{Q_s}$	SVR = Systemic vascular resistance MAP = Mean arterial pressure CVP = Mean central venous pressure (RA) Q_s = Systemic blood flow	• Neonate: 10-15 units • Infancy to adulthood: 20 units • 800-1500 $\frac{\text{dynes} \times \text{sec}}{\text{cm}^5}$ (equation multiplied by 80)

TABLE 11-2. Cardiac catheterization data

Abbreviation	Stands for (units)	How derived	Normal values	Comments
Q_s	Systemic blood flow (L/min)	$\frac{\dot{V}O_2}{SaO_2 - MVO_2}$	2.5-4.5 $L/min/m^2$	• Cardiac output decreases with age and decreases 10% from the supine to the sitting position.
Q_p	Pulmonary blood flow (ml/kg/min)	$\frac{\dot{V}O_2}{PVO_2 - PaO_2}$	2.5-4.5 $L/min/m^2$	• $Q_p = Q_s$ if no shunting is present. • $Q_p > Q_s$ if left-to-right shunts are present. • $Q_p < Q_s$ if right-to-left shunts are present.
$\dot{V}O_2$	Oxygen consumption (L/min)	Calculated by using a Douglas bag to collect and measure O_2 and CO_2 in expired gas and comparing these values to those of ambient air	5-8 ml/kg/min	• $\dot{V}O_2$ is heart rate and age dependent. • For calculations, F_EO_2 and F_IO_2 must be room air or 100% O_2 and be carried to four decimal places.
CaO_2	Systemic arterial oxygen content (ml/L)	Calculated from PaO_2, SaO_2, Hgb	15-20 ml/L	• This value may be 1%-2% less than $CpvO_2$ secondary to drainage of the coronary venous blood through the Thebesian veins.
$CmvO_2$	Mixed venous oxygen content (ml/L)	Calculated from $PmvO_2$, $SmvO_2$, Hgb	14-15 ml/L	• In the absence of intracardiac shunts, this equals PaO_2. In the presence of intracardiac shunt, it can be measured from the right atrium or SVC.
$CpvO_2$	Pulmonary venous oxygen content (ml/L)	Calculated from $PpvO_2$, $SpvO_2$, and Hgb	20-21 ml/L	• High pulmonary blood flows, as with ASD, VSD, will decrease the value. • Since it depends on $\dot{V}/\dot{Q}$, lung disease can affect the value depending on where sampling occurs.
$CpaO_2$	Pulmonary artery oxygen content (ml/L)	Calculated from $PpaO_2$, $SpaO_2$, and Hgb	14-15 ml/L	• The value should be the same as that taken in the RV. A 3% step up or more between the PA and RV is significant. In DORV or VSD, a step up is seen in the PA secondary to their subpulmonic nature.

Continued.

TABLE 11-2. Cardiac catheterization data—cont'd

Abbreviation	Stands for (units)	How derived	Normal values	Comments
PAP	Pulmonary artery pressure (mm Hg)	Measured	Newborn: $\frac{65\text{-}80}{35\text{-}50}$ Child: $\frac{15\text{-}25}{10\text{-}16}$	• Increases with left-to-right shunting.
LAP	Mean left atrial pressure (mm Hg)	Measured	Newborn: 3-6 Child: 5-10	• A dominant V wave is related to increased pulmonary blood flow.
PCWP	Pulmonary capillary wedge pressure (mm Hg)	Measured	Newborn: 6-9 Child: 8-11	• PCWP shows damping of the a and v waves and has a mean level of 2-3 mm Hg higher than the pulmonary venous pressure.
SVR	Systemic vascular resistance $\left(\frac{\text{dynes} \times \text{sec}}{\text{cm}^5}\right)$	$\frac{MAP - CVP}{Q_s} \times 80$	800-1500	• SVR is lower in the newborn because arterial pressure is lower • At 12-18 months, SVR gradually rises to adult levels.
PVR	Pulmonary vascular resistance $\left(\frac{\text{dynes} \times \text{sec}}{\text{cm}^5}\right)$	$\frac{PAP\text{-}LAP(PCWP) \times 80}{Q_p}$	150-250	• The value is considerably higher in the neonate up to 2 months of age.
Q_p/Q_s	Ratio of pulmonic to systemic blood flow	$\frac{SaO_2 - SmvO_2}{SpvO_2 - SpaO_2}$ *or* $\frac{CaO_2 - CmvO_2}{CpvO_2 - CpaO_2}$	1/1	• A ratio of 2:1 implies a left-to-right shunt equal to systemic blood flow. A ratio of 4:1 implies a left-to-right shunt three times greater than systemic blood flow. • A ratio of 0.8:1 indicates a pulmonary blood flow 20% less than systemic blood flow (i.e., a right-to-left shunt).

AVA	Aortic valve area (cm^2)	$\frac{Q(ml/sec)}{44.5 \times \sqrt{\Delta P}}$	2.6-3.5 cm^2 in adults	• Neonatal AS is determined by the presence of a critical gradient across the valve, rather than determination of valve area. • Treatment is seldom required before the fourth decade (adult values). • <0.7 cm^2 can account for symptoms of heart failure, angina, and syncope. • <0.4 cm^2, or a gradient of 50 mm Hg with a normal cardiac output, is considered critical. • 44.5 is also used for calculations of the pulmonic valve.
MVA	Mitral valve area (cm^2)	$\frac{Q}{31.5 \times \sqrt{\Delta P}}$	4-6 cm^2 in adults	• ≤1 cm^2 usually leads to symptoms. • 1.5-2.5 cm^2 will precipitate symptoms with moderate to severe exercise.
F	Flow (ml/sec)	$\frac{\text{CO (ml/min)}}{\text{Diastolic filling pressure (sec/min)}}$ *or* Systolic ejection period (sec/min)	Variable, depending upon preload, afterload, and contractility	• For the mitral valve, flow is calculated during diastole. • For the aortic valve, flow is calculated during systole.
ΔP	Mean pressure gradient across the valvular orifice (mm Hg)	Difference between simultaneously measured pressures in two chambers	Minimal gradients should be present across normal valves	• Critical stenosis is implied by the following gradients: • Aortic: >40 mm; justifies operative intervention • Pulmonic: 10-15 mm.

CLASSIFICATION OF CONGENITAL HEART DISEASE

1. Lesions with increased pulmonary blood flow
   - Atrial septal defect
   - Ventricular septal defect
   - Patent ductus arteriosus
   - Endocardial cushion defect
   - Aortopulmonary window
2. Lesions with decreased pulmonary blood flow (cyanotic)
   - Tetralogy of Fallot
   - Pulmonary atresia
   - Tricuspid atresia
   - Ebstein's anomaly
3. Complex shunts (mixing of pulmonary and systemic circulation)
   - Truncus arteriosus
   - Transposition of the great arteries
   - Total anomalous pulmonary venous drainage
   - Hypoplastic left heart syndrome
   - Double outlet right ventricle
4. Obstructive lesions
   - Aortic stenosis
   - Mitral stenosis
   - Pulmonic stenosis
   - Coarctation of the aorta
   - Cortriatriatum
   - Interrupted aortic arch
5. Lesions causing airway obstruction
   - Double aortic arch
   - Anomalous pulmonary artery

CLASSIFICATION OF CONGENITAL HEART DISEASE

See box above.

Simple Shunts

To understand the pathophysiology of shunt lesions, it is important to know how flow, pressure, and resistance equate in the cardiovascular system. The relationship is shown by the following equation:

$$Q = \frac{P}{R}$$

where

Q = Blood flow (cardiac output)
P = Pressure within a given chamber or vessel
R = Vascular resistance of the pulmonary or systemic bed

That is, the cardiac output of the right ventricle is dependent on the pressure generated in the ventricle and the resistance to flow provided by the pulmonary outflow tract and vasculature. An analogous situation can be applied to the left ventricle and outflow to the aorta. If these two systems are linked by a shunt, flow across the shunt will be determined by the pressure generated across the shunt and the resistance to flow. A left-to-right shunt exists because higher left-side pressures increase flow across the shunt in the face of relatively lower pulmonary vasular resistance (e.g., VSD). A shunt can be right to left if pulmonary resistance becomes higher than systemic (e.g., pulmonic stenosis). To some degree, the bidirectionality of a shunt can be manipulated by raising or lowering pulmonary or systemic vascular resistance.

Simple shunts occur between the pulmonary and systemic circulation when a disruption takes place between the two systems (e.g., ASD, VSD, PDA). The magnitude of shunt flow across an ASD or VSD is determined by the size of the orifice and the resistance to flow. Small ASDs and VSDs are known as restrictive shunts because the amount of flow is limited by the small size of the defect. Large ASDs, VSDs, and PDAs are known as nonrestrictive shunts because the large size of the defect and relatively lower PVR increase the magnitude of the shunt.

Obstructive Lesions

Obstructive lesions (AS, PS, coarctation of the aorta) result in pressure overloading of the corresponding ventricles and provide resistance to flow.

Complex Shunts

Complex shunts occur with an obstructive lesion on one side of the heart and subsequent shunting to the opposite side through an associated defect (ASD, VSD, or PDA). The magnitude and direction of shunt flow are determined by the degree of obstruction to flow and the relative resistances of the pulmonary and systemic circuits. Mixing of the pulmonary and systemic circulation occurs at either the atrial or ventricular level.

LEFT-TO-RIGHT SHUNTS

The following defects increase pulmonary blood flow:

- ASD
- VSD
- PDA
- AV canal
- Aortopulmonic window

For descriptions of these defects, as well as intraoperative techniques and anesthetic management for them, see Management of Specific Left-To-Right Shunts.

Pathophysiology

Increased pulmonary blood flow results from higher left-sided pressures on the one hand and, on the other, decreased resistance by the right ventricular outflow tract and pulmonary vasculature. CHF or pulmonary edema result from increased pulmonary blood flow and can inhibit oxygen diffusion causing hypoxemia and cyanosis.

Eisenmenger's Syndrome

Left-to-right shunts can reverse as a result of elevated pulmonary vascular resistance (PVR). In approximately 50% of patients with untreated VSD and 10% of patients with untreated ASD, PVR increases in response to long-standing increased pressure and volume in the pulmonary vasculature. Eventually the shunt reverses and becomes right to left when PVR exceeds left-sided pressure. Eisenmenger's syndrome is a right-to-left shunt with cyanosis in a patient who has pulmonary hypertension and a history of septal defect or PDA.

Therapeutic Maneuvers

The following therapies can be used to decrease pulmonary blood flow or minimize CHF in patients with left-to-right shunts:

1. *Indomethacin*. The patent ductus arteriosus (PDA) will usually close within 24 hours after initiation of indomethacin therapy (0.1-0.3 mg/kg IV or NG). Complications include platelet and renal dysfunction, which reverses after cessation of the drug. The use of indomethacin is contraindicated in necrotizing enterocolitis, hyperbilirubinemia (>10 mg/100 ml), renal dysfunction (BUN >29 mg/100 ml, creatinine > 1.6 mg/100 ml), and clotting abnormalities.
2. *Digoxin/diuretic*. This regimen is employed for CHF and atrial dysrhythmias. It can be ineffective in premature infants and cause digitoxicity and electrolyte abnormalities.
3. *PA Banding*.
   a. Restriction of pulmonary circulation is achieved by placing a surgical band around the main pulmonary artery, which increases resistance to blood flow and reduces the magnitude of the left-to-right shunt. The goal is to decrease the pulmonary pressure distal to the band to 33% to 50% of aortic pressures.
   b. Improved systemic blood flow after successful banding will be indicated by a slight decrease in CVP and a rise in aortic pressure. A rise in CVP, along with cyanosis, bradycardia, and desaturation are suggestive of too tight a band (too little pulmonary blood flow).
   c. Since the band is placed while the patient is under general anesthesia with positive pressure ventilation (which increases pulmonary resistance and decreases flow) and increased F_IO_2 (which decreases pulmonary resistance and increases flow), the pulmonary artery pressures obtained in the operating room may change postoperatively when spontaneous ventilation is resumed.
   d. Placement of a pulmonary artery band in small children is a temporizing measure to avoid definitive repair (usually a VSD or AV canal).
   e. Resistance to flow may increase significantly with time because the band does not grow with the child. Initiation of positive pressure ventilation in a child with an unrepaired shunt and long-standing PA band may increase resistance sufficiently to reverse the shunt (right to left), creating an Eisenmenger's syndrome with rapid desaturation and cyanosis.

Anesthetic Management

Premedication

The goal is to sedate the patient without hemodynamic or respiratory compromise. In children less than 1 year of age premedication usually is unnecessary. If a low cardiac output or CHF is present, dosages should be reduced or premedication withheld (see also Chapter 4). Otherwise, the following dosages are usually given.

Good cardiac function and no cyanosis

- Pentobarbital 2-5 mg/kg PO, PR, IM
- Morphine 0.1 mg/kg + scopolamine 0.01-0.02 mg/kg IM
- Morphine 0.1 mg/kg + pentobarbital 2-4 mg/kg IM
- Meperidine 3 mg/kg + pentobarbital 3-5 mg/kg PO
- Diazepam 0.1-0.5 mg/kg PO
- Midazolam 0.08 mg/kg IM

Poor cardiac function, CHF, or cyanosis

- No premedication is given if the patient is severely compromised.
- Giving one half the doses recommended above may be considered if the child is in mild CHF.

Induction Techniques

1. The goal of induction is to decrease the amount of left-to-right shunting and maintain systemic blood flow.
   Methods for reducing blood flow include the following:
   - *Inhalation agents*. These reduce SVR and improve systemic flow.
   - *Narcotics*. With deeper planes of anesthesia, SVR will decrease.
   - *Inspired F_IO_2*. Since oxygen is a direct pulmonary vasodilator, decreasing F_IO_2 helps to limit pulmonary blood flow.
   - *Positive pressure ventilation*.The heightened resistance to cardiac flow caused by increasing intrapulmonary pressure assists in decreasing pulmonary blood flow.
   - *Nitrous oxide*. Nitrous oxide probably increases PVR and should help in limiting the amount of shunt. It is wise to avoid N_2O in situations with a long-standing left-to-right shunt, large Q_p/Q_s, or documented pulmonary hypertension because shunt reversal could occur.
2. The choice of induction technique (IV versus inhalation) is not critical if myocardial function is preserved. In the failing heart, narcotic techniques may cause less myocardial depression and hemodynamic changes. Ketamine is contraindicated because it raises SVR and PVR and may increase the left-to-right shunt.
3. Some pharmacokinetics are affected by left-to-right shunts.
   - A left-to-right shunt can speed anesthetic induction by inhalation agents if systemic blood flow (i.e., cardiac output) is reduced, causing a decrease in the rate of transfer of the anesthetic to the brain.
   - IV agents may have slower onset times because of continuous dilution in the pulmonary circulation. If more drug is given to hasten onset, side effects of overdose may appear when distribution finally occurs.

4. All patients should receive endocarditis prophylaxis (see Appendix D for standard treatment protocols).
5. Meticulous removal of all air bubbles from intravenous lines is mandatory to prevent air emboli crossing the shunt and entering the systemic circulation.

Postoperative Problems

After surgical closure, the following problems may be encountered in the postoperative period:

- SVT and AV conduction disturbances are common in the early postoperative period. Conduction delays may persist indefinitely.
- If PVR was elevated before surgery, the increase in RV afterload after closure may not be tolerated and maneuvers to decrease PVR may be necessary (100% O_2, vasodilators, isoproterenol).
- Postoperative valvular incompetence is possible in canal defects.
- Prolonged postoperative ventilation is usually not necessary for simple, asymptomatic ASD secundum closures. Patients with failure to thrive, CHF, or malnourishment usually require mechanical ventilation postoperatively.

Management of Specific Left-to-Right Shunts

Atrial Septal Lesions

Patent foramen orale (PFO)

DESCRIPTION

- Functional closure occurs at birth with anatomic closure at 2 to 3 months.
- It is incidentally found during 40% of VSD closures.
- An isolated PFO is asymptomatic; patency may allow for paradoxic emboli.

ANESTHETIC CONSIDERATIONS

- These generally do not require repair.
- If the patient has recurrent paradoxic emboli, the PFO can be closed during cardiac catheterization with percutaneous placement of an umbrella occluder.

ASD (secundum defect)

DESCRIPTION

- 80% of all ASDs are the secundum type defect; they occur predominantly in females at a ratio of 2:1.
- A fixed split S_2 and systolic murmur is heard at the LLSB.
- Secundum defects are asymptomatic until early adulthood, when pulmonary hypertension and Eisenmenger's syndrome develop (rare). If large, they can cause symptoms of dyspnea, fatigue, and atrial arrhythmias.
- ASD closure is recommended at 4-5 years of age to prevent development of pulmonary hypertension.

ANESTHETIC CONSIDERATIONS

- Anesthetic considerations are those for a left-to-right shunt (see p. 221).
- Early extubation in the operating room is possible for uncomplicated ASD closures.
- Many of these simple ostium secundum defects can be repaired with percutaneous umbrella occluders during catheterization.

Sinus venosus defect

DESCRIPTION

- This is a rare defect near the RA-SVC junction frequently associated with partial anomalous pulmonary venous return (PAPVR).
- An atrial defect (ASD) actually allows for mixing and helps to maintain oxygenation.
- ECG: RBBB and first-degree AV block.
- Catheterization: increased venous saturation in the RA.

ANESTHETIC CONSIDERATIONS

- Anesthetic considerations are those for a left-to-right shunt (see p. 221).

Endocardial Cushion Defects

DESCRIPTION

- These result from the failure of the endocardial cushions and septum primum to fuse.
- They are frequently associated with clefts in the anterior leaflet of the mitral valve causing mitral regurgitation and early cardiac failure.
- They are a common lesion in children with Down's syndrome.

ANESTHETIC CONSIDERATIONS

- Most patients have large left-to-right shunts and are symptomatic in infancy.
- Premedication should be avoided if significant CHF exists.
- A PA band is frequently placed in infancy.

Complete AV canal

DESCRIPTION

- Failure of both cushion fusion and septal-cushion fusion results in a single A-V valve with 5 to 6 leaflets.
- CHF, pulmonary hypertension, pneumonia, and failure to thrive are common.
- Mitral regurgitation is present in 50% of patients.
- Catheterization: increased venous saturation at atrial and ventricular levels.

ANESTHETIC CONSIDERATIONS

- SVT and AV conduction disturbances are common. Postoperative valvular incompetence can occur.
- If preexisting pulmonary HTN exists, then the increase in RV afterload postclosure may not be well tolerated and maneuvers to decrease PVR are necessary (100% O_2, pulmonary vasodilators, spontaneous ventilation).
- PA banding in early infancy is common.

Ventricular Septal Lesions (VSD)

See box on the next page for catheterization data.

Supracristal defects

- The defect lies just below the aortic annulus and above the crista supraventricularis.
- The right coronary cusp of the aortic valve may lack support.

Infracristal defects

- Commonly referred to as a membranous defect.
- This is the most common form of VSD (80%).
- It is found beneath the crista supraventricularis in the membranous septum.

Canal type
- The VSD that is associated with an AV canal.
- It lies very high in the septum.

Muscular defects
- Lying lower in the muscular septum, it is believed to be caused by excessive absorption of septal tissue during septal formation.
- The defect may contain multiple small holes ("Swiss cheese").

Anesthetic considerations
- The anesthetic considerations are as for left-to-right shunts.
- The surgical incision site plays a large role in postpump considerations. The RA is incised with membranous types, the RV with supracristal types, and the LV with muscular defects. If a ventriculostomy is necessary, then ischemia is not uncommon and inotropes may be required to support cardiac function.
- Heart block, from AV node or His bundle dysfunction, can result from direct injury to the conduction tissue or transiently from edema. Therefore, placement of epicardial pacing wires is essential.
- Hemodynamically significant shunts may remain in up to 6% to 10% of patients. Residual shunt can be identified by transesophageal echocardiography postbypass, or transthoracic echocardiography in the postoperative period.
- Aortic insufficieny can result from a suture catching a valve leaflet during the repair.

CATHETERIZATION DATA FOR VENTRICULAR SEPTAL LESIONS

- $Q_p/Q_s < 1.5$ In 20% to 50% of cases, these small defects close spontaneously before age 5. Since flow is limited, life expectancy is normal.
- $Q_p/Q_s = 1.5\text{-}3$ In moderate defects, PVR may be elevated and RVH develop.
- $Q_p/Q_s = 3.5\text{-}5$ If large unrestricted defects can be treated medically, their size will decrease proportionately with heart growth.

Arterial Lesions

Patent ductus arteriosus

DESCRIPTION
- A persistent fetal communication from the main pulmonary artery to the descending aorta.
- Incidence is 1 in 2,000 live births with a female-to-male predominance of 2:1. Common in premature infants.
- Symptoms include tachypnea, FTT, and CHF.
- Runoffs in the pulmonary circulation with a large PDA lowers aortic diastolic pressure leading to end organ ischemia.

ANESTHETIC CONSIDERATIONS
- Invasive pressure monitoring is not essential. A blood pressure cuff and pulse oximeter may be sufficient to monitor systemic pressure.

- Adequate vascular access is essential. Hemorrhage due to the loss of vascular control is possible.
- Although either IV or inhalation agents are usually well tolerated, decreasing SVR with isoflurane may help decrease left-to-right shunting.
- A rise in afterload postclosure can require vasodilator therapy.
- Postoperative respiratory support (mechanical ventilation) is generally required in neonates and small infants.
- Endocarditis prophylaxis is required (see Appendix D).

Aortopulmonary windows

DESCRIPTION

- This lesion is rare and results in communication between the great arteries above their origin.
- Rapid equilibration between pulmonary and systemic pressures occurs.
- LVH, RVH, and left atrial enlargement may be present on ECG.

ANESTHETIC CONSIDERATIONS

- Deep hypothermia and total circulatory arrest are usually required for repair.

RIGHT-TO-LEFT SHUNTS

Defects that decrease pulmonary blood flow include the following:

Tetralogy of Fallot
Tricuspid atresia
Tricuspid stenosis
Pulmonary stenosis
Ebstein's anomaly

For descriptions of these defects, as well as intraoperative techniques and anesthetic management for them, see Management of Specific Right-to-Left Shunts.

Pathophysiology

All lesions that produce a right-to-left shunt contain not only a connection between the right and left heart, but also must offer increased resistance to blood flow through the pulmonary vasculature. Children with these lesions have marked hypoxemia and cyanosis.

Therapeutic Maneuvers

Goals of Therapy

The goals of therapy are to decrease pulmonary resistance to promote pulmonary blood flow, or increase systemic vascular resistance to increase pressure into the pulmonary vasculature. If Flow equals Pressure/Resistance ($Q=P/R$), then flow into the pulmonary artery is increased by decreasing resistance or increasing pressure.

Prostaglandin E_1 (PGE_1)

Infusion rates of 0.03-0.10 μg/kg/min will maintain patency of the PDA, thereby increasing pulmonary blood flow. PGE_1 is shown to be most effective in neonates less than 96 hours old and weighing less than 4 kg. Maximum effect is obtained in 30 minutes. Complications of use include vasodilation, hypotension, bradycardia, arrhythmias, apnea or hypoventilation, seizure-like activity, and hyperthermia.

Palliative Shunts

See Table 11-3 for types of palliative shunts.

1. If flow to the pulmonary artery is anatomically obstructed, it may be impossible to therapeutically alter pulmonary or systemic vascular resistance sufficiently to overcome hypoxia. In this situation, the placement of a surgical shunt is indicated to increase pulmonary blood flow distal to the obstructing lesion. Shunt placement decreases hypoxemia and prepares the pulmonary artery for future anatomic repair by stimulating its growth.
2. Complications of shunts include kinking or thrombosis; unilateral shunting to one lung resulting in pulmonary edema; arm ischemia; Horner's syndrome; SVC syndrome; and chylothorax.
3. Shunts placed under positive pressure ventilation offer less resistance to flow when spontaneous ventilation is resumed postoperatively. Although it is desirable to maximize shunt size to increase pulmonary blood flow, postoperative pulmonary edema may result when positive pressure ventilation is discontinued if the shunt placed is too large.

Premedication

1. The goal of premedication for a child with right-to-left shunting is to prevent crying and agitation that will aggravate shunting, hypoxemia, and cyanosis. Recommendations for premedication follow.

- Morphine (0.1-0.2 mg/kg) + pentobarbital (2-4 mg/kg) IM *or*
- Meperidine (3 mg) + pentobarbital (2-4 mg) PO

2. Morphine helps to decrease PVR and relax the infundibular outflow tract (as in tetralogy of Fallot).
3. The child is transported with oxygen to increase pulmonary vasodilation.
4. A nurse or physician should accompany the child to the operating room.

Induction Techniques

1. The goal of induction is to improve pulmonary blood flow to reduce hypoxemia and cyanosis.
2. Pharmacokinetics are altered in right-to-left shunts. Limited pulmonary blood flow can prolong an inhalation induction. Because less anesthetic is absorbed from the lung, less is available to the brain. IV drug doses should be reduced during induction because dilution in the pulmonary circulation is bypassed and distribution into the systemic and cerebral circulation occurs much sooner.
3. Prophylaxis for endocarditis is recommended (Appendix D).
4. Meticulous removal of air bubbles from all intravenous lines is essential with right-to-left shunts. An air bubble can easily pass from the right side of the heart into the systemic or cerebral circulation.

TABLE 11-3. Surgical shunts for cyanotic lesions

Procedure	Indication	Description	Complications
Rashkind-Miller	TOGA	• Balloon atrial septostomy	• Hemorrhage
Blalock-Hanlon	TOGA	• Open atrial septostomy	• Right pulmonary veins are clamped during excision of atrial septum, which can cause hemorrhage into right lung
Blalock-Taussig	Cyanotic Lesions TOF PA TA	• Subclavian artery is transected and anastomosed to a branch of the pulmonary artery	• Ischemia to extremity on side of shunt • Stenosis of the shunt • Too much pulmonary blood flow (rare)
Potts	Cyanotic Lesions TOF PA TA	• Anastomosis between descending aorta and left pulmonary artery	• Difficult to predict flow through shunt; too much pulmonary flow can result
Waterston	Cyanotic Lesions TOF PA TA	• Anastomosis between ascending aorta and right pulmonary artery	• Difficult to predict flow through shunt; too much pulmonary flow can result
Central	Cyanotic Lesions	• A gortex graft is placed between the ascending aorta and main pulmonary artery	• Difficult to predict flow through shunt; too much pulmonary flow can result
Glenn	Cyanotic Lesions TOF Ebstein's anomaly PA TA	• Side to side anastomosis between SVC and distal end of transected right pulmonary artery	• Creates a low-pressure conduit; high intrathoracic pressures (i.e., positive pressure ventilation) can reverse the shunt • Pulmonary hematoma and hemorrhage

5. Techniques for induction include the following:
   - *Continuation of PGE_1 infusion*. Any infant who is dependent on the patency of the ductus for oxygenation should be maintained on the infusion up to cardiopulmonary bypass.
   - *Oxygen*. High levels of inspired oxygen will dilate the pulmonary vasculature, decrease resistance, and improve flow through the lungs.
   - *Ketamine*. Ketamine raises both SVR and PVR and is ideal for lesions where pulmonary flow is determined more by fixed obstruction than by dynamic pulmonary vascular resistance. Its analgesic and sedative effects are also useful to calm a crying child while maintaining spontaneous ventilation, which preserves lower intrapulmonary pressures.
   - *Morphine*. Morphine is an ideal agent for lesions with dynamic outflow obstruction, such as infundibular spasm in tetralogy of Fallot. Children who suffer from hypercyanotic spells or who have shown clinical improvement on propranolol are good candidates for morphine.
   - *Beta blockade*. Treatment with propranolol for children over 6 months of age with tetralogy of Fallot keeps the infundibulum relaxed and the heart slow for adequate flow across the stenotic pulmonary valve. In the operating room, esmolol would be a better choice because of its short duration of action.
   - *Inhalation agents*. As with morphine, children with dynamic outflow obstruction are better candidates for inhalation agents. Halothane, which maintains a slow heart rate, depresses the myocardium (relaxing the infundibulum), and has the least drop in SVR, is the agent of choice.
   - *Hydration*. Adequate right-sided filling pressures are needed to overcome obstruction to pulmonary outflow. Adequate hydration is also necessary in the child with polycythemia secondary to long-standing hypoxemia. Dehydration increases the risk of cerebral vascular accidents and other sequelae of thrombotic events. Intravenous fluids should be started if prolonged fasting is anticipated.
   - *Nitrous oxide*. N_2O will constrict the pulmonary vasculature and worsen preexisting cyanosis. Its use is not recommended for cyanotic lesions.
   - *Positive pressure ventilation*. Positive pressure ventilation can further limit pulmonary circulation. Spontaneous ventilation or gentle assisted ventilation during induction is advised. Once hemodynamics are stable and anesthesia has been induced, the effect of positive pressure ventilation at low pressure with no PEEP can be evaluated. Muscle relaxation should not be instituted until the effects of positive pressure ventilation on oxygen saturation are known.
   - *Rapid heart rates*. An increased heart rate will decrease filling time across the obstructed pulmonary artery. Vagolytic agents (e.g., atropine) should be avoided whenever possible.

Management of Specific Right-to-Left Shunts

Tetralogy of Fallot (TOF)

Description

- TOF comprises 10% of all CHD. Four anomalies make up the tetrad.
  1. RV outflow tract obstruction (infundibular stenosis, pulmonic stenosis, or supravalvular stenosis)

2. Subaortic VSD
3. Overriding aorta
4. RVH

- Palliative shunts are used to improve pulmonary blood flow and encourage growth of the pulmonary arteries if they are atretic. Primary pulmonary artery reconstruction is an alternative to shunt placement. Technical advances have made complete repair possible at an earlier age.
- Hypercyanotic spells (Tet spells) occur because of low PaO_2, low pH, and/or infundibular spasm. Episodes manifest as cyanosis and hyperventilation and occur with feeding, crying, defecation, or stress.
- Long-standing hypoxemia results in high hematocrits. Hematocrits below 60% are desirable to reduce the incidence of thrombotic events.
- ECG: RVH, right axis deviation.
- Catheterization: details anatomy, step up in saturation from RA to RV, step down from LA to LV.

Anesthetic considerations

- The induction technique should consider the nature of the RV outflow obstruction, that is, fixed or dynamic (see section on induction techniques).
- Induction should maintain SVR and lower PVR (fentanyl, ketamine, sufentanil). Halothane is useful to relax infundibular obstruction.
- Hypercyanotic spells can occur while under anesthesia (see Table 11-4 below).

TABLE 11-4. Treatment of hypercyanotic spells

Treatment	Effect
100% O_2	• Acts as a specific pulmonary vasodilator, decreasing PVR
Volume: bolus (10 ml/kg)	• Opens the right ventricular outflow tract
Morphine sulfate (0.1 mg/kg)	• Sedation, decreases PVR
Ketamine	• Increases SVR, sedation
Phenylephrine Infusion (2-5 μg/kg/min) Bolus (10 μg/kg)	• Increases SVR
Propranolol	• Decreases HR, improving flow across an obstructed valve • Decreases RV infundibular spasm
Halothane	• Decreased RV outflow obstruction • Decreases HR
Thiopental	• Negative inotropy
Squatting	• Increases SVR
Anesthetic agents contraindicated or not useful	
Atropine	• Increases HR, resulting in decreased blood flow across the pulmonary stenosis
N_2O	• Increases PVR
Isoflurane, enflurane	• Decreases SVR
Epinephrine	• Positive inotropy, chronotropy
Dopamine	• Positive inotropy, chronotropy
Halothane (in patients with extreme RV failure)	• Negative inotropy

- Heart block or conduction abnormalities are common after complete repair (VSD closure).
- RV failure and need for inotropic support should be anticipated after right ventriculotomy.
- Persistent collaterals can produce pulmonary steal syndrome.
- Palliative shunts must be ligated before initiating bypass for complete repair.
- Endocarditis prophylaxis is necessary (see Appendix D).

Pulmonary Stenosis (PS)

Description

- As an isolated defect, PS occurs in 10% of patients with CHD. PS is most commonly associated with Noonan's syndrome.
- If stenosis is severe, RV pressures may exceed LV pressures. Right-to-left shunting will occur across any septal defect.
- Infants with critical PS show symptoms of cyanosis, acidosis, and poor perfusion within 24 to 48 hours.
- Oxygenation in a neonate depends upon the presence of a PDA.
- Symptoms of moderate stenosis appear at 2 to 3 years of age as fatigue and dyspnea.
- SEM is heard at the second left ICS.
- There is a high association of hypoplastic RV with a VSD.
- A significant valvular gradient is one greater than 50 mm Hg.

Anesthetic considerations

- A PGE_1 infusion should be administered to newborns with critical PS to maintain the patency of the PDA for oxygenation.
- Adequate fluid hydration is necessary to keep the RVOT as open as possible.
- Tachycardia should be avoided to minimize myocardial oxygen consumption and increase flow across the stenosis.
- Inotropic support is often necessary after a right ventriculotomy.
- Conduction abnormalities are common in the postbypass period. External pacing wires are essential.

Ebstein's Anomaly

Description

- Redundancy and downward displacement of the tricuspid valve create atrialization of the RV with tricuspid incompetence.
- An ASD is common with right-to-left shunting.
- 5% to 10% of patients will have an accessory bundle of Kent associated with Wolff-Parkinson-White syndrome (WPW).

Anesthetic considerations

- Heavy premedication is indicated. Any large increases in heart rate (HR) will augment the tricuspid insufficiency.
- Inhalation agents are poorly tolerated because of depressed cardiac function.
- Oxygen saturation monitoring with pulse oximetry may be hampered by the absence of a quiet venous bed because of TR.
- IV induction with fentanyl, vecuronium, and benzodiazepines is well tolerated.

- Conduction abnormalities are common in the postbypass period. External pacing wires are essential.

Tricuspid Atresia (TA)

Description

- TA occurs in 1.5% to 3.0% of all CHD cases. TA is always associated with an ASD. The RV is hypoplastic or absent. Some degree of pulmonic stenosis and a VSD are also common features.
- In 90% of children there will be cyanosis with limited pulmonary blood flow.
- The presence of a large VSD may indicate left-to-right shunt and CHF.
- ECG: right atrial enlargement and LV dominance.

Anesthetic considerations

- Patency of the ductus arteriosus is necessary for pulmonary perfusion. Neonates will need a PGE_1 infusion.
- Usually repair is staged with initial placement of a palliative shunt.
- Preoperative hydration is critical to keep the RVOT open and to lower high hematocrits. Hematocrits should not exceed 60%.
- Induction technique depends upon the nature of the shunting. Most will have right-to-left shunting with cyanosis.
- Avoid excessive increases in heart rate and myocardial contractility.

Tricuspid Stenosis

Description

- Isolated tricuspid stenosis is very rare.
- Patients with an ASD will be cyanotic as a result of right-to-left shunting.
- Patients with no associated ASD are cyanotic and show symptoms of RV failure, liver congestion, and ascites.

Anesthetic considerations

- Anesthetic considerations are those for reduced pulmonary perfusion (see tricuspid atresia and pulmonary stenosis).

COMPLEX CONGENITAL HEART DISEASE
Pathophysiology

Complex shunts generally result in the mixing of pulmonary and systemic blood flow at either the atrial or ventricular level (mixing lesions). The children are cyanotic and commonly have CHF. Many of these lesions have simultaneous right-to-left and left-to-right shunting.

Preoperative review of the most recent cardiac catheterization reports is essential. Degree of shunting, chamber pressures, pressure gradients, and function of any palliative shunts will direct the anesthetic management.

Induction Technique

The choice of appropriate technique and agents depends largely upon the nature of the lesion. If right-to-left shunting is predominant, the induction technique should employ those strategies used for right-to-left shunts. The same principle holds for lesions with predominantly left-to-right shunting.

Children with CHF as a result of large mixing lesions are best managed with narcotics, oxygen, and relaxants to minimize myocardial depression and hemodynamic changes.

Types of Complex CHD (Mixing Lesions)

Transposition of the Great Arteries (TOGA)

Description

- A parallel circulation is created by the aorta originating anteriorly from the RV and the pulmonary artery arising from the LV.
- Classification is based on whether the aorta is to the right (type D) or left (type L) of the pulmonary artery.
- Of patients with this condition, 50% have a VSD.
- Mixing of pulmonary and systemic circulation is necessary to sustain life.
- Presence of a PFO or PDA is variable.
- Progression of pulmonary vascular disease is common if unrepaired.

Anesthetic considerations

- Rashkind balloon septostomy of the atrial septum is usually done in the neonatal period if mixing is inadequate. If possible, the patent ductus is maintained with PGE_1.
- Senning and Mustard procedures create an atrial baffle, which diverts pulmonary venous return to the right side of the heart and aorta. Obstruction of the pulmonary veins with intrapulmonary hemorrhage can occur. Inotropic support is indicated because the RV will be functioning as the systemic pump.
- The switch procedure is now done with increased frequency. The coronary arteries are reimplanted; careful monitoring for ischemia is required.
- Acidosis is corrected and hydration maintained preoperatively.
- Fentanyl, sufentanil, and ketamine are well tolerated.
- High inspired F_IO_2 is indicated to preserve left-to-right shunting. N_2O is avoided.
- Atrial dysrhythmias and conduction disturbances are common postoperatively.

Truncus Arteriosus (TA)

Description

- TA is a failure of separation between the systemic and pulmonary circulations. The truncus is one large rudimentary vessel arising from both the RV and LV.
- Three types exist:
  1. The truncus divides into an aorta and main pulmonary artery.
  2. The pulmonary arteries arise posteriorly from the truncus.
  3. The pulmonary arteries arise laterally from the truncus.
- The truncus overrides a large VSD.
- CHF and pulmonary overperfusion are common.

Anesthetic considerations

- Mortality is greater than 80% if surgery is not performed within the first year of life.
- Positive pressure ventilation is well tolerated. In general, however, methods used to decrease pulmonary perfusion, as in left-to-right shunts, do not apply, because this is a mixing lesion. Persistent efforts to lower pulmonary flow may result in RV overload and failure.
- Postoperative complications include residual VSD, conduit obstruction (CVP monitoring will help with this diagnosis), pulmonary HTN, and RV failure.

Anomalous Pulmonary Venous Return

Description

- Four sites of drainage exist:
    1. Supracardiac—pulmonary veins drain into the SVC, creating a left-to-right shunt (pulmonary recirculation).
    2. Infracardiac—pulmonary veins drain into the portal or hepatic system.
    3. Cardiac—pulmonary veins drain into the RA or coronary sinus.
    4. Mixed.
- An ASD is part of the complex and is necessary for blood to reach the left side of the heart. Some degree of pulmonary venous obstruction also exists, causing pulmonary congestion.
- In a partial anomaly, there is a step-up in saturation in the RA.
- In a total anomaly, there is mixing of all systemic and pulmonary blood flow.
- Pulmonary hypertension is common.
- Airway obstruction can occur.

Anesthetic considerations

- A partial anomalous pulmonary venous return (PAPVR) is managed like an ASD.
- A total anomalous pulmonary venous return (TAPVR) may require inotropic support for the RV and measures to lower PVR.
- Obstruction, kinking, or thrombosis of the pulmonary vein to LA anastomosis may occur.

Hypoplastic Left Heart Syndrome

Description

- The LV may be hypoplastic or absent.
- Associated anomalies include aortic valve atresia with a hypoplastic aorta and atresia of the mitral valve.
- Severe CHF is also present.
- Mortality is high within the first month of life (95%).
- Systemic blood flow depends on the patency of the ductus arteriosus.

Anesthetic considerations

- Repair consists of a modified Fontan procedure (RA to distal PA conduit) and redirection of the pulmonary venous return to the RV, which will supply the aorta. The proximal portion of the PA is anastomosed to the atretic aorta to supply systemic perfusion from the RV.
- Inotropic administration is required to support the RV because it will supply systemic circulation.

Double Outlet Right Ventricle (DORV)

Description

- Both great arteries arise from the RV; a VSD is always present.
- Often there is some degree of pulmonic stenosis.

Anesthetic considerations

- Management depends on the amount of pulmonary blood flow. Some children have a high Q_p/Q_s ratio and are managed like VSDs. Others have considerable RVOT obstruction and are managed like TOFs.

TABLE 11-5. Surgical procedures for correction of congenital heart disease

Eponym of procedure	Disease to be corrected	Technique	Anesthetic considerations
Norwood	Hypoplastic left heart syndrome	*Stage 1:* 1. Reconstruction of the aorta from a transected pulmonary artery, the proximal portion connected with the ascending aorta, the distal portion connected with the systemic circulation by a Blalock-Taussig shunt 2. A near total atrial septectomy *Stage 2:* Modified Fontan procedure	• See specifics under Hypoplastic left heart syndrome.
Fontan	• Tricuspid atresia • Single ventricle • Pulmonary atresia • Hypoplastic left ventricle	1. Conduit (valved) from the right atrium to the main or right pulmonary artery 2. Closure of the ASD	• PVR is minimized both before and after bypass to ensure pulmonary blood flow. • Cardiac output is optimized by increasing filling pressures (RAP < 20 mm Hg if possible). • Residual right-to-left shunts can be seen postrepair. • Conversion is made to spontaneous ventilation and extubation as soon as possible to minimize intrapulmonary pressures. • Normal sinus rhythm is essential because the atrial kick pumps the blood through the conduit.

Jatene	Transposition of the great arteries (TOGA)	1. Anatomic correction by division of the great arteries with reattachment to their correct ventricular outflow 2. Coronary reimplantation	• Care should be taken to avoid increasing PVR; PDA patency should be maintained with prostaglandins. • Inhalation inductions are slowed secondary to low effective pulmonary blood flow. • Myocardial depression and bradycardia are poorly tolerated. • LV failure is possible after correction if it is inadequately prepared to pump systemic pressures. • Coronary insufficiency postrepair can lead to ischemia.
Rastelli	• TOGA with VSD and LV outflow obstruction • Double outlet right ventricle	1. Oversewing of the main pulmonary artery 2. Conduit from the RV to the distal main pulmonary artery 3. Closure of the VSD such that the LV outflow is to the aorta	• As with the Jatene procedure. • Obstruction to LV outflow after correction may require pressor support. • Conduit obstruction resulting in diminished pulmonary blood flow is possible. • Heart block is a problem in the recovery phase.
Blalock-Hanlon	TOGA	1. Open atrial septectomy 2. Clamping of the right pulmonary veins during the excision	• As with the Jatene procedure. • Clamping of the pulmonary vein can lead to hemorrhage into the right lung.
Damus-Kaye-Stansel	• TOGA with poor coronary anatomy for the Jatene procedure • Double outlet right ventricle	1. Pulmonary artery cut with proximal end anastomosed to side of aorta establishing left ventricle to aortic flow 2. Valved conduit from RV to distal pulmonary artery establishes pulmonary flow	• As with the Jatene and Rastelli procedures.

Continued.

TABLE 11-5. Surgical procedures for correction of congenital heart disease—cont'd

Eponym of procedure	Disease to be corrected	Technique	Anesthetic considerations
Danielson	Ebstein's anomaly	1. Plication of atrialized portion of RV, bringing anterior and posterior portions of the tricuspid valves back to the normal annulus	• Myocardial and depressive effects of inhalation agents are to be avoided. • Tachycardia is poorly tolerated because it decreases diastolic filling time and increases RA pressures, resulting in a greater right-to-left shunt. • Minimizing PVR enhances pulmonary blood flow. • Supraventricular arrhythmias are common.
Mustard	TOGA	1. After excision of interatrial septum, an interatrial baffle using pericardium or synthetic material is created, directing pulmonary venous blood across tricuspid valve into RV, with systemic venous blood passing below baffle through mitral valve	• As with procedures for TOGA. • Postrepair the RV becomes the pump for systemic blood flow and can be dysfunctional. • Systemic or pulmonary venous obstruction can result from improper placement of the baffle. • Dysrhythmias, which are commonly atrial, occur postrepair.
Senning	TOGA	1. As for Mustard procedure except autologous tissue is used with theoretical advantage that it can grow with the heart	• As with the Mustard procedure.

OBSTRUCTIVE LESIONS

Pathophysiology

Obstructive lesions (valvular, vascular, or other deformities) cause decreased perfusion and pressure overload of the corresponding ventricle. CHF is a consistent finding in this group of anomalies.

Induction Technique

The pressure gradient across an obstructive lesion will define anesthetic management.

- Lesions with a large pressure gradient (> 50 mm Hg) and CHF are best managed with narcotics (fentanyl or sufentanil) to maintain a slow heart rate. Tachycardia will increase myocardial demand and decrease flow across the obstruction.
- Inhalation agents can precipitously decrease SVR and further augment a large gradient, limiting flow beyond that lesion. Also undesirable are the negative inotropic effects.
- Patients with smaller pressure gradients (< 40 mm Hg) and good perfusion beyond the obstruction may tolerate an inhalation induction.

Types of Obstructive Lesions

Coarctation of the Aorta

Description

- Two types exist:
  1. *Preductal*—narrowing of the aortic isthmus. Other anomalies occur in 90% of patients. A PDA is necessary to perfuse the lower body.
  2. *Postductal*—patients are asymptomatic until ductal closure. Extensive collaterals via the intercostal or mammary arteries develop to supply the lower body.
- CHF in infancy and HTN in the upper extremities are classic findings.
- The risk of cerebral aneurysm is greater for these children.

Anesthetic considerations

- Surgery is indicated when the pressure gradient exceeds 40 mm Hg or systolic blood pressure is greater than 180 mm Hg.
- PGE_1 infusions are used with preductal coarctation to keep the ductus arteriosus patent for perfusion to the lower body.
- Endocarditis prophylaxis is necessary (Appendix D).
- Inhalation agents that lower blood pressure by vasodilation are useful.
- Preductal placement of intraarterial catheters are most accurate. If possible, two arterial catheters, one preductal, the other postductal, are ideal for blood pressure management and assessment of perfusion to upper and lower extremities. Pre- and postductal oximetry is helpful.
- HTN persists postoperatively and requires both vasodilator therapy and beta blockade.
- Cooling to 33° C aids in preservation of spinal cord function if cross-clamping of the aorta is necessary during repair. Evoked potentials may be used to monitor spinal cord function if compromise to the spinal arteries is anticipated.

Interrupted Arch

Description

- This lesion involves failure of the fourth to sixth aortic arches to fuse and results in dependence on a PDA for perfusion to the lower body.
- Other commonly associated anomalies are a VSD, aortopulmonic window, and truncus arteriosus.
- Three types exist:
  1. Type A—interruption distal to the left subclavian
  2. Type B—interruption between left carotid and left subclavian (most common)
  3. Type C—interruption between the innominate artery and the left carotid
- Closure of the PDA leads to metabolic acidosis and renal failure.

Anesthetic considerations

- PGE_1 infusion is necessary to maintain patency of ductus.
- Considerations are similar to those for coarctation.

Aortic Stenosis

Description

- Three types of AS exist:
  1. Valvular—stiff, thickened bicuspid valve fused at the commissures (80% of all AS)
  2. Subvalvular—eventually turbulence develops beyond the initial obstruction, causing thickening of valve leaflets and incompetence (10% of AS)
  3. Supravalvular—associated with Williams syndrome; tortuous coronary arteries with a predilection for early atherosclerosis evolving because of proximal location to the obstruction and subjection to high pressures
- Syncope, angina, and CHF are common symptoms.
- ECG shows LVH.

Anesthetic considerations

- Valvular and supravalvular obstruction do not tolerate myocardial depressants or tachycardia. Hypotension can be catastrophic because coronary perfusion will markedly decrease.
- Narcotics are the preferred anesthetic technique.
- Subvalvular stenosis can behave like idiopathic hypertrophic subaortic stenosis. Hypovolemia, hypotension, tachycardia, and vasodilation augment the obstruction and worsen perfusion. Beta blockers improve flow.
- Endocarditis prophylaxis is necessary (Appendix D).

Mitral Stenosis

Description

- This is a rare lesion in children, more common in males.
- Pulmonary vascular disease and cor pulmonale can develop secondary to elevated LA pressures.
- Ischemia and fibrosis lead to LV dysfunction in severely obstructed valves.

Anesthetic considerations

- Endocarditis prophylaxis is needed (Appendix D).
- Maintenance of sinus rhythm and a normal or lower HR will optimize LV filling.
- Anticholinergics and pancuronium should be avoided.
- A high preload is necessary for perfusion across the stenotic valve. Dehydration is poorly tolerated.
- Halothane and nitrous oxide may be acceptable, but sicker children will require fentanyl or sufentanil for minimal cardiac depression.
- Reduction of PVR and SVR postoperatively may be needed.

Cortriatriatum

Description

- The LA is partitioned into two chambers. A superior chamber receives the pulmonary venous return, and an inferior chamber communicates with the mitral valve. The chambers are connected by fenestrations in a partitioning membrane.
- Hemodynamic changes are similar to those in mitral stenosis. Pulmonary HTN and RV failure develop within the first year of life.

Anesthetic considerations

- Anesthetic management is similar to that for mitral stenosis.

LESIONS INVOLVING THE AIRWAY

Pathophysiology

- Vascular rings and a double aortic arch result from the failure of the embryologic fourth to sixth aortic arches to regress.
- The anomalies encroach upon the trachea and/or esophagus, causing symptoms to emerge usually before 1 year of age, including stridor, dysphagia, recurrent respiratory tract infections, cyanosis, and reflex apnea (respiratory arrest precipitated by irritation to an area of tracheomalacia).
- Treatment is rarely necessary if symptoms are not present in infancy because the rings become insignificant with the growth of the child.

Anesthetic Management

- Surgical repair is generally performed through a left thoracotomy.
- Induction is likely to aggravate preexisting airway obstruction and should be approached with caution.
- Atropine helps to reduce secretions.
- Patients with tracheomalacia may sustain airway collapse with increased negative intrathoracic pressures.
- Muscle relaxants should not be used until after the airway is secured. For this reason, an inhalation induction maintaining spontaneous ventilation is best.
- Massive bleeding may occur during resection, and vascular access should be appropriate. An arterial catheter and central venous access are usually indicated.
- Preexisting tracheomalacia will persist postoperatively and may worsen with edema. Prolonged mechanical ventilation should be anticipated.

ACQUIRED HEART DISEASE

Rheumatic Heart Disease (RHD)

Description

- RHD is associated with group A β-hemolytic streptococcal infections of the upper airway and affects young children more commonly in the winter and spring.
- Clinical manifestations include carditis, polyarthritis, chorea, subcutaneous nodules, and erythema marginatum. In 76% of the cases, carditis appears within the first week of onset of the disease and may be treated with corticosteroids.
- Patients with recurrent attacks of infection or those with severe carditis may go on to develop rheumatic heart disease. The mitral valve is involved 85% of the time, the aortic valve 54%, and the tricuspid and pulmonary valves less than 5% of the time. Patients are predisposed to endocarditis.

Anesthetic Considerations

- Anesthetic considerations are based on the specific cardiac involvement. Patients rarely require valvular replacement before adulthood.

Kawasaki Syndrome

Description

- Mucocutaneous lymph node syndrome is an acute febrile exanthem of children, which is manifested by fever, conjunctival injection, oral erythema with crusting of the lips, induration of the hands and feet followed by erythema and desquamation of the soles and palms, a diffuse erythematous rash, and lymphadenopathy.
- Cardiac involvement occurs 20% of the time, manifested by pericarditis during the first and second weeks and coronary aneurysms between the second and sixth weeks. The majority of the aneurysms involve the left and right coronary arteries, and 99% of them can be detected by echocardiography.
- Sequelae include pericardial effusion with decreased LV function and CHF, aneurysmal thrombosis or rupture leading to infarction, and arrhythmias.

Anesthetic Considerations

- Children requiring anesthesia should be managed like adults with coronary artery disease.
- Tachycardia and myocardial depression are to be avoided.
- A calibrated ECG to follow ST segment changes is indicated.

Takayasu Disease

Description

- A rare form of arteritis that occurs with strikingly greater frequency among females, Takayasu disease involves the aorta and the proximal portions of its branches leading to occlusion.

- The disease may begin in childhood with symptoms of hypertension, cardiomegaly, dyspnea, ocular disturbances, and marked weakening of the pulses in the upper extremities.
- Slow progression occurs even with treatment (steroids and cytotoxic drugs). Survival ranges between 1 and 20 years from the onset.

Anesthetic Considerations

- Anesthetic considerations include control of hypertension and avoidance of myocardial ischemia.

CARDIOMYOPATHIES

Idiopathic Hypertrophic Subaortic Stenosis (IHSS)

Description

- IHSS results from muscular growth of the LV outflow tract.
- Symptoms of dyspnea, angina on exertion, and orthopnea are most consistently present. Sudden death occurs in 3% to 4% of cases.
- Patients often have some degree of mitral valve incompetence resulting in a decrease in LV compliance.
- Surgical repair is indicated if the gradient between the LV and the aorta is over 40 mm Hg.

Anesthetic Considerations

- The mainstays of treatment are beta blockade (negative inotropy to reduce outflow stenosis and slow heart rate) and maintenance of adequate preload and afterload. Filling volumes must be monitored so that hypovolemia, hypotension, reflex tachycardia, and vasodilation can be avoided.
- Preoperative anxiety should be tempered by a generous premedication.
- Halothane and fentanyl are usually very well tolerated, but ketamine is not.
- Sinus rhythm should be maintained.
- Regional anesthesia is contraindicated because of the decreased afterload and preload.

Carnitine Deficiency

Description

- Carnitine is important in the transport of long-chain fatty acids into mitochondria. If deficient, cardiac enlargement and CHF result.
- The deficiency responds well to L-carnitine therapy, which may improve LV function.

Anesthetic Considerations

- Narcotics, which have little effect on myocardial contractility, are usually selected.
- Inhalation agents are best avoided.
- Volume replacement must be sufficient to maintain cardiac output without resulting in pulmonary edema.

ANESTHETIC MANAGEMENT OF NONCARDIAC SURGERY IN CHILDREN WITH CHD

1. A recent history and physical examination results (particularly growth percentiles, exercise tolerance, and degree of cyanosis or CHF), list of medications, and current laboratory values should be available to the anesthesiologist.
2. The most recent cardiac catheterization and echocardiographic data should be reviewed. Anesthetic management is determined through the following:
   - Q_p/Q_s (type and degree of shunt)
   - Pressure gradients
   - Myocardial contractility
   - Function of palliative shunts
   - Anatomy
3. Appropriate premedication is ordered based on age of patient, presence of CHF or cyanosis, and degree of respiratory dysfunction.
4. Antibiotic prophylaxis is necessary (Appendix D).
5. All air bubbles are meticulously removed from intravenous lines.

MONITORING FOR OPEN HEART SURGERY

Noninvasive

- ECG: calibrated, at least leads II and V_5, monitor and diagnostic mode, variable sweep controls. (See Chapter 5.)
- A precordial stethoscope is vital during induction for continuous monitoring of breath sounds and heart tones.
- Pulse oximetry allows for continuous monitoring of oxygen saturation. It is useful to have more than one probe on the patient should one fail during the operation, and to monitor pre- and postductal saturations when indicated.
- An automated blood pressure cuff is useful even if an intraarterial catheter is used.
- Core temperature is monitored by esophageal and rectal probes. It is useful to monitor brain temperature during deep hypothermic circulatory arrest, using tympanic membrane or nasopharyngeal probes.

Invasive

Arterial Catheters

Arterial catheters provide beat-to-beat pressure monitoring and allow for blood gas and laboratory determinations. The sites of these include the following:

Radial artery (preferred site)

1. Allen's test will check for adequacy of collateral blood flow.
2. The wrist is placed in extension.
3. A 22- or 24-gauge catheter is used in neonates and toddlers (under 5 years). A 20-gauge catheter is preferable for older children.

4. The skin is punctured with a 20-gauge needle to decrease skin resistance.
5. The catheter should enter the skin at a 15- to 25-degree angle until the artery is punctured, when the angle is decreased to 10 degrees for catheter insertion.
6. The catheter is then flushed with heparinized saline (1 unit/ml) through a T-piece connector and attached to a calibrated transducer.
7. Complications include hand ischemia, thrombosis, infection, central air emboli, and exsanguination if unrecognized disconnection occurs.

Umbilical artery. This site is often used in the critically ill newborn. (See Chapter 2 for technique.)

Femoral artery. The femoral artery can be cannulated percutaneously or by cutdown, but carries a higher risk of contamination than more peripheral locations.

Dorsalis pedis artery (DPA). Collateral flow can be determined by compression of the DPA simultaneously with the posterior tibial artery (PTA), noting blanching of the great and second toes, with subsequent return of color on release of the PTA.

Central Venous Pressure Monitoring

Central venous pressure monitoring allows for pressure monitoring and for rapid administration of fluids or drugs to the central circulation. Approaches include the following:

Internal jugular vein (Fig. 11-1)

1. The patient is positioned supine, the neck extended with a roll under the shoulders.
2. The right internal jugular vein is the preferred site because it provides an almost straight line into the RA.
3. The neck is prepared and draped sterilely, and the patient is placed in the Trendelenburg position with the head turned to the left.
4. The internal jugular vein is cannulated by inserting the needle from a standard pediatric CVP kit at the apex of the triangle where the two heads of the sternocleidomastoid (SCM) muscles meet, at an angle of 25 to 30 degrees, aiming toward the ipsilateral nipple. Alternatively, the catheter can be inserted anteriorly to the SCM midway between the sternal notch and the mastoid, pointing toward the ipsilateral nipple at an angle of approximately 30 degrees.
5. The catheter should be transduced to ensure that it is in the vein. Inadvertent carotid artery cannulation is possible in patients with large mixing lesions because right-sided and left-sided pressures may be nearly identical and cyanosis alters the normal color of arterial blood.
6. After transducing, the guidewire is inserted with the J curving medially and posteriorly.
7. The platysma should be cut where the wire enters the skin, and the dilator introduced.

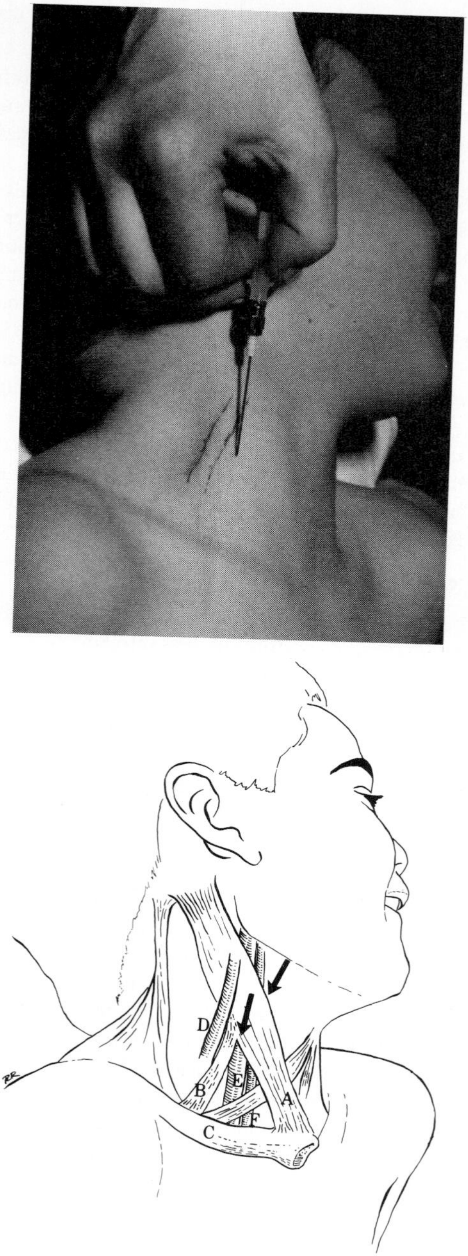

Fig. 11-1. The internal jugular vein can be cannulated inserting a needle at the apex of the triangle of the two heads of the sternocleidomastoid *(SCM)* and aiming for the ipsilateral nipple (*lower arrow and photograph*).
The vein can also be located by inserting the needle anteriorly to the SCM at a point halfway between the mastoid process and sternal notch aiming at the ipsilateral nipple *(higher arrow)*. (Legend: *A* = medial head of the SCM; *B* = lateral head of the SCM; *C* = clavicle; *D* = external jugular vein; *E* = internal jugular vein; *F* = carotid artery.)

8. Next the catheter itself is introduced over the wire.
9. The catheter is sutured in place, and a sterile dressing applied.
10. Complications include pneumothorax, carotid artery puncture, hematoma formation with compression of the airway, puncture and cannulation of the vertebral artery, arrhythmias, air emboli, and hemothorax.

External jugular vein (EJ)

1. The EJ is a superficial vessel and is cannulated with the catheter parallel to the skin, similarly to veins on the extremities.
2. A slightly larger roll under the shoulders for more extreme head extension may be necessary to place the catheter against the skin and avoid the mandible.
3. Since the catheter is placed under direct vision, it need not be transduced. The risk of inadvertent arterial cannulation are avoided.
4. The guidewire is inserted with the curve (J) pointed medially and posteriorly to facilitate passage under the clavicle.
5. A small skin cut will ease insertion of the dilator. The plastysma lies deep to the EJ distal to the point of catheter insertion. Passage through the platysma is facilitated by dilation, not by cutting.
6. Filling the catheter with saline or water before insertion decreases the chance that air bubbles will enter the central circulation.

Umbilical vein. The catheter should be documented to be above the liver in the IVC or RA (see Chapter 2 for insertion techniques).

Femoral vein. This vein is cannulated by either percutaneous or cutdown techniques.

Left Atrial Pressure Monitoring

A left atrial catheter placed by the surgeon after thoracotomy or sternotomy allows for monitoring of left-sided filling pressures. Percutaneous placement of pulmonary artery catheters is often not possible in small pediatric patients, but may be placed by the surgeon under direct vision.

Transesophageal Echocardiography

The use of transesophageal echocardiography allows for evaluation of chamber size, anatomic defects, myocardial function, directional flow of blood, and adequacy of repair. Adult probes can probably be used safely in children over age 3, although the time period that the probe can be left in the esophagus and the incidence of complications are not well understood. Pediatric probes are available.

CARDIOPULMONARY BYPASS

Goals

1. Adequate perfusion of the patient's organs without using the heart as a pump
2. Maintenance of CVP for effective drainage into the extracorporeal circuit
3. Maintenance of normal PaO_2, pH, and $PaCO_2$

Cannulation

Venous

Usually two separate cannulae are placed, one in the SVC and one in the IVC. Any major vein can be used, the femoral vein being the most common alternative to central vein cannulation.

Arterial

Usually a single cannula in the anterior aspect of the ascending aorta is placed. If an interrupted aortic arch is present, cannulation of both the proximal and distal ends of the aorta is performed. The femoral artery can be used if necessary.

Oxygenators

- Membrane oxygenators permit gas exchange through a synthetic membrane. They offer the advantage over bubble oxygenators (see following) of improved platelet survival and fewer microemboli. They are more costly, difficult to set up, and it is more difficult to remove air bubbles from the circuit.
- Bubble oxygenators permit gas exchange by bubbling the gas flow through the blood, defoaming and filtering the blood, then transfusing it back to the patient. Advantages include simplicity in the setup and the prime, and the capacity to oxygenate a large volume of blood. Disadvantages include hemolysis, thrombocytopenia, and platelet dysfunction, especially when perfusion is necessary for more than 2 hours.

Prime

Each circuit has its own obligatory prime volume: that volume of solution necessary to fill the circuit and ensure that no air is pumped. The volume varies from 750 to 1,200 ml in most circuits. The Cobe Variable Prime Membrane Lung allows different amounts of priming volumes depending on the size of the child: 290 ml for neonates and up to 420 ml for larger children.

Hemodilution results from a volume of priming solutions considerably greater than the patient's blood volume. In addition, most primes are hyponatremic, hypocalcemic, hypomagnesemic, hypocarbic, acidotic, and hypoosmolar. Common sequelae of CPB include hypoproteinemia, thrombocytopenia, anemia, hypocoagulability, and hypothermia. To avoid extreme hemodilution in small children, a combination of blood and plasma is used.

Flow

Flow is measured by an electromagnetic flowmeter on the arterial side of the circuit. The rate is higher in pediatric cases because of higher metabolic demands and a pristine vascular tree. Flows as high as 150 to 175 ml/kg/min are common.

Anticoagulation

Anticoagulation is effected with 4 mg/kg of IV heparin. An activated clotting time (ACT) of 300 to 400 sec is adequate to assume CPB, but values greater than 400 are necessary to ensure no microscopic evidence of aggregates. The ACT should be checked every 30 minutes while on CPB.

Hypothermia

- Moderate hypothermia provides temperatures between 25° and 30° C.
- Profound hypothermia provides temperatures between 15° and 20° C. A combination of this temperature and circulatory arrest has the advantage of providing a bloodless field, decreased blood trauma, and enhanced myocardial protection. Circulatory arrest can be maintained for up to 1 hour without significant neurologic sequelae. Trickle flow (very low pump flows) is more commonly used than complete circulatory arrest.
- Surface cooling can be accomplished with the room temperature reduced to 22° C, a cooling blanket at 15° C, ice packed around the head, an unheated breathing circuit, and intravenous fluids.
- The effects of hypothermia are as follows:
  1. Hypothermia acts on the heart to maintain ATP stores but also leads to arrhythmias, bradycardia, and decreased contractility and compliance.
  2. It decreases the cerebral metabolic rate, as well as total body oxygen consumption.
  3. Increased blood glucose occurs secondary to decreases in insulin levels, increases in ACTH, cortisol, epinephrine, and norepinephrine. Gluconeogenesis in the liver usually persists during moderate hypothermia.
  4. Hypothermia leads to intense vasoconstriction and poor rheologic characteristics because of the increased viscosity of blood; thus the need for hemodilution and systemic heparinization.

Perfusion during CPB

- Perfusion should be adequate to maintain a normal metabolic state with a urine output of 2 to 3 ml/kg.
- The mixed venous blood gas is a reliable indicator of perfusion.
- Hypotension and hypertension may indicate inadequate perfusion.
- Causes of inadequate perfusion include inadequate venous return or inadequate arterial flow (may reflect improper cannula size), hypovolemia, inadequate flow rate, and peripheral resistance abnormalities.
- If perfusion pressure seems too low for the age and perfusion rate, the possibility of substantial aortopulmonary communication should be considered (undiagnosed shunt). All known shunts should be ligated before bypass.

Anesthesia and CPB

- Hypothermia decreases anesthetic requirements.
- Priming solutions cause marked dilution of drugs, which necessitates the administration of additional doses in the postbypass period.
- A volatile anesthetic vaporizer can be inserted into the gas delivery system. Isoflurane is an attractive choice because of its effect on cerebral EEG activity and reduction of peripheral vasomotor tone.

Rewarming

1. Ice bags are removed.
2. The operating room is warmed.
3. The heating blanket is warmed to 37° C.
4. The use of nitroprusside or droperidol (75-100 μg/kg) helps to ensure even warming by vasodilatation.
5. Upon completion of rewarming, differences between core and peripheral blood temperatures (esophageal and rectal) should be no greater than 1° or 2°. Otherwise, increased organ damage and coagulopathies may result.
6. Sinus rhythm should be established. Cardioversion or pacing may be required.

Discontinuation of CPB

1. Monitors are recalibrated.
2. Adequate hematocrit level, ABGs, and electrolyte balance are ensured.
3. Ventilation with 100% oxygen is resumed.
4. Inotropic and vasodilator drugs in bolus and infusion doses are made available.
5. Difficulties in discontinuation from bypass may be due to inadequacy of the repair, a lengthy bypass period, or preexisting myocardial damage.

ARRHYTHMIAS

See Table 11-6.

Causes

In general, arrhythmias can be caused by electrolyte disturbances, acid/base abnormalities, hypoxemia, hypercarbia, autonomic imbalance, surgical trauma to the conduction system, improper development of the conduction system, and aberrant pathways in the conduction system (as in Wolff-Parkinson-White syndrome).

Diagnosis

Accurate and rapid diagnosis of the dysrhythmia is essential. Lead II is often the best lead for the evaluation of P waves, but with tachyarrhythmias the rates are often too rapid for easy analysis. Atrial epicardial electrograms or esophageal electrocardiography are both valuable tools for diagnosis of these types of arrhythmias.

TABLE 11-6. Common pediatric arrhythmias

Arrhythmia	Causes	Diagnosis	Treatment
Asystole	Hypoxia Ischemia Direct myocardial injury Severe electrolyte disturbances Succinylcholine	Isoelectric ECG without complexes	• Adequate oxygenation • Epinephrine IV/ETT/intracardiac • Atropine • Isoproterenol
Sinus bradycardia	Hypoxia Direct injury Increased ICP Acidosis Vagal stimulation	Heart rate: <100 1st year of life <80 ages 1-5 <60 over 5 years of age	• Adequate oxygenation is first ensured • Drug therapy as in asystole
Sick sinus	Direct injury Cardiomyopathy Ischemia Myocarditis Digitalis toxicity Congenital anomalies • ASD • L-TOGA • Kawasaki disease • Ebstein's anomaly	• Sinus bradycardia or sinus arrest with nodal or ventricular escape rhythms giving rise to tachyarrhythmias • Stokes-Adams attacks	• Permanent pacemaker
First-degree A-V block	Digitalis Inferior wall infarction Hyperkalemia Acute rheumatic fever Calcium channel blocker toxicity	PR > .20 msec	• Rarely requires treatment

Continued.

TABLE 11-6. Common pediatric arrhythmias—cont'd

Arrhythmia	Causes	Diagnosis	Treatment
Second-degree heart block			
Mobitz I	Inferior wall infarction Digoxin excess	Progressive lengthening of PR interval until one P wave is not conducted	• Rarely requires treatment
Mobitz II	Conduction pathology distal to bundle of His Anterior wall infarction	PR intervals are constant before a dropped beat occurs	• Permanent pacemaker may be required because progression to complete AV block is frequent
Complete heart block	Digitalis toxicity Congenital Acquired connective tissue disease in mother Cardiac tumors Myocarditis L-TOGA Asplenia or polysplenia syndrome Endocardial fibroelastosis	• Atria and ventricles beat independently • Rate of atria is faster than that of ventricle • PR interval constantly changes	• Isoproterenol • Permanent pacemaker
Atrial fibrillation	Rheumatic heart disease Mitral valve prolapse Ebstein's anomaly Cardiomyopathy	Rapid irregular ventricular rate; absent P waves	• Synchronized cardioversion • Digoxin • Propranolol • Verapamil
Atrial flutter	Direct injury Rheumatic heart disease Mitral valve prolapse Pericarditis WPW	Sawtooth pattern between normal QRS	• Digoxin • Overdrive pacing • Propranolol • Cardioversion • Verapamil

Paroxysmal atrial tachycardia	Often seen in healthy individuals	Three or more consecutive premature atrial contractions	• Vagal maneuvers • Propranolol • Verapamil • Edrophonium
Supraventricular tachycardia	Reentry phenomenon through the A-V node or accessory pathways Ebstein's anomaly Infection Fever WPW	• Regular RR interval • Narrow QRS • Rate 200-300 in infants, 150-250 in older children	• Vagal maneuvers • Propranolol • Verapamil • Phenylephrine
Premature ventricular contractions	Ischemia Irritability Metabolic disturbances Cardiac tumors IHSS Long QT Cardiomyopathy	• Wide QRS ($\geq$ .12 sec) • T wave and QRS usually point in opposite directions • Often followed by a compensatory pause	• Lidocaine • Bretylium • Phenytoin • Procainamide • Synchronized cardioversion .5-2 Joules/kg (if hypotensive)
Long QT syndrome	Congenital form associated with deafness and sudden death Familial tachycardia in which QT prolongation occurs only with excessive exercise and not at rest Acquired causes: • Infarction • Myocarditis • Mitral valve prolapse • Head injury • Cervical injury	Depends on heart rate: normally, QT prolongation does not exceed half the PR interval if HR < 80	• Beta blockade • Digoxin • Calcium channel blocker • Bretylium • Phenobarbital • Left stellate ganglion block • Acquired are treated with isoproterenol, correction of disturbance

Continued.

TABLE 11-6. Common pediatric arrhythmias—cont'd

Arrhythmia	Causes	Diagnosis	Treatment
	• Adrenal insufficiency • Amyloidosis • Hypothermia • Hypocalcemia • Hypokalemia • Hypomagnesemia • Antiarrhythmic drugs		
Wolff-Parkinson-White syndrome (WPW)	Accessory bundle of Kent	• Delta wave • PR $<$ .12 sec • Type A: R wave in V_1 • Type B: S wave in V_1	• Propranolol • Quinidine • Procainamide • Cardioversion
Torsade de pointes	Electrolyte disturbances Drug toxicity • Quinidine • Disopyramide	QRS twists and turns in opposite directions	• Overdrive atrial pacing

BIBLIOGRAPHY

Cumming GR and Carr W: Relief of dyspnoeic attacks in Fallot's tetralogy with propranolol, Lancet 1:519-22, 1966.

Freed MD and others: Prostaglandin E in infants with ductus arteriosus dependent congenital heart disease, Circulation 64:899-905, 1981.

Greeley WJ and Reves JG: Transesophageal atrial pacing for the treatment of dysrhythmias in pediatric surgical patients, Anesthesiology 68:282-85, 1988.

Greeley WJ and others: Comparative effects of halothane and ketamine on systemic arterial oxygen saturation in children with cyanotic heart disease, Anesthesiology 65:666-68, 1986.

Greeley WJ and others: Intraoperative esophageal electrocardiography for dysrhythmia: analysis and therapy in pediatric cardiac surgical patients, Anesthesiology 65:669-72, 1986.

Greeley WJ and others: Intraoperative hypoxemic spells in tetralogy of Fallot: an echocardiographic analysis of diagnosis and treatment, Anesth Analg 68:815-19, 1989.

Hickey PR: Anesthesia for children with heart disease. In Ryan JF and others: A practice of anesthesia for infants and children, New York, 1986, Grune & Stratton.

Hickey PR and Crone RK: Cardiovascular physiology and pharmacology in children: normal and diseased pediatric cardiovascular systems. In Ryan JF and others, editors: A practice of anesthesia for infants and children, New York, 1986, Grune & Stratton.

Hickey PR and Wessel DL: Anesthesia for treatment of congenital heart disease. In Kaplan JA, editor: Cardiac anesthesia, ed 2, Philadelphia, 1987, WB Saunders Co.

Hickey PR and others: Pulmonary and systemic hemodynamic effects of nitrous oxide in infants with normal and elevated pulmonary vascular resistance, Anesthesiology 65:374-78, 1986.

Hickey PR and others: Pulmonary and systemic hemodynamic responses to fentanyl in infants, Anesth Analg 64:483-86, 1985.

Hickey PR and others: Pulmonary and systemic hemodynamic responses to ketamine in infants with normal and elevated pulmonary vascular resistance, Anesthesiology 62:287-93, 1985.

Hollinger I: Diseases of the cardiovascular system. In Katz R and Steward D, editors: Anesthesia and uncommon pediatric diseases, Philadelphia, 1987, WB Saunders Co.

Laishley RS, Burrows FA, and Lerman J: Effect of anesthetic induction regimens on oxygen saturation in cyanotic congenital heart disease, Anesthesiology 65:673-77, 1986.

Lake CL: Pediatric cardiac anesthesia, Norwalk, Conn, 1988, Appleton & Lange.

Lewis AB and others: Side effects of therapy with prostaglandin E, in infants with critical congenital heart disease, Circulation 64:893-98, 1981.

Lister G and Pitt BR: Cardiopulmonary interactions in the infant with congenital cardiac disease, Clin Chest Med 4:219-32, 1983.

Prielipp RC, Rosenthal MH, and Pearl RG: Hemodynamic profiles of prostaglandin E_1, isoproterenol, prostacyclin and nifedipine in vasoconstrictor pulmonary hypertension in sheep, Anesth Analg 67:722-29, 1988.

Shaddy RE and others: Continuous intravenous phenylephrine infusion for treatment of hypoxemic spells in tetralogy of Fallot, J Pediatr 114:468-70, 1989.

Shulman ST, Amrin D, and Risno A: Prevention of bacterial endocarditis, Circulation 70:1123A-27A, 1984.

Strong MJ, Keats AS, and Cooley DA: Arterial gas tensions under anaesthesia in tetralogy of Fallot, Br J Anaesth 39:472-79, 1967.

Tanner GE and others: Effect of left to right, mixed left to right and right to left shunts on inhalational anesthetic induction in children, Anesth Analg 64:101-7, 1985.

12

ANESTHETIC MANAGEMENT OF CHILDREN WITH HEMATOLOGIC DISORDERS

Harvey Stern

There was a young man from Bohemia
Whose blood was filled with leukemia
He turned and he spat
When they gave him cisplat
And his kidneys complained of uremia.
DIXON HILL

ANEMIA

The oxygen dissociation curve is shifted to the right in most types of anemia. The decreased oxygen affinity permits more oxygen to be released at higher O_2 tensions, permitting increased oxygen extraction without compromising the tissue tension of oxygen. Red cells of patients with anemia generate more 2,3-diphosphoglycerate, which combines with deoxygenated hemoglobin and decreases the affinity of oxygen. Transfusion is indicated when physiologic compensation for anemia is unlikely.

Physiologic Anemia

Normal Neonate

1. Term infants have a higher hemoglobin and hematocrit than older children.
2. During the first week of life the hemoglobin level begins to decrease, continuing for the first 6 to 8 weeks of life. Hemoglobin levels rarely drop below 9 g/dl.

3. Erythropoiesis ceases when the O_2 saturation rises at birth. Stimulation of bone marrow by erythropoietin resumes when the hemoglobin falls to 10 to 11 g/dl at 8 to 12 weeks of age.
4. Decreased fetal red cell survival (45 to 70 days) contributes to anemia.
5. The expansion of blood volume that accompanies rapid growth in the first 3 months of life also contributes to physiologic anemia.

Premature Infant

The premature infant has a more pronounced fall in hemoglobin level with a nadir that may be reached by the fifth week of life.

1. In infants weighing less than 1200 g at birth the hemoglobin may drop to 8 g/dl or lower.
2. In smaller preterm infants the rate and degree of hemoglobin drop may be more severe.

Treatment

Physiologic neonatal anemia usually requires no treatment other than adequate nutrition.

Aplastic Anemia

Aplastic anemia is characterized by a marrow that is mostly devoid of hematopoietic cells and by a peripheral pancytopenia. The marrow retains its architecture but is replaced by large amounts of fat.

Congenital Aplastic Anemia

1. Usually associated with a complex of other anomalies of the skeletal, integumentary, renal, and cardiac systems
2. An autosomal recessive trait with variable expression

Characteristics of Acquired Aplastic Anemia

1. It may result from drugs, toxins, or infections.
2. The agent most commonly responsible is chloramphenicol, accounting for up to half of the cases.
3. Drug-related aplasia may be either dose dependent or idiosyncratic. (See the box on the next page for implicated drugs.)
4. Inhalation of hydrocarbons (such as "glue sniffing") also may be associated with aplastic anemia.
5. It also may occur during viral hepatitis.

Treatment

1. Transfusions may be indicated if hemoglobin is less than 9 g/dl.
2. Corticosteroids
3. Androgens

Survival

1. The 10-year survival rate is 40% to 50% in the congenital cases and about 10% in the acquired cases. Demise is usually secondary to hemorrhage or sepsis.

DRUGS ASSOCIATED WITH APLASTIC ANEMIA

Dose-Related

Chloramphenicol
Alkylating agents
Antimetabolites (folic acid antagonists, purine and pyrimidine analogues)
Mitotic inhibitors
Anthracyclines
Inorganic arsenicals

Idiosyncratic

Chloramphenicol
Phenylbutazone
Phenytoin
Gold compounds
Organic arsenicals
Quinacrine
Insecticides

Anesthetic Considerations

1. Preoperative assessment of other congenital lesions should be made. Coexistence of congenital heart disease requires prophylactic antibiotics (Appendix D).
2. Any infections present should be treated.
3. A hematologist should be consulted, and a complete blood count and coagulation studies should be obtained, unless the urgency of the operation necessitates otherwise.
4. If severe neutropenia is present, broad spectrum antibiotics should be employed.
5. Blood transfusions may be necessary, but they may further depress erythropoiesis.
6. Platelets should be available if thrombocytopenia is present.
7. Intramuscular injections should be avoided because of the likelihood of thrombocytopenia. Premedication should be given orally.
8. If the patient has been on chronic steroids a stress dose is warranted (hydrocortisone, 4 to 8 mg/kg in three divided doses).
9. Nitrous oxide should be avoided because it can depress the bone marrow. Air oxygen mixtures may be employed.
10. Securing the airway should be as atraumatic as possible to avoid excessive bleeding.
11. Postoperative supplemental oxygen may be required.
12. Analgesics may be given orally or intravenously.

Chronic Renal Failure (CRF)

1. Patients with CRF who have plasma creatinine concentrations greater than 3.5 mg/dl usually will have a normochromic normocytic anemia. Hemoglobin concentrations as low as 5 to 8 g/dl may accompany CRF.

2. The anemia reflects both decreased erythrocyte production and survival. Decreased erythrocyte production most likely is caused by lowered erythropoietin production in the presence of elevated BUN levels. Erythrocyte survival time is shortened by 50%, reflecting erythrocyte membrane fragility. A hemorrhagic tendency may further exacerbate this anemia.
3. The anemia in CRF is usually well tolerated because of its slow onset. However, the decreased oxygen-carrying capacity can still cause tissue hypoxia. Increased tissue perfusion from decreased blood viscosity can offset the decreased O_2 carrying capacity. In addition, release of oxygen from hemoglobin to the tissues is facilitated by a shift of the oxyhemoglobin dissociation curve to the right, resulting from metabolic acidosis and increased levels of 2,3-DPG.
4. Usually it will not be necessary to transfuse these patients, although the patient's hemoglobin level, overall status, and surgical blood loss must be considered.

Iron Deficiency Anemia

1. Iron deficiency anemia (see the box below for accompanying physiologic changes) is the most common hematologic disease in pediatric patients.
2. Low birth weight and perinatal hemorrhage are associated with decreased iron stores and hemoglobin mass in the newborn. As hemoglobin decreases during the first 8 to 12 weeks of life, iron is reclaimed and stored. This stored iron is usually ample for hematopoiesis during the first 6 to 9 months of life. In low–birth weight infants or in the context of perinatal bleeding, stored iron may be depleted earlier.
3. Iron deficiency is more common from 9 to 24 months of age, and relatively infrequent after 2 years of age. The occurrence in older children may indicate blood loss (frequently GI).
4. Clinical symptoms include pallor, irritability, anorexia, tachycardia, cardiac dilatation, and systolic murmurs.

PHYSIOLOGIC CHANGES IN IRON DEFICIENCY ANEMIA

↓ Iron stores
↓ Serum ferritin (<10 ng/ml)
↓ Serum iron
↑ Total iron-binding capacity (>350 μg/dl)
↑ Free erythrocyte protoporphyrins (accumulation of heme precursors)
↑ Hypochromia
↑ Microcytosis
↔, ↑ Reticulocyte count

Treatment

Therapy consists of oral administration of ferrous salts.

1. Optimal replacement is with 6 mg/kg/24 hr of elemental iron. Ferrous sulfate is 20% and ferrous gluconate is 10% to 12% elemental iron by weight.

2. Bone marrow may respond within 2 days, and increases in hemoglobin may be seen from 4 to 30 days after beginning iron therapy.
3. Blood transfusion is necessary only when the anemia is very severe or when there is superimposed infection that may interfere with the response to therapy.

Anesthetic Considerations

1. Elective surgery should be delayed until the anemia is evaluated and treated. Urgent cases may require preoperative blood transfusions.
2. Premedications that can cause significant respiratory depression should be avoided.
3. An elevated cardiac output caused by anemia may slow induction of anesthesia with inhalation agents.
4. Intraoperatively, adequacy of oxygenation should be assessed with oximetry and arterial blood gas analysis.
5. Local or regional techniques may be used, as associated coagulopathy is rare.

Hemolytic Anemia

1. Hemolytic anemias are characterized by shortened red blood cell (RBC) survival time. RBCs are normally in the circulation for 100 to 120 days. The senescent cells (about 1%) are replaced daily by the bone marrow. With decreased red cell survival time, bone marrow activity increases. Erythropoietic elements of the marrow may become hyperplastic, causing the marrow to expand the medullary spaces. Radiographic changes may be seen, especially in the skull, metacarpals, and phalanges.
2. Laboratory findings include elevated unconjugated (indirect) bilirubin that usually does not result in jaundice in the presence of normal hepatic function. Plasma hemoglobin concentration increases and plasma haptoglobin decreases because it combines with free hemoglobin and is cleared from the circulation.
3. Bone marrow may be stimulated to increase its output as much as 6- to 8-fold. Patients with hemolytic anemia may have aplastic crises or periods of transient bone-marrow failure. Life-threatening anemia may occur, but these periods are self-limited, lasting for 10 to 14 days. These aplastic crises usually are associated with infections. (See Anesthetic Considerations for aplastic anemia on 256.)

Spherocytosis

General Characteristics

1. Hereditary spherocytosis is a structural abnormality in erythrocytes characterized by spheroidal shape and deficiency in red cell membrane surface area.
2. The disease is one of autosomal dominant inheritance.
3. These cells are trapped in the spleen, where they meet their demise. Red cell survival rates are almost normal in patients after splenectomy.

Clinical Symptoms

1. Anemia, jaundice, and splenomegaly are the usual initial clinical symp-

toms. Anemia usually is not severe because of normoblastic hyperplasia of the bone marrow.

2. Compensation by the bone marrow may be interrupted temporarily by episodes of marrow failure referred to as an "aplastic crisis," most commonly precipitated by infection.
3. Marrow failure with a more gradual onset may be secondary to folate deficiency, as folate utilization is increased in this disorder.
4. Anemia also can occur because of an accelerated rate of hemolysis, though this is less common than aplastic crises.

Treatment

Splenectomy is the treatment of choice, especially in children and young adults. Infection is a major concern in these patients after splenectomy. Postsplenectomy survival is essentially normal.

Glucose 6-Phosphate Dehydrogenase (G-6-PD) Deficiency

Patients with G-6-PD deficiency may have episodic hemolytic anemia. Hemolysis usually is associated with stress, especially during administration of certain drugs, with infection, during the newborn period, and, in some people, with exposure to fava beans. The drugs listed in the box below should be avoided.

DRUGS ASSOCIATED WITH HEMOLYTIC ANEMIA IN G-6-PD DEFICIENCY

- Analgesics
  Phenacetin
  Aspirin
- Sulfonamides and sulfone
- Antimalarials
- Miscellaneous
  Nitrofurantoin
  Chloramphenicol
  Naphthalene
  Methylene blue
  Nalidixic acid
  Ascorbic acid

Nitrous Oxide and Megaloblastic Anemia

1. Nitrous oxide has been associated with the inhibition of methionine synthetase activity, which may impair DNA synthesis, inactivate vitamin B_{12}, and result in megaloblastic anemia.
2. The changes are related to the duration of N_2O exposure (may occur after only 1 to 2 hours) and are more common in sick patients than in patients who had uncomplicated surgery.
3. Folinic acid may be used to prevent bone-marrow toxicity, but even with folinic acid administration, N_2O should be avoided in patients with depressed bone marrow.

ONCOLOGY AND CHEMOTHERAPEUTIC AGENTS

1. Childhood neoplasms that infiltrate bone marrow are primarily acute leukemias, most commonly acute lymphoblastic leukemia. Leukemias comprise about one-third of all childhood malignancies. There is a pre-

disposition towards white female children, and peak incidence is at about 2 to 4 years of age.

2. Treatment consists of steroids and cytotoxic agents, often with adjunctive radiotherapy to reduce the likelihood of meningeal metastases. Treatment may extend over a number of years. Cytotoxic agents may have diverse adverse systemic effects (Table 12-1).
3. Severe anemia requiring blood transfusion may be present secondary to the disease process or to the therapy. Thrombocytopenia also can occur and may necessitate the temporary cessation of therapy. Intramuscular drug administration should be avoided because of possible thrombocytopenia.
4. Bacterial and fungal infections may occur, requiring antibiotics and immunoglobulins.
5. Radiotherapy and chemotherapy can cause nausea and vomiting. Preoperatively, antiemetics (such as metoclopramide) and H_2 blockers should be considered.

TABLE 12-1. Adverse effects of cytotoxic agents

Group	Subgroup	Generic name (brand)	Adverse effects
Alkylating agents	Nitrogen mustards	• Mustargen • Cyclophosphamide (Cytoxan) • Alkeran • Melphalan • Chlorambucil (Leukeran)	Nausea Alopecia Hemorrhagic cystitis Marrow suppression Inhibition of plasma cholinesterase
	Alkyl sulfonates	Busulfan	Myelosuppression Skin pigmentation Pulmonary fibrosis
	Nitrosoureas	• CCNU (CeeNU) • BCNU (BiCNU)	Delayed myelosuppression Nausea Alopecia Pulmonary fibrosis
Antimetabolites	Folic acid analogues	Methotrexate	Myelosuppression Renal damage
	Pyrimidine analogues	• 5-fluorouracil • Cytosine arabinoside	Anorexia Nausea Stomatitis Diarrhea Myelosuppression
	Purine analogues	6-mercaptopurine	Myelosuppression Bile stasis Nausea Vomiting Hepatocellular dysfunction

TABLE 12-1. Adverse effects of cytotoxic agents—cont'd

Group	Subgroup	Generic name (brand)	Adverse effects
Naturally occurring products	Vinca alkaloids	Vinblastine (Velban)	Myelosuppression Nausea Local phlebitis Depression Constipation
		Vincristine (VCR, Oncovin)	Peripheral neuropathy Autonomic neuropathy Alopecia
	Antibiotics	Doxorubicin (Adriamycin)	Myelosuppression Alopecia Nausea Vomiting Myocardial damage (doses >500 mg/m^2)
		Daunorubicin (Daunomycin)	Cardiotoxicity Myelosuppression Nausea Vomiting Alopecia
		Bleomycin (Blenoxane)	Fever Alopecia Skin and nail changes Acute pulmonary edema (hypersensitivity) Pulmonary fibrosis (usually over 300 U/m^2, enhanced by high F_IO_2) Minimal myelosuppression
		Dactinomycin (Actinomycin D)	Myelosuppression Nausea Vomiting Local inflammation
		Mithramycin (Mithracin)	Fall in elevated Ca^{++} levels Nausea, vomiting Myelosuppression Hepatotoxicity Nephrotoxicity

Continued.

TABLE 12-1. Adverse effects of cytotoxic agents—cont'd

Group	Subgroup	Generic name (brand)	Adverse effects
		Mitomycin C (Mutamycin)	Myelosuppression Nausea Local inflammation
	Enzymes	L-asparaginase (Elspar)	Nausea Hepatotoxicity Pancreatitis Urticaria Anaphylaxis Decreased fibrinogen
Synthetics	Platinum coordination complexes	Cisplatin, DDP (Platinol)	Nausea Vomiting Renal damage Ototoxicity Peripheral neuropathy
	Substituted urea	Hydroxyurea (Hydrea)	Myelosuppression Nausea Alopecia Skin atrophy Teratogenesis
	Methylhydrazine derivative	Procarbazine (Matulane)	Nausea Myelosuppression CNS depression Peripheral neuropathy

HEMOGLOBINOPATHIES

Over 100 different inherited hemoglobinopathies have been described. Altered hemoglobin structure often results in dysfunction.

Sickle Cell Disease

General Characteristics

1. Hemoglobin S is the result of valine substituted for glutamic acid at position 6 on the β-chain of hemoglobin. This error is transmitted by a single gene, and the homozygote has more hemoglobin S than the heterozygote. The severity of the disease is proportional to the amount of hemoglobin S present and also is related to other factors (amount of Hb A, fetal Hb, and interaction with β-thalassemia).
2. The gene for Hb S occurs in 10% of the blacks in North America, and is also seen in Hispanics.
3. Heterozygotes usually have sickle cell trait but rarely present serious clinical problems.

Physiology

Homozygotes, with a high proportion of Hb S, have sickled red blood cells when the hemoglobin is deoxygenated. Sickling leads to increased hemolysis and formation of sickle cell aggregates. These aggregates may cause microembolic vasoocclusion with subsequent organ ischemia and infarction.

Clinical Manifestations

1. The hemolytic anemia may be severe because of rapid clearance of sickled cells.
2. Splenomegaly, jaundice, bone marrow hyperplasia, and reticulosis are common. Autosplenectomy may occur by 4 to 5 years of age because of splenic infarction.
3. The lungs, bones, brain, and liver are also susceptible to infarction. CNS disturbances may include seizures and impairment of intellect.
4. Death may occur from peripheral circulatory failure (peak age of 6 to 18 months), which has presenting symptoms of cough, fever, diarrhea, vomiting, pallor, and drowsiness.
5. During childhood, acute episodes of vasoocclusion, or sickling crises, develop. Pain, especially in the limbs, may necessitate hospitalization. These patients may show symptoms such as pyrexia, tachycardia, and mild dehydration that worsens vascular sludging. Aplastic crises or episodes of bone-marrow hypoplasia may occur, and infections may be a recurring problem.
6. The kidney is particularly vulnerable to infarction, with loss of function accompanying severe pain. Renal function may be compromised, though progression to significant renal disease is uncommon during childhood.
7. Growth problems, leg ulcers, and priapism leading to impotence may be seen in adolescents.
8. Chest pain and cough may indicate a syndrome involving unilateral or bilateral lung consolidation.
9. Chronic treatment consists of transfusions, hydration, antibiotics, and in some patients, splenectomy.

Anesthetic Management

1. These patients may come to the operating room for removal of pigment gallstones, drainage or shunting in priapism, grafting for leg ulcers, cautery for epistaxis, or with pain from vasoocclusive disorders that can mimic osteomyelitis or abdominal emergencies, in addition to requiring surgery for lesions unrelated to sickle cell disease.
2. Vascular stasis is a particular hazard to these patients. The propensity to vascular stasis is caused by the increased viscosity of blood with sickle cells, which may be worsened by intraoperative hypothermia, diminished perfusion from low cardiac output, dehydration, and hypovolemia. Use of tourniquets should be avoided.
3. Hypoxia also can trigger sickling crises. Although pulse oximetry may be valid with oxyhemoglobin S, it is totally inaccurate with deoxygenated, polymerized Hgb S. It is safer to decrease hemoglobin S by exchange transfusions than to rely on the accuracy of pulse oximetry to alert the

anesthetist to patient hypoxia. For elective surgery, hemoglobin S should be less than 30% after exchange transfusion and overall hemoglobin should be greater than 10 g/dl.

4. Spinal anesthesia has been in disfavor with some because of the potential for hypotension and decreased tissue perfusion.
5. These surgical patients will benefit from the intensive-care setting postoperatively. Hypoxia must be avoided. Aseptic techniques should be strictly observed in intravenous cannulation and administration of drugs. Adequate hydration must be maintained. Postoperative pain should be reduced to avoid increases in catecholamines and decreased regional perfusion. Patient-controlled analgesia is ideal for older children (see Chapter 22).

Thalassemia

General Characteristics

1. Thalassemia syndromes are a group of common hereditary anemias characterized by reduced production of one or more of the normal globin chains of hemoglobin. The thalassemia is characterized by the hemoglobin chain that is produced at a reduced rate.
2. Production of α- and β-globulins usually is coordinated to produce balanced tetramers. Unbalanced synthesis leads to anemia because there is less functional hemoglobin present.
3. Hemolysis and severe anemia may develop if accumulation of the unaffected globin chain damages the red cells.

α-Thalassemia

1. This disease occurs primarily in people of Mediterranean, African, or Asian descent but is not limited to those groups. Its geographic distribution may suggest a protective effect against malaria.
2. Clinical severity of the disorder is related to abnormalities in one to four of the α-globin genes giving rise to four clinical syndromes.
   a. The silent carrier state has three functioning α-genes and is difficult to detect clinically.
   b. α-Thalassemia trait has two functioning α-globin genes and results in a mild anemia similar to iron deficiency anemia.
   c. Hemoglobin H disease (named after hemoglobin H, a tetramer of 4 β-globin chains) has one functioning α-globin gene and presents with a mild-to-moderate hemolytic anemia. Hemoglobin levels will range from 5 to 10 g/dl. Hemoglobin H comprises 5% to 30% of the hemoglobin in the erythrocyte. It has a markedly increased O_2 affinity, with a reduction in release of O_2 to the tissues. These red cells will hemolyze easily as a result of hemoglobin H oxidation. Patients may have splenomegaly, or skeletal changes from marrow hyperplasia. Exposure to oxidant drugs (see the box on the next page) may accelerate hemoglobin H oxidation and precipitate a hemolytic crisis.
   d. Homozygous α-thalassemia has no functioning α-globin chains and is a fatal disease.

DRUGS WITH OXIDANT PROPERTIES

Prilocaine	Vitamin K	Penicillamine
Benzocaine	Methylene blue	Nitrofurantoin
Phenacetin	Quinidine	Sulfones
Aspirin	Nitroprusside	Antimalarials
Acetaminophen	Sulfonamides	Chloramphenicol
Amyl Nitrate		

β-Thalassemia

1. β-thalassemia syndromes produce severe hemolytic anemias.
2. It was described originally in people of Mediterranean descent but it is found in people of almost any background.
3. As with α-thalassemia, β-thalassemia may be a result of many different genetic defects.
4. Homozygous β-thalassemia also is known as thalassemia major or Cooley's anemia. These patients have a severe hemolytic anemia. Most patients require chronic transfusions to survive. Homozygous individuals usually have splenomegaly and bone marrow hyperplasia and may be folate deficient. Hypersplenism may be treated by splenectomy. In patients who are transfused frequently, iron overload may be the predominant problem. Iron toxicity may cause liver dysfunction, pancreatic injury with glucose intolerance, and cardiomyopathy. Congestive heart failure is the most common cause of death.
5. β-thalassemia intermedia describes the less-severe form of homozygous disease (often found in blacks), characterized by less hemolysis and infrequent transfusion requirements.
6. Thalassemia minor causes less-severe anemia because there is one normal β-gene and the δ- (hemoglobin A2) and γ- (fetal hemoglobin F) genes are able to compensate. Clinically these patients appear to have iron deficiency anemia. Transfusions or splenectomy rarely are needed.

Anesthetic Considerations

1. The primary anesthetic concerns for thalassemia patients is level of anemia and oxygen-carrying capacity. Many of these patients have hypersplenism and coagulation defects. Preoperatively, CBC, platelets, and coagulation studies including bleeding time should be obtained. Transfusion may be necessary in the severely anemic patient. A total hemoglobin of 8 to 10 g/dl should be sufficient for surgery (exception: Hemoglobin H, see no. 6 at the top of the next page.)
2. Patients who have had frequent transfusion should be evaluated for signs of iron toxicity.
3. Bone marrow hyperplasia can cause overgrowth of the maxilla, causing difficult laryngoscopy.
4. Patients who have had a splenectomy will have decreased resistance to certain infections.

5. The anesthetic technique should encompass high concentrations of inspired oxygen, normocapnia to improve oxygen delivery, and decreased myocardial and tissue demand (e.g., avoiding tachycardia).
6. Hemoglobin H does not allow effective oxygen delivery to the tissues. The amount of hemoglobin H must be subtracted from the total hemoglobin when assessing need for transfusion. Oxidant drugs should be avoided because they will accelerate the rate of hemoglobin H oxidation and the rate of hemolysis.

COAGULOPATHIES

See Fig. 12-1 on opposite page for coagulation cascade.

Hemophilia

General Characteristics

1. Hemophilia is an X-linked recessive trait.
2. It affects only males but is carried by heterozygous females.
3. Hemophilia A, a deficiency of factor VIII, is clinically indistinguishable from hemophilia B, a factor IX deficiency that is much rarer.
4. A level of factor VIII activity below 3% is seen with severe hemophilia.
5. In some patients (5% to 10%) a milder form of hemophilia is seen with factor VIII activity of 5% or more.
6. Factor VIII deficiency also is seen in von Willebrand's disease.

Clinical Manifestations

1. Severe hemophilia usually involves a bleeding tendency in the first year of life, sometimes at circumcision.
2. Hemarthroses may be seen in the first few years of life.
3. Spontaneous hemorrhages occur during childhood, especially in the deeper tissues such as the psoas muscle, retroperitoneal space, joints, and bladder (hematuria).
4. Milder hemophilia may show excessive bleeding only after surgery or dental extraction.
5. Detection may follow screening coagulation tests in small children. Clotting time may be prolonged with a normal bleeding time.

Anesthetic Management

1. Factor VIII levels should be replenished before surgery, in consultation with the patient's hematologist. Factor VIII activity should be greater than 20% of normal (see the box on p. 268 for sources of factor VIII and relative activity). One unit of factor VIII is the activity present in 1 ml of fresh pooled normal plasma. A formula to determine the number of units of factor required is:

$$\frac{\text{body weight (kg)} \times \text{percent desired increase in activity}}{1.5}$$

That is, 1 U/kg body weight increases the factor VIII concentration by 1.5%. If the desired increment in factor VIII activity is 40% in a 20-kg child the units of factor VIII needed are 20 × 40/1.5 = 533 U (533 ml pooled normal plasma).

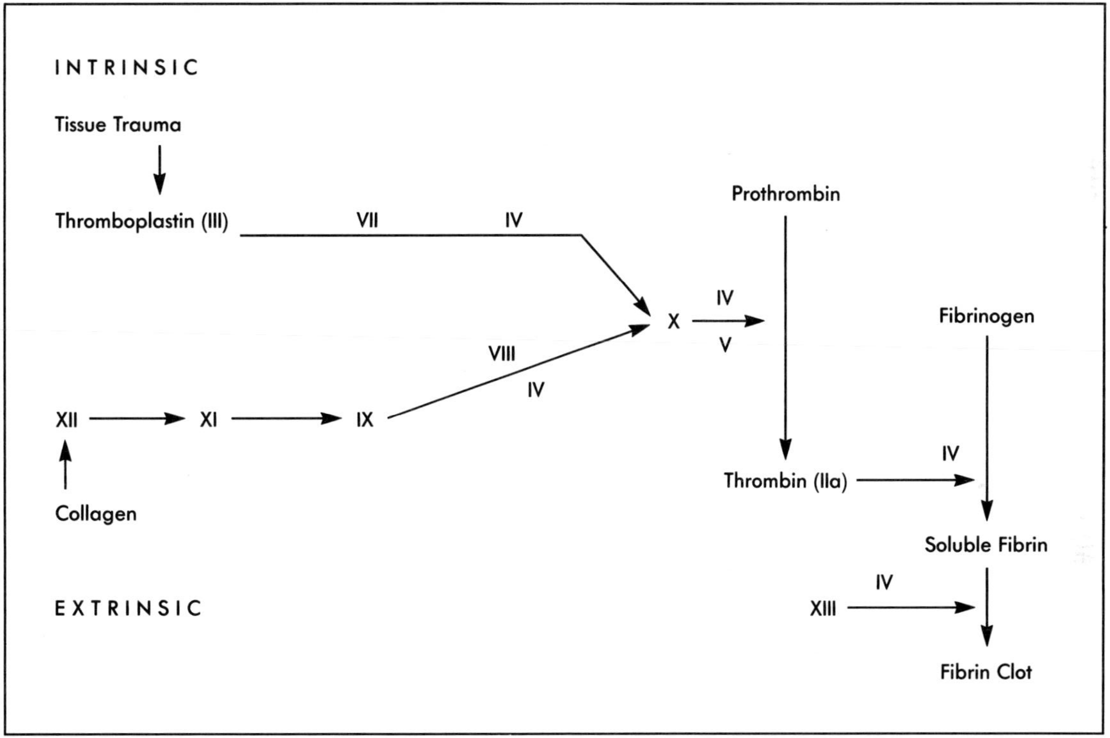

Fig. 12-1. The coagulation cascade. Intact intrinsic and extrinsic pathways leading to a common final pathway are necessary for normal coagulation.

Sources of factor VIII	Activity
FFP	0.7 μ/ml
Dried factor VIII fraction	25 μ/ml (after reconstitution)
Cryoprecipitate	75-100 μ/bag
Desmopressin (DDAVP)	Increases factor VIII level in blood 300% to 600% (only useful in mild cases)

2. Intramuscular injections are contraindicated. Venous cannulation should be done cautiously to preserve future access and avoid hematoma formation.
3. Patients should be tested for factor VIII antibody. All elective procedures in patients with antibody should be avoided. Sometimes porcine sources of factor VIII will suffice, but it is important to be ready to treat anaphylaxis.
4. Because hemophiliacs frequently have had multiple transfusions of blood products they are at increased risk for harboring hepatitis B antigen or human immunodeficiency virus.
5. Preoperative anemia can be treated with transfusion, but it is still important to correct the bleeding tendency by factor VIII infusion. Emergently, if factor VIII is not available, fresh frozen plasma (20 ml/kg) should be given preoperatively.
6. The anesthesiologist should avoid any procedures that may lead to hemorrhage. Instrumentation of the upper airway should be minimized. Nasal intubation should be avoided.

von Willebrand's Disease

General Characteristics

1. von Willebrand's disease is an autosomal dominant coagulation defect affecting both sexes. The specific defect probably is caused by the deficiency of a protein known as von Willebrand's factor, which is important for factor VIII activity and platelet function.
2. Patients have decreased factor VIII, with an increased bleeding time and impaired platelet function.
3. Patients can have epistaxis, mucosal bleeding, increased bruising, or excessive bleeding at surgery.

Treatment

1. Treatment before surgery includes cryoprecipitate administration to supply factor VIII and von Willebrand's factor (factor VIII concentrates alone are not effective).
2. Desmopressin (DDAVP) also will stimulate the release of von Willebrand's factor. The DDAVP dose for adults and children is 0.3 μg/kg over a 15- to 30-minute period.

Idiopathic Thrombocytopenic Purpura (ITP)

General Characteristics

A severe deficiency of circulating platelets is typical of ITP despite adequate quantities of megakaryocytes in the marrow. It is likely that an immune mechanism is responsible for the thrombocytopenia. Platelet antibodies rarely are detected, but high levels of IgG have been found bound to platelets.

Clinical Manifestations

1. Seventy percent of patients have an antecedent viral infection present 1 to 4 weeks before the onset of purpura.
2. Patients will have widespread purpura and petechiae. There may be nasal or oral bleeding, hematuria, or GI bleeding.
3. Diagnosis is based on history, clinical picture, CBC, and a bone marrow biopsy.

Treatment

1. Mild cases with a platelet count above 25,000 and without significant clinical bleeding may resolve spontaneously within a few weeks.
2. ITP may be more severe and persistent, requiring steroid therapy. Ten percent of ITP patients will require splenectomy.

Anesthetic Management

1. Stress doses of steroids may need to be given in patients who have been treated with steroids (hydrocortisone 4 to 8 mg/kg in three divided doses).
2. Intramuscular injections are contraindicated.
3. Regional techniques should be avoided.
4. Platelet concentrates should be available and given in doses of 1 U/5 kg (0.2 U/kg) to correct thrombocytopenia when indicated. ABO cross-matching is necessary. Microfilters may remove platelets and should not be used. If a splenectomy is being performed, platelets should not be given until the splenic pedicle is clamped.
5. After splenectomy, antibiotics may prevent overwhelming infection.
6. Sterile technique in the operating room should be meticulous to avoid infection in the splenectomy and postsplenectomy patient.

Polycythemia

Etiology

1. The diagnosis of polycythemia is made where there is a concentration of hemoglobin that is consistently higher than 22 g/dl in neonates and higher than 17 g/dl in children.
2. Polycythemias are extremely rare in children except when they are associated with chronic arterial desaturation. Renal hypoxia results in increased production of erythropoietin, stimulating increased production of red blood cells. Cardiovascular anomalies involving right-to-left shunts and pulmonary diseases resulting in impaired oxygenation are the most common causes of secondary polycythemia.
3. Living at high altitudes can also cause secondary polycythemia. Hemoglobin level will increase about 4% for each rise of 1000 m in altitude.

4. The etiology of neonatal polycythemia includes fetal hypoxia, intrauterine transfusion, or twin-to-twin transfusion. If polycythemia is severe the neonate may have seizures, heart failure, respiratory distress and thrombosis of peripheral blood vessels or the renal vein, brain damage, and necrotizing enterocolitis.

Clinical Manifestations

1. Clinical findings may include cyanosis, digital clubbing, and hyperemia of sclerae and mucous membranes.
2. Above a hematocrit of 70% there is a marked increase in blood viscosity, hindering perfusion to tissues.
3. In severe cases of polycythemia the usual postnatal fall in hemoglobin is absent. Anemia will develop months later; with iron therapy, the hematocrit may rise to 75% or more.

Treatment

If the hematocrit is above 60% to 70%, partial exchange transfusion should be performed with fresh frozen plasma or albumin. A guide for transfusion is:

$$Vol_E = \frac{BV \times (Hct_o - Hct_d)}{Hct_o}$$

where

Vol_E = volume of exchange
BV = blood volume
Hct_o = observed hematocrit
Hct_d = desired hematocrit

IMMUNODEFICIENCY (AIDS)

Multiple congenital and acquired diseases may result in varying degrees of immunodeficiency (see the box on the next page). However, human immunodeficiency virus (HIV) is now a leading cause of immunodeficiency in the infant and the child. Conservative estimates project that there will be 3000 children with AIDS in the United States by 1991. In the majority of HIV infected children the virus apparently is transmitted from mother to child, although it may be transmitted by sexual contact, blood transfusion, or inoculations by body secretions.

Laboratory Diagnosis

Serodiagnosis in the infant can be difficult. Infants may have placental transfer of maternal antibodies to HIV. Passively acquired antibodies may persist for months to over a year, and may result in false-positive diagnostic tests. A seropositive child less than 15 months of age must have other clinical or laboratory evidence of HIV infection to be considered infected (Fig. 12-2). Conversely, a child infected with a virus may not exhibit antibody response for months, resulting in false-negative initial diagnostic tests. The interval from infection to seroconversion in children is unknown.

DISEASES ASSOCIATED WITH IMMUNODEFICIENCY

Primary immunodeficiencies

- Panhypogammaglobulinemia (Bruton disease)
- Selective deficiency of IgA
- Selective deficiency of IgM
- IgG subgroup deficiency
- DiGeorge syndrome
- Nezelof syndrome
- Cartilage-hair hypoplasia
- Combined immunodeficiency disease
- Omenn disease
- Wiskott-Aldrich syndrome
- Ataxia-telangiectasia
- Chronic mucocutaneous candidiasis
- Graft-versus-host disease

Secondary immunodeficiencies

- Adenosine deaminase deficiency
- Nucleoside phosphorylase deficiency
- Loss of immunologic materials
  - Nephrotic syndrome
  - Protein-losing enteropathy
  - Loss from lymphatic system
- Viral infections
- Nutritional deficiency
- Chemical or physical immunosuppression
- Blood transfusions

Physiology

1. The HIV virus infects the helper-inducer subset of T-lymphocytes, as well as the monocyte-macrophage lineage. This causes suppression of helper T-cell numbers and function and an increase in suppressor T-cells.
2. Early B-cell dysfunction in children who lack preexisting antibodies results in more problems with bacterial infections than are manifested in adult patients. Defective B-cell function also leads to impaired antibody production.

Clinical Manifestations

1. Craniofacial abnormalities suggest early antenatal infection including microcephaly, box-like forehead, ocular hypertelorism, nasal and ocular anomalies, and patulous lips.
2. Congenitally infected children usually become symptomatic by 4 to 6 months of age and may have lymphadenopathy and hepatomegaly at birth or even opportunistic infections in the first month of life.
3. Children are more likely than adults to develop serious bacterial infection, which is the most common initial manifestation, including *Streptococcus, Haemophilus, Staphylococcus, Salmonella,* and *Pseudomonas.*

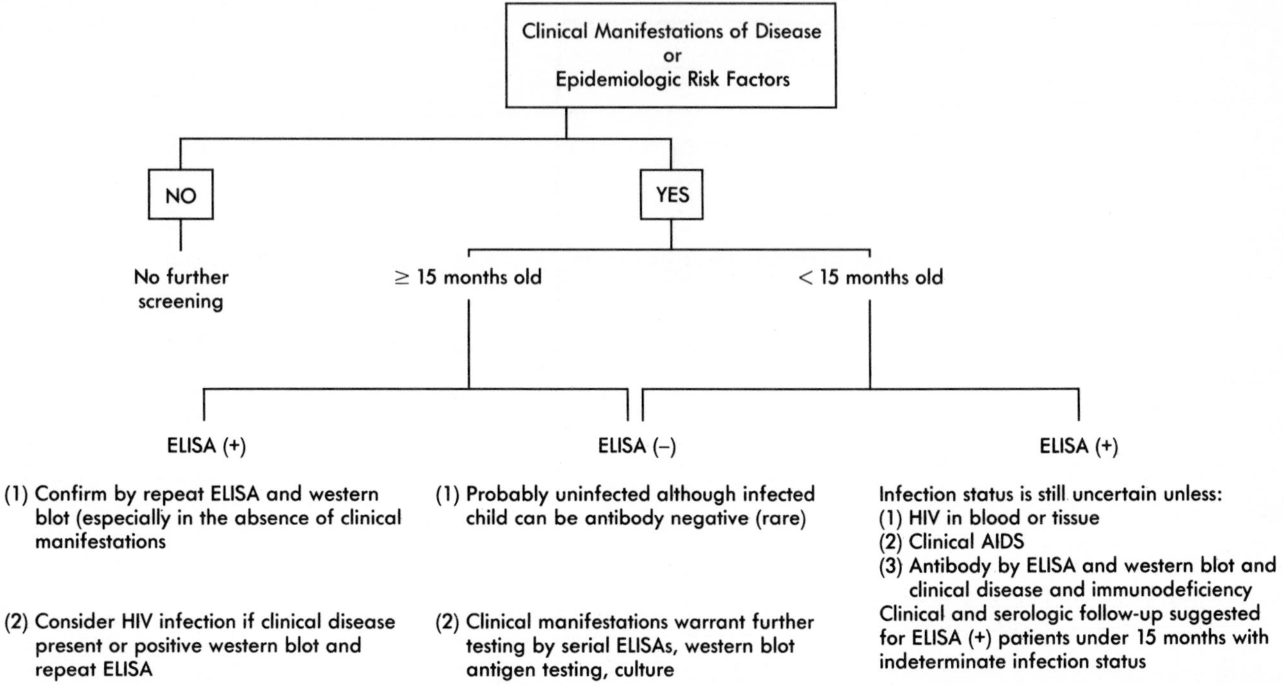

Fig. 12-2. Testing for HIV infection in children. (Adapted from Falloon J and others: Human immunodeficiency virus infection in children, J Pediatr 114:1-30, 1989.)

4. HIV-infected children frequently develop a characteristic encephalopathy that causes developmental delays, behavioral abnormalities, paresis or palsy, and ataxia. Seizures are not typical.
5. Unlike adults, lymphocytic interstitial pneumonitis (LIP) occurs in about half of the children with AIDS. Although the prognosis is better than for children with pneumocystis, hypoxemia can occur with progressive pulmonary dysfunction.
6. *Pneumocystis carinii* pneumonia presents more acutely with fever, dyspnea, cough, hypoxemia, and rales/rhonchi on auscultation.
7. Nonopportunistic viral infections such as varicella, herpes zoster, and rubeola can cause severe morbidity.
8. Kaposi's sarcoma is very rare in children.
9. Abnormalities of all organ systems can be present including:
   a. Hepatitis
   b. Azotemia
   c. Cardiomyopathy
   d. Retinal perivasculitis
   e. Anemia, neutropenia, thrombocytopenia, and coagulopathy
   f. Nonspecific findings including failure to thrive, weight loss, diarrhea, fever, and dermatitis

Drug Therapy

AZT (Azidothymidine)

1. Nucleoside analogue antiretroviral
2. Good absorption orally
3. Satisfactory CNS penetration
4. Toxic effects include macrocytosis, anemia, neutropenia, pancytopenia, headache, nausea, myalgia, and neurologic symptoms

Trimethoprim-Sulfamethoxazole

1. Used to treat *Pneumocystis* pneumonia
2. Toxic effects include leukopenia, rash, thrombocytopenia, fever, and hepatitis

Pentamidine

1. Used to treat *Pneumocystis* if patient cannot tolerate trimethoprim-sulfamethoxazole
2. Toxic effects include azotemia, leukopenia, thrombocytopenia, hypoglycemia and diabetes, hepatitis, hypotension, and sterile abscesses (if given intramuscularly)

Anesthetic Management

1. The anesthesiologist should assume that all patients potentially are infected with the virus and practice appropriate precautions.
2. Care should be exercised to avoid introducing bacteria into the patient's system during venous cannulation and airway management.
3. Anesthetic care should be dictated by the patient's condition. Nutritional deficits or mild anemia may require few changes in the planned anesthetic.

Conversely, it is not unusual for patients in extremis, particularly with *Pneumocystis carinii* pneumonia, to present for biopsy or placement of indwelling central venous catheter. "Do not resuscitate" decisions made by primary-care physicians and families to avoid prolonged intubation may be impossible to follow during general anesthesia. Management plans and anesthetic morbidity need to be discussed in detail with the family, primary physicians, and surgeons before entering the operating room.

BIBLIOGRAPHY

Berger JJ, Modell JH, and Sypert GW, editors: Megaloblastic anemia and brief exposure to nitrous oxide—a causal relationship, Anesth Analg 67:197-98, 1988.

Bunn HF: Disorders of hemoglobin. In Wilson JD and others, editors: Harrison's principles of internal medicine, ed 12, New York, 1988, McGraw Hill.

Cooper RA and Bunn HF: Hemolytic anemias. In Wilson JD and others, editors: Harrison's principles of internal medicine, ed 12, New York, 1988, McGraw Hill.

Cote CJ: Blood replacement and blood product management. In Ryan JF and others, editors: A practice of anesthesia for infants and children, Orlando, Fla, 1986, Grune & Stratton.

Falloon J and others: Human immunodeficiency virus infection in children, J Pediatr 114:1-30, 1989.

Gibson JR: Anesthetic implications of sickle cell disease and other hemoglobinopathies. In Barash P, editor: American Society of Anesthesiologists Refresher Course, vol 14, Philadelphia, 1986, JB Lippincott Co.

Hain WR: Diseases of blood. In Katz J and Steward DJ, editors: Anesthesia and uncommon pediatric diseases, Philadelphia, 1987, WB Saunders Co.

Keifer JC, Russell GB, and Snider MT: Pulse oximetry inaccuracy with sickle hemoglobin: is it due to different absorption spectra? Anesthesiology 71(3):A370, 1989.

Keitt AS: Introduction to the anemias. In Wyngaarden JB and Smith LH: Cecil textbook of medicine, ed 18, Philadelphia, 1988, WB Saunders Co.

Keitt AS: Anemia due to bone marrow failure. In Wyngaarden JB and Smith LH: Cecil textbook of medicine, ed 18, Philadelphia, 1988, WB Saunders Co.

Kushner JP: Hypochromic anemias. In Wyngaarden JB and Smith LH: Cecil textbook of medicine, ed 18, Philadelphia, 1988, WB Saunders Co.

Pearson HA: Diseases of the blood: developments of the hematopoietic system. In Nelson WE, editor: Textbook of pediatrics, ed 13, Philadelphia, 1987, WB Saunders Co.

Rubin P: Clinical oncology: a multidisciplinary approach, ed 6, Rochester, NY, 1983, American Cancer Society.

Stoelting RK and Dierdorf SF, McCammon RL: Anesthesia and co-existing disease, ed 2, New York, 1988, Churchill Livingstone.

Williams WJ, editor: Hematology, ed 3, New York, 1983, McGraw Hill.

13

ANESTHETIC MANAGEMENT OF PEDIATRIC NEUROLOGIC DISORDERS

Cindy W. Hughes

Jack and Jill went up the hill,
to fetch a pail of water;
Jack fell down and broke his crown,
And Jill came tumbling after.
ANON

INTRACRANIAL DYNAMICS

The management of neurosurgical problems in infants and children is based upon an understanding of intracranial physiology and the differences between children and adults.

Increased Intracranial Pressure (ICP) in Children

1. The normal ICP in children is ≤15 mm Hg; the same as in adults.
2. Increased ICP is often difficult to diagnose in infants and young children, because open suture lines increase the compliance of the cranial vault. When pressures are sufficiently high and sustained there will be bulging of the fontanelle and eyes. Eventually there will be an increase in head circumference and the presence of "sunset eyes."
3. Neurologic signs of ICP are diffuse and nonspecific. The child is either increasingly irritable or increasingly sedate. There is a slowing of motor responses to both painful and nonpainful stimuli.
4. Because of open sutures the typical Cushing response to raised ICP (hypertension, bradycardia, and dilated pupils) usually is not present in infants. Papilledema is also unusual, despite high intracranial pressures.

5. To diagnose increased ICP in infants and children a CT scan of the head is essential because of the vague neurologic symptoms and inconsistency of the usual physical signs. The scan reveals diffuse edema, small obliterated ventricles, midline shift, and masses.

Control of ICP

The intracranial vault contains the brain parenchyma and fluid. The three fluid compartments are the interstitial fluid (80%), blood (10%) and cerebrospinal fluid (CSF; 10%). ICP is controlled by the manipulation of these three fluid compartments.

Cerebrospinal Fluid

Production. CSF is produced in the choroid plexus and renewed five times a day. An adult will produce as much as 750 ml/day. Production in children varies with age and pathophysiology. Infants may produce 100 ml/day.[1]

Production of CSF is not affected by changes in ICP. It can be decreased by certain drugs: furosemide, steroids, and acetazolamide. These drugs, however, only have a temporary effect upon production.

Reabsorption. Reabsorption of CSF occurs in the arachnoid villi. Although the arachnoid villi can compensate and increase CSF reabsorption during periods of increased ICP, the process is limited. Intracranial hemorrhage, infection, and many central nervous system congenital malformations decrease the rate of CSF absorption.

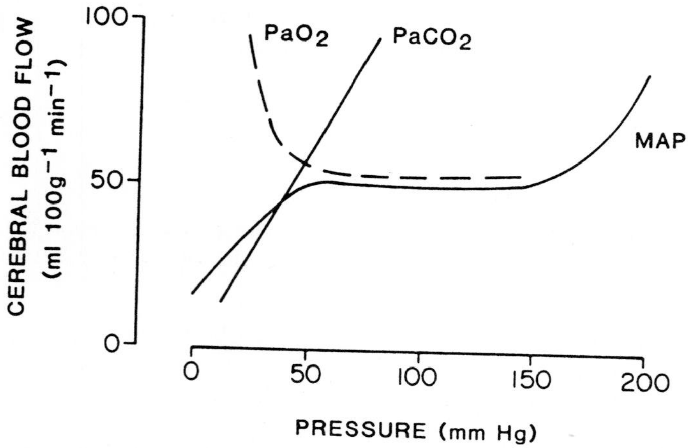

Fig. 13-1. Cerebral blood flow is influenced by arterial oxygenation (PaO_2), alveolar ventilation ($PaCO_2$), and mean arterial pressure (MAP). (Stoelting RK; Central nervous system. In *Pharmacology and physiology in anesthetic practice,* Philadelphia, JB Lippincott, 1987, p 587, with permission.)

Cerebral Blood Flow (CBF)

Physiology. CBF determines the level of cerebral blood volume (CBV) at any given time. The blood flow depends upon metabolic demand or cerebral metabolic rate of oxygen consumption ($CMRO_2$). The local pH of brain tissue (concentration of H^+ ions) can be a reflection of acidosis, ischemia, or hypercarbia. A decrease in pH causes an increase in CBF and thus CBV. *Autoregulation.* The central nervous system is one of the three tissue beds that can autoregulate its blood flow in order to maintain cerebral perfusion over a wide range of blood pressures (MAP = 50 to 150 mm Hg). Cerebral blood flow is also very reactive to changes in $PaCO_2$; they are correlated linearly between 20 and 80 mm Hg (Fig. 13-1).[2]

The figures for cerebral autoregulation in children are unknown, but it is considered an intact mechanism at even very low blood pressures. As in adults, the CBF is very sensitive to changes in $PaCO_2$ between 20 and 80 mm Hg.

The immature autonomic nervous system of the premature infant results in impaired myogenic control of arteriolar resistance. Cerebral perfusion in these children depends upon systemic blood pressure. Therefore they are prone to intracerebral hemorrhages when stressed or hypertensive.

Lowering ICP

(See the box below.)

MANEUVERS TO LOWER ELEVATED ICP

Hyperventilation

PCO_2 25-30 mm Hg
CBF decreases 4% for each 1 mm Hg decrease in PCO_2
Cerebral ischemia is associated with a PCO_2 <20 mm Hg

Diuretics

Furosemide 0.5-1.0 mg/kg IV
Mannitol 0.5-1.0 g/kg IV

Steroids

Hydrocortisone 1.0-1.5 mg/kg/dose IV
Dexamethasone 0.5-1.5 mg/kg IV (loading dose)
0.25-0.5 mg/kg/dose IV (maintenance)

CSF drainage

HR, BP, and pupils are monitored carefully during removal of CSF.

Position

Elevate head of bed 30-45 degrees.

1. *Hyperventilation.* In children, lowering PCO_2 affects cerebral autoregulation and decreases the CBF by arteriolar vasoconstriction. The effects of lowered PCO_2 in neonates are not well described. The effects of hyperventilation last longer in a child than in an adult (6 hours).[3]
2. *Diuretics.* Furosemide decreases the production of CSF, the amount of interstitial fluid, and the circulating blood volume.

   Osmotic diuretics such as mannitol decrease the amount of interstitial fluid and the circulating blood volume.

3. *Removal of CSF*. The rapid removal of CSF by subarachnoid or ventricular drainage in the presence of elevated ICP can result in herniation of the cerebellar tonsils.
4. *Steroids*. Steroids restore the integrity of the blood-brain barrier in abnormal/ischemic tissue and decrease production of CSF.
5. *Position*. Raising the head of the patient by 30 to 45 degrees facilitates jugular venous drainage, decreasing venous congestion and CBV.

PREOPERATIVE ASSESSMENT
Physical Examination

1. A complete history and physical examination focusing on the neurologic defects should be performed. Many neurologic defects are associated with other problems (e.g., meningomyelocele and Arnold-Chiari syndrome, craniosynostosis and Apert's syndrome or Crouzon's disease).
2. Signs or symptoms of raised ICP are noted, including nausea, vomiting, hypertension, increased head circumference, and lethargy or irritability. All neurologic deficits should be documented before the administration of anesthesia or onset of surgical procedures. The presence of raised ICP or substantial neurologic impairment will influence induction techniques and agents, airway management, and the choice of muscle relaxants.
3. The patient should be examined for an intact gag reflex and swallowing mechanism. Airway protection may be limited in patients with hypotonia, a history of aspiration pneumonia, and bulbar symptoms.

Premedication
Indications

Indications for premedication include the presence of vascular anomalies (arteriovenous malformation [AVM] or aneurysm). These children need to be as sedate as possible without depressing ventilation. Appropriate drug choices include hypnotics, barbiturates and benzodiazepines (Table 13-1). Narcotics are usually avoided.

Contraindications

Premedication usually is *contraindicated* when it depresses ventilation, which can markedly increase ICP, or if it alters neurologic assessment.

TABLE 13-1. Premedication for children with intracranial vascular anomalies

Drug	Dose	Route
Diazepam	0.2 mg/kg	PO
Midazolam	0.06-0.08 mg/kg	IM
Pentobarbital	4-5 mg/kg	PO/IM
Chloral hydrate	20-50 mg/kg	PO
Methohexital	20-30 mg/kg	PR

MONITORING

ASA Standards

1. The noninvasive monitoring of a pediatric patient for a neurosurgical procedure should meet the ASA standards of monitoring, which include the following:
   - ECG
   - Blood pressure cuff
   - Pulse oximeter
   - Auscultation of heart and breath sounds
   - Temperature monitoring
   - Monitoring of expired gas for CO_2
2. Invasive monitoring with an arterial catheter is recommended for:
   - Close hemodynamic control of blood pressure
   - Frequent sampling of blood for arterial blood gasses ($PaCO_2$), hematocrit, and electrolytes
   - The transducer level should be adjusted depending on the patient's head level; the lateral corner of the eye is used as a landmark when the patient's head is elevated during the procedure.
3. A precordial doppler is recommended for procedures done in the sitting position to detect possible air emboli.
4. Cerebral evoked potentials (mapping) are monitored during selected procedures.
5. Urinary output should be measured during major intracranial operations, when diuretics are employed, when a lengthy operation is planned, and when major blood loss and volume replacement are anticipated.

POSITIONING

Sitting Position

The sitting position is used rarely in young children, because it does little to improve the surgical exposure. Use of the sitting position for older children necessitates monitoring for venous air emboli with a precordial doppler and placement of a central venous catheter for extraction of air.

Prone Position

The prone position commonly is used for spinal procedures (e.g., repair of meningomyelocele and release of tethered cord). Attention to endotracheal tube placement and patency is essential in this position. Some advocate the use of a nasotracheal or wire-reinforced tube. Pressure on the posterior pharynx and larynx caused by the natural curve of the endotracheal tube can lead to postoperative airway edema and obstruction.

AGENTS FOR INDUCTION AND MAINTENANCE OF ANESTHESIA

1. Laryngoscopy and endotracheal intubation can increase ICP if either coughing or hypertension and tachycardia occur. This response can be attenuated by several agents (Table 13-2).
2. It is ideal to insert an IV before induction when increased ICP is sus-

TABLE 13-2. Agents for induction and maintenance of anesthesia in patients with elevated intracranial pressure

Drug	Effects
Intravenous agents	
Barbiturates	Lower ICP by producing dose-dependent depression of CBF and $CMRO_2$ up to a maximum of 40% to 50% of normal, correlating with a quiet EEG
Lidocaine	Can decrease the response to intubation if given intratracheally or intravenously several minutes before intubation as an adjunct to induction
Benzodiazepines	Evidence is controversial regarding the effects on CBF and $CMRO_2$, but both most likely are decreased; Probably best used as a premedicant
Etomidate	Can produce up to a 50% decrease in CBF and $CMRO_2$ with EEG suppression similar to barbituates; Not widely used in pediatrics; Can suppress adrenal function
Ketamine	Generally contraindicated because it causes cerebral stimulation; Increases ICP, CBF, and $CMRO_2$
Opioids	Increase cerebrovascular resistance and decrease CBF and $CMRO_2$ (Fentanyl >morphine >meperidine); Very high doses of fentanyl and sufentanil have precipitated seizures in animal models
Inhalation agents	
Halothane	Increases ICP by increasing CBV by direct cerbrovasodilation; Decreases CSF production, but increases resistance to absorption
Enflurane	Increases ICP by cerebrovasodilation and by increasing CSF production and resistance to CSF absorption; May lower seizure threshold at >2 MAC in the face of hyperventilation
Isoflurane	Produces little change in CBF at 1 MAC; More depression of $CMRO_2$ than halothane; Less impairment of autoregulation than halothane
Nitrous Oxide	May increase ICP; Elevations of ICP can be attenuated with thiopental and hyperventilation; Should be discontinued before closure of the dura so that it does not cause expansion of closed, air-filled spaces

pected. However, it is not clear if placing an IV in a crying, struggling child is a better technique when ICP is elevated than a calm, controlled inhalation induction.

3. Controlled ventilation with a $PaCO_2$ between 25 to 30 mm Hg is critically important in the child with elevated ICP regardless of agents selected.

CHOICE OF MUSCLE RELAXANTS

Succinylcholine (Depolarizing Relaxant)

Succinylcholine administration should be avoided unless a rapid-sequence induction is indicated. It is contraindicated in muscular dystrophies, multiple sclerosis, spinal cord injuries, encephalitis, crush injuries, and burn injuries because of the risk of hyperkalemia.

Increases in ICP have been reported with succinylcholine, although these effects are attenuated by induction doses of thiopental (5 to 10 mg/kg) or pretreatment with nondepolarizing relaxants.[4]

Nondepolarizing Relaxants

1. Relaxants provide a motionless field for difficult surgical dissections.
2. Anesthetic requirements are minimal after skin incision and craniotomy; relaxants assure absence of movement even when anesthetic doses are reduced.
3. If a preexisting neurologic deficit exists, the neuromuscular blockade monitor should be placed on an unaffected limb.
4. Pancuronium may elevate ICP by increasing heart rate and blood pressure.
5. Curare and atracurium release histamine, causing vasodilation, increased CBV, and decreased cerebral perfusion pressure (CPP).
6. Laudanosine, a metabolite of atracurium, may cause cerebral stimulation, although it is probably unimportant clinically.
7. Vecuronium, devoid of hemodynamic effects, is an ideal relaxant for intracranial procedures. An infusion may be used for lengthy cases.

No Relaxants

The surgical team may request that no muscle relaxants be used, particularly during procedures on the spinal cord, when nerve function needs to be assessed intraoperatively (e.g., meningomyelocele, release of tethered cord).

The endotracheal tube can be secured with a short-acting agent (e.g., atracurium or vecuronium) and reversed before the operation and testing of nerve function. Relaxants may be avoided by inducing and intubating only with inhalation agents.

ANESTHETIC MANAGEMENT OF COMMON PEDIATRIC NEUROSURGICAL PROCEDURES

Dysraphism (Meningomyelocele, Encephalocele)

1. Adequate preoperative hydration is imperative, especially if a CSF leak exists.
2. All antibiotics should be continued.
3. Preexisting neurologic deficits should be documented.
4. The use of succinylcholine may precipitate hyperkalemia, because these infants frequently have lower motor neuron involvement.
5. The trachea may be intubated with the child awake, in the lateral position. If the defect is too large to be supported safely, the infant can be held during intubation.
6. The operation is performed in the prone position, necessitating careful padding of pressure points and a secure airway.
7. The surgeon may request that no muscle relaxant be given so that nerve function can be tested.
8. These infants will be kept in the prone position postoperatively and may require prolonged mechanical ventilation.

Hydrocephalus

1. Operations for obstructive hydrocephalus include ventriculoperitoneal shunt, ventriculoatrial shunt, ventriculopleural shunt, or fourth ventriculostomy.
2. Communicating hydrocephalus is usually corrected with a lumboperitoneal shunt.
3. These children are at risk for developing meningitis/encephalitis; careful aseptic technique should be used during venous cannulation and administration of intravenous drugs.
4. Patients are also susceptible to hypotension during CSF drainage. Blood pressure should be monitored closely and accurately.
5. Ventriculoatrial shunts pose an increased risk of air emboli. Methods to decrease the size and incidence of air emboli include the following:
   - Avoiding the use of N_2O
   - Maintaining intravenous hydration to ensure that the hydrostatic pressure in the venous circulation is high
   - Controlled positive pressure ventilation to keep venous pressure high
6. Ventriculoatrial shunts require atrial catheter placement, often under ECG guidance. The catheter should be filled with saline, and have a sterile ECG lead placed on the distal end. The P wave will be upright and get progressively larger as the proximal end of the saline-filled catheter passes through the coronary sinus. The P wave becomes biphasic in the atrium.
7. Most children can be awakened in the operating room after placement of a CSF shunt and do not require prolonged mechanical ventilation.

Craniosynostosis

1. Craniosynostosis is often found in children with dysmorphic syndromes (Apert's and Crouzon's) which are also associated with a difficult airway.
2. An increased incidence of elevated ICP is associated with craniosynostosis.
3. Craniosynostectomy often results in significant and rapid blood loss. A large-bore IV catheter is essential for volume replacement. An arterial catheter should be considered for blood pressure monitoring and following the hematocrit and blood gases.
4. Patients should be observed in the ICU after surgery because of the high risk of subdural or epidural hematoma formation.
5. Unless other medical problems are present, these children usually do not require prolonged ventilation.
6. Narcotics and sedatives should be used judiciously so as not to obscure the postoperative neurologic examination.

Aneurysms and Arteriovenous Malformations

1. Children with intracerebral vascular lesions should be premedicated before arrival in the operating room to minimize the risk of bleeding or rupture of the aneurysm caused by crying and struggling.
2. A variety of induction techniques can be used to keep the child calm. A steal induction, inhalation induction, intravenous induction, or rectal

administration of methohexital are all acceptable methods as long as coughing, which can lead to vessel rupture, is avoided.
3. The placement of at least two large-bore IV catheters will be helpful for volume resuscitation if profuse bleeding occurs.
4. An arterial catheter for blood pressure monitoring and obtaining laboratory data is essential. This can be placed after the child has been induced and the airway secured.
5. The trachea should be intubated after a muscle relaxant has been given to avoid any coughing during endotracheal tube insertion.
6. A hypotensive technique may help reduce bleeding (see Chapter 14).
7. Tracheal extubation should be accomplished with minimal coughing or bucking to decrease the risk of bleeding or rupturing sutures. Methods used to achieve a quiet extubation include the following:
   - Deep extubation (not appropriate for an infant or small toddler)
   - Extubation of the trachea while maintaining tight hemodynamic control with vasodilator agents
   - Administration of lidocaine before extubation to depress airway reflexes
8. Narcotics and sedatives should be used judiciously so that the child can cooperate fully with a neurologic examination in the postoperative period.

Intracranial Tumors

1. Signs or symptoms of raised ICP and any neurologic deficits should be documented.
2. The age, neurologic status, ICP, and associated medical conditions will determine the most appropriate induction technique including the following:
   - Inhalation
   - Intravenous
   - Rectal
3. As previously mentioned, muscle relaxants and maintenance anesthesia will provide a motionless field during tumor resection.
4. Placement of an arterial catheter is needed for the following:
   - Tight hemodynamic control
   - Obtaining laboratory data (blood gases, hematocrit, electrolytes)
5. Methods to lower ICP should be employed if raised ICP is present (see the box on p. 277).
6. Jugular venous drainage may be impaired by high peak inspiratory pressures.
7. Urine output should be monitored with an indwelling Foley catheter. When the urine output exceeds 10% of the child's estimated blood volume (EBV) after administration of diuretics, it should be replaced with dextrose 5% and 0.2% normal saline (D_5.2NS) in addition to routine maintenance fluids.
8. Many children can be awakened at the end of the procedure. Having the child alert in the postoperative period permits close monitoring of the neurologic status.
9. Prolonged intubation/ventilation may be necessary after posterior fossa

tumor resections in the prone position. The airway may be compromised by edema or loss of airway reflexes.

SEIZURE DISORDERS

Classification (See the box below)

Seizures are the clinical manifestation of a disorder of brain metabolism, infection, scarring, edema, tumor, or vascular anomaly. The seizure itself represents an excessive and usually self-limited neuronal discharge. Epilepsy is a common childhood problem, and approximately 50% of childhood epilepsy is idiopathic, with many clinical forms in existence.

INTERNATIONAL CLASSIFICATION OF EPILEPTIC SEIZURES[5]

I. Partial Seizures (beginning focally)
  A. Elementary symptomatology (generally without impairment of consciousness)
    1. With motor symptoms
    2. With special sensory or somatosensory symptoms
    3. With autonomic symptoms
    4. Compound forms
  B. Complex symptomatology (generally with impairment of consciousness)
    1. With impairment of consciousness only
    2. With cognitive symptomatology
    3. With affective symptomatology
    4. With "psychosensory" symptomatology
    5. With "psychomotor" symptomatology
    6. Compound forms
  C. Partial seizures secondarily generalized
II. Generalized seizures (bilaterally symmetrical and without focal onset)
    1. Absences (petit mal)
    2. Infantile spasms
    3. Clonic seizures
    4. Tonic seizures
    5. Tonic-clonic seizures (grand mal)
    6. Myoclonic
    7. Atonic seizures
III. Unclassified epileptic seizures

Common Disorders

See Table 13-3 for old and new terminology.

Febrile Seizures

A febrile seizure is a generalized, brief tonic-clonic (grand mal type) seizure that occurs during a high fever, most commonly in the 3-month to 6-year age group. Approximately 2% to 5% of all children experience a febrile seizure. Most febrile seizures are benign, although 33% may have a second episode. The treatment of febrile seizures is controversial, and it is not uncommon to find a child on prophylactic therapy.[6]

Neonatal Seizures

Neonatal seizures are usually seen in the setting of prenatal asphyxia, birth injury, hypocalcemia, hypoglycemia, or secondary to an intraventricular hemorrhage in a premature infant. The seizure presents as a subtle change in behavior such as eye fluttering, sucking, drooling, tonic posturing, or apnea. Electroencephalogram (EEG) and CT scan help to confirm the diagnosis.

The prognosis of neonatal seizures largely depends upon the underlying etiology. The outcome cannot be predicted based on borderline abnormal EEGs. Infants whose serial EEGs are normal tend to have only minor sequelae.[7]

Infantile Spasms

Infantile spasms are a generalized seizure disorder occurring during the first year of life. A brief flexion contracture of the head, neck, and upper extremity with extension of the extremities (i.e., "jack-knife" spasms) are most common. Invariably, either poor motor function or mental retardation also will be present. Unfortunately, infantile spasms respond poorly to conventional epileptic therapy.[7]

Absence Seizures (Petit Mal)

Petit mal seizures usually develop in children before 10 years of age, but are rare in children less than 3 years old. The child stares blankly for brief periods and is unaware of these lapses in time. The three-per-second spike pattern is a hallmark EEG finding for this seizure disorder.[5]

Tonic-Clonic Seizures (Grand Mal)

Grand mal seizures are usually characterized by a loss of consciousness followed by a "cry" during rhythmic tonic contraction of chest-wall muscles. Respiratory stridor, cyanosis, and urinary incontinence commonly occur. The seizure is followed by a postictal period of confusion or sleep.

The onset of seizures in adults (after the age of twenty) must be studied for an underlying etiology. Although most grand mal seizures in children are idiopathic a complete diagnostic evaluation should be undertaken.

TABLE 13-3. Commonly used terminology and new classifications

Old classification	New classification
Petit mal seizures	Absence seizures
Grand mal seizures	Tonic-clonic seizures
Psychomotor seizures	Complex partial seizures
Temporal lobe seizures	Complex partial seizures
Minor motor seizures	Atonic or akinetic seizures
Focal motor seizures	Simple partial seizures
Jacksonian seizures	Simple partial seizures

ANTIEPILEPTIC AGENTS

The agents used in the treatment of epilepsy generally fall into one of the following categories: barbiturates, benzodiazepines, succinimides, and hydantoins. Their ability to prevent or reduce excessive neuronal discharge lies in a number of neurophysiologic effects: reduction of Na^+ or Ca^{++} fluxes, reduction of evoked responses, and potentiation of presynaptic or postsynaptic inhibition.[9]

ANESTHETIC IMPLICATIONS OF EPILEPSY

1. The child with epilepsy requires a thorough preoperative history and physical examination with careful scrutiny for many of the common side effects of anticonvulsant therapy (Table 13-4). A complete blood count with differential and liver function tests often are indicated.

TABLE 13-4. Anticonvulsant therapy

Drug (brand name)	Side effects
Phenytoin (Dilantin)	Nystagmus Megaloblastic anemia Gum hyperplasia Hirsutism Encephalopathy
Phenobarbital (Luminal)	Impaired development of fine motor skills Sedation, nystagmus
Primidone (Mysoline)	Marked sedation
Carbamazepine (Tegretol)	Ataxia Anorexia Diplopia Vertigo Hepatic dysfunction Leukopenia
Ethosuximide (Zarontin)	GI upset Headaches, dizziness Leukopenia Photophobia
Valproic acid (Depakene, Epilim)	GI upset Thrombocytopenia Acute hepatic failure Alopecia
Clonazepam (Clonopin)	Hyperactivity Irritability Belligerence

2. All anticonvulsant drugs should be continued in the perioperative period to maintain adequate blood levels and seizure control.
3. A candid discussion with the parents concerning the need to continue anticonvulsant therapy (despite an otherwise NPO status) and the potential for postoperative seizures should take place.
4. Accelerated or altered biotransformation of volatile anesthetic agents due to enzyme induction by chronic anticonvulsant therapy may be an important consideration when choosing agents.
5. Practically, all anesthetic agents can be used safely in the child with epilepsy. Controversy surrounds certain agents such as methohexital, meperidine, fentanyl, ketamine, and enflurane (Table 13-5). In general, most anesthetic agents cause EEG-wave slowing and decrease $CMRO_2$.

TABLE 13-5. Anesthetic agents and seizures

Drug	Implications in the seizure patient
Barbiturates	Dose-related effect upon the EEG Isoelectric EEG at high doses Methohexital may lower seizure threshold
Ketamine[10]	Hallucinogenic and convulsant properties can be seen on EEG; however, a predominance of theta activity and loss of alpha rhythm is seen with subsequent doses of ketamine and deeper planes of anesthesia; may actually raise seizure threshold Severe myoclonus in infants with myoclonic encephalopathy Although studies have shown no seizures in patients with known seizure disorders, it may be best to choose an alternative agent that is not as controversial
Benzodiazepines	Primarily used for sedation, anxiolysis, and amnestic properties Significantly raise seizure threshold
Narcotics	Meperidine's metabolite normeperidine is a well-recognized cerebral irritant; its use with MAO inhibitors is contraindicated because of seizures Several case reports of grand mal seizures following fentanyl have been reported; EEG studies have not corroborated these findings[11,12]; the use of fentanyl is not contraindicated in a child with seizures
Halogenated agents	Increased and altered biotransformation by liver enzymes may be of concern Enflurane and concomitant hypercarbia can cause audiogenic seizures Isoflurane may produce spikes on EEG without seizures Halothane has no epileptogenic potential
Atracurium	Laudanosine, a product of degradation, may cause cerebral excitation that does not appear to be clinically significant[4]

SURGERY FOR SEIZURE CONTROL[13]

Population

1. Patients with frequent seizures with life impairment
2. Patients who have demonstrated refractoriness to medical therapy
3. Patients for whom therapeutic agents have unacceptable toxicity
4. Older children or adolescents who can cooperate with the extensive preoperative evaluation (prolonged EEG recordings, mapping, neuropsychological testing) and an operative procedure under local anesthesia with minimal sedation.

Anesthetic Management

Initial anesthetic management includes preoperative evaluation of seizure disorder, neurologic deficits, medications, and side effects from medical therapy (including evaluation of hematologic and hepatic function).

Conscious Patient

1. Infiltration of long-acting local anesthesia by the surgeon
2. Monitored sedation carefully titrated to maintain patient cooperation (see Table 20-4 on Drugs for Monitored Sedation in Chapter 20)
3. Ability to treat acute seizure activity and manage airway

General Anesthesia

1. Requires use of electrocorticography.
2. Anesthesia may be induced with a short-acting barbiturate and maintained with N_2O, fentanyl, and muscle relaxants.
3. Low concentrations of volatile agents may be used and discontinued during recording of the seizure focus.
4. Anticonvulsant therapy should be resumed immediately after seizure resection because the incidence of seizure activity is often initially increased.

REFERENCES

1. Rosman N: Increased intracranial pressure in children, Pediatr Clin North Am, 21:483-99, 1974.
2. Rockoff MA: Pediatric neurosurgical anesthesia. In Ryan JF and others: A practice of anesthesia for infants and children, ed 1, Orlando, Fla, 1986, Grune & Stratton.
3. Bruce D: Management of severe head injuries. In Cottrell JE and Turndorf H, editors: Anesthesia and neurosurgery, St Louis, 1983, CV Mosby Co.
4. Hoffman WE and Grundy BL: Neuroanatomy and neurophysiology. In Barash PG, Cullen BF, and Stoelting RK, editors: Clinical anesthesia, Philadelphia, 1989, JB Lippincott Co.
5. Zion T: Diagnosis and pharmacologic therapy of epilepsy. In Fishman MA: Pediatric neurology, Philadelphia, 1986, Grune & Stratton.
6. Fishman M: Febrile seizures. In Fishman MA: Pediatric Neurology, Philadelphia, 1986, Grune & Stratton.
7. Glaze D: Neonatal seizures. In Fishman MA: Pediatric Neurology, Philadelphia, 1986, Grune & Stratton.

8. Menkes J: Seizure disorders. In Current pediatric therapy, Chicago, 1983, WB Saunders.
9. Rall TW and Schleifer LS: Drugs effective in the therapy of the epilepsies. In Goodman and Gilman: The pharmacologic basis of therapeutics, ed 8, New York, 1990, Pergamon Press.
10. Corssen G, Little SC, and Tanakoli M: Ketamine and epilepsy, Anesth Analg 53:319-35, 1974.
11. Tommasino C, Maekawa T, and Shapiro HM: Fentanyl induced seizures activate sub-cortical brain metabolism, Anesthesiology 60:283, 1984.
12. Murkin JM and others: Absence of seizures during induction of anesthesia with high dose fentanyl, Anesth Analg 63:489, 1984.
13. Cucchiara RF, Blach S, and Steinkeler JA: Anesthesia for intracranial procedures. In Barash PG, Cullen BF, and Stoelting RK, editors: Clinical anesthesia, Philadelphia, 1989, JB Lippincott Co.

14

ANESTHETIC MANAGEMENT OF PEDIATRIC MUSCULOSKELETAL DISORDERS

Karen M. Kabat

Children, you are very little,
And your bones are very brittle
If you would grow great and stately,
You must try to walk sedately.
ROBERT LOUIS STEVENSON
GOOD AND BAD CHILDREN

SCOLIOSIS

Scoliosis is the lateral curvature and rotation of the spine (see Table 14-1 below for classification of scoliosis). Severity of the curve is determined by the degree of angulation measured on the x-ray by the Cobb Method. Curves

TABLE 14-1. Classification of scoliosis

Type	Age	Sex	Associated problems
Congenital	Birth	M = F	Results from vertebral abnormalities (e.g., hemivertebra)
Idiopathic:			
• Infantile	Birth-2 yr	M > F	May have mental retardation, congenital anomalies, inguinal hernias 80% to 90% resolve spontaneously
• Juvenile	3-6 yr 7-10 yr	M > F F > M	Rarely self-resolving
• Adolescent	Postpuberty	F > M	Curve may progress if > 60° at spinal maturation

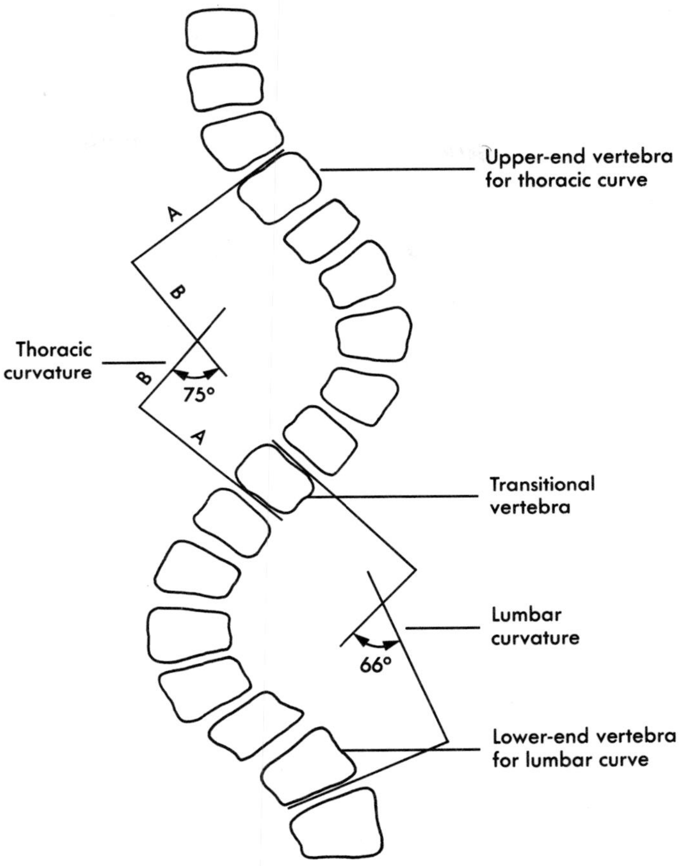

Fig. 14-1. Cobb Method of measuring degree of spinal angulation in scoliosis. Lines are drawn parallel to the upper border of the highest vertebral body and lower border of the lowest vertebral body of the curve *(A)*. Lines drawn perpendicularly to A will intersect *B*, forming an angle equal to the degree of curvature. (Adapted from Bernstein RL: Anesthetic management of patients with scoliosis, ASA Refresher Courses, vol 16, Chapter 2, Philadelphia, 1988, JB Lippincott.)

of less than 20 degrees usually cause few physiologic effects and therefore rarely require operative intervention (see Fig. 14-1 for technique of curve measurement).

Physiologic Effects

As the curvature increases, rotation results in narrowing of the chest cavity, causing a restrictive pulmonary process. With spinal curvatures of less than 65 degrees, lung volumes may be normal. As the degree of curvature increases the lung volume and compliance of the lungs and chest wall decreases. When the curvature approaches 65 degrees and there is a long history of scoliosis, pulmonary hypertension may develop.

CARDIORESPIRATORY EFFECTS OF SCOLIOSIS

- Ventilation/perfusion abnormality
  - ↑ Alveolar-arterial oxygen gradient (A-aDO_2)
  - ↑ Dead space (V_D/V_T)
- Total lung volume (TLV)
  - ↓ Vital capacity (VC)
  - ↓ Functional residual capacity (FRC)
- ↓ PaO_2, normal $PaCO_2$ (may increase with advanced disease)
- ↓ Ventilatory response to CO_2
- Pulmonary hypertension, cor pulmonale (secondary to chronic hypoxia and low lung volumes)
  - Right ventricular enlargement
  - Right atrial enlargement
  - Pulmonic insufficiency
- Tracheal shortening or distortion, pulmonary artery kinking

Criteria for Prolonged Postoperative Mechanical Ventilation

1. VC $<$ 50% predicted value (functional VC $<$ 2.0 L)
2. Elevated baseline $PaCO_2$ ($>$45 mm Hg)
3. Decreased baseline PaO_2
4. Pulmonary hypertension

Operative Treatment

Anterior Approach (Luque instrumentation)

This approach is used mainly when posterior fusion is not possible (e.g., spinal cord defects). The technique requires a thoracotomy with division of the diaphragm to gain access to the vertebrae. Bleeding, postoperative pain control, and respiratory dysfunction are significant problems. One-lung ventilation should be considered to improve surgical exposure.

Posterior Approach (Harrington rod placement and spinal fusion)

This technique involves placement of a hook into the facet joint of the upper and lower vertebra to hold a distraction rod along the concave aspect of the curve. A compression rod may be placed similarly on the convex side. Vertebrae are decorticated and spinous processes, intraspinal ligaments, and facet joints are obliterated. Bone graft, usually from the iliac crest, is used to fuse the spine. The procedure may be lengthy, requiring multiple transfusions. Recovery is prolonged.

Fixed, rigid curves may first require an anterior approach for discectomy before attempting distraction by the posterior approach. Both procedures may be done during the same operation or in two separate staged operations.

Anesthetic Management

Positioning

The Renton-Hall operation frame provides four padded supports—paired and V-shaped. The upper support should be at the anterior/lateral part of the thorax, while the lower supports the anterior/lateral aspects of the pelvis.

This minimizes abdominal pressure and inferior vena cava (IVC) compression so that functional residual capacity remains near normal. IVC compression can lead to blood diversion into the vertebral venous system, resulting in increased bleeding. Maintenance of FRC minimizes atelectasis. Care should be taken to pad the legs and avoid knee contact with the table.

Blood Loss

Blood loss usually is dependent on venous engorgement of the vertebrae and the extent and difficulty of the operative procedure, not the severity of the curve. Blood loss can be minimized by the following:

1. Correct positioning with minimal pressure on the IVC.
2. Infiltration of the operative site with large volumes of dilute epinephrine solution (1:500,000). On the rare occasion when larger epinephrine doses are used (greater than 1.5 μg/kg or 0.15 ml/kg of 1:100,000 solution) then prophylactic β-blockade may be indicated.
3. Hyperventilation to $PaCO_2$ of 25 to 30 mm Hg can cause peripheral vasoconstriction that reduces blood loss. However, a low $PaCO_2$ decreases spinal cord blood flow thus making ischemia possible.
4. Autologous storage for intraoperative transfusions.
5. Hemodilution.
6. Use of cell saver–retrieved blood.
7. Controlled hypotension
   a. Controlled hypotension is a technique that may reduce blood loss and decrease operative time. When utilizing this technique, arterial monitoring is essential for beat-to-beat observation of blood pressure because cardiopulmonary resuscitation would be nearly impossible in the prone position. After determining the patient's baseline mean arterial pressure a decrease of 25% to 30% generally is well tolerated if gradual in onset (over 10 to 15 minutes). This technique allows time for cerebral, renal, and coronary vascular beds to dilate and maintain adequate perfusion.
   b. Hyperventilation with hypotension may lead to spinal cord ischemia. The F_IO_2 should be increased to compensate for physiologic shunting and a near-normal $PaCO_2$ maintained. Assessment of arterial blood gases can reveal adequate oxygenation/ventilation and possible metabolic acidosis secondary to low perfusion or nitroprusside toxicity.
   c. Agents used to induce controlled hypotension include the following:
      1. Sodium nitroprusside (SNP)
         - Onset is within 30 seconds after starting infusion
         - The infusion rate is titrated easily to the desired level of hypotension
         - Combination with a β-blocking agent (propranolol or esmolol) prevents reflex tachycardia (which increases oxygen consumption) and decreases the amount of drug required to produce the desired level of hypotension
         - Maximum dose limit is 8 to 10 μg/kg/min

- Tachycardia, tachyphylaxis, and acidosis may indicate early toxicity and suggest use of an alternative drug
- SNP can increase intracranial pressure

2. Nitroglycerin
   - Causes decreases in preload and cardiac output
   - Reflex tachycardia can be limited by β-blockade
   - Usual dosage range is 1 to 10 μg/kg/min
3. Trimethaphan
   - Infusion maximum is 100 μg/kg/min
   - Avoids reflex tachycardia because of ganglionic blocking activity
   - Slower onset than sodium nitroprusside
   - Slight reverse-Trendelenburg is needed to enhance hypotensive effect
   - Causes pupillary dilation
4. Inhalation agents (halothane, enflurane, isoflurane)
   - For desired level of hypotension, cardiac depression may be significant
   - Onset is slower than nitroprusside

Monitoring Spinal Cord Function

Intraoperative "Wake-Up" Test

This test requires that patients move their extremities on command after placement of the distraction rod to test gross spinal motor function. The patient must be cooperative; preoperative discussion is essential. The test should not be considered for use in uncooperative patients, the mentally retarded, young children, paraplegics, or the hearing-impaired.

Nitrous-narcotic (balanced) technique. To awaken the patient, approximately half the calculated neuromuscular reversal dose is given and titrated over 5 minutes until spontaneous respiration returns. If spontaneous respirations do not occur in the presence of adequate twitch response, small amounts of naloxone (20-μg aliquots) should be titrated slowly. At this point, nitrous oxide is discontinued and the airway should be monitored closely. Extubation may occur or the rod may dislodge if there is excessive movement. The patient is asked to move his or her hands and feet sequentially. Absence of movement or weakness of one or both feet indicates that rod adjustment is necessary. After the test is completed, thiopental should be given to induce rapid loss of consciousness and amnesia.

Inhalation technique. If an inhalation agent is being used, the agent should be discontinued at least 10 minutes before planned awakening. The patient should be reanesthetized using a rapid-acting intravenous induction agent with amnestic properties (i.e., thiopental) after the test is completed.

Somatosensory Corticol Evoked Potentials (SSEP)

This technique involves electrical stimulation of at least two peripheral nerves from surface electrodes, one above the lesion and one below the lesion. The nerves used most frequently are the posterior tibial and median.

Surface electrodes are placed over the contralateral cortex of the respective somatosensory areas preoperatively. Many ambient conditions affect SSEPs, including inhalation agents, nitrous oxide, etomidate, large doses of thiopental, incomplete muscle relaxation, hypotension, hypothermia, and hypoxia. Although this test may help predict postoperative outcome, SSEPs monitor dorsal column function (not motor function), so that postoperative neurological defects may result without significant intraoperative SSEP changes.

Dysplastic Disease of Bone and Cartilage

See Table 14-2 on pp. 296-297.

JUVENILE RHEUMATOID ARTHRITIS

Juvenile rheumatoid arthritis (JRA) or Stills disease is an autoimmune disease associated with chronic nonsuppurative inflammation of synovium and connective tissue.

Incidence

1. Females affected more commonly than males
2. Rarely occurs in children younger than 6 months
3. Usually occurs between 1 and 3 years of age

Physiologic Manifestations

Airway

1. Temporomandibular joint involvement limits aperture.
2. Extreme mandibular hypoplasia occurs because of growth impairment.
3. Narrowing of the glottis, anterior fixation of the cords, and rotation of the larynx are common.
4. Cervical spine inflammation results in limitation of neck movement. Subluxation of atlantoaxial joint occurs more commonly after 5 years of age and may result in cord compression, quadriplegia, and possibly death.

Respiratory

Common findings include the following:

1. Pleural effusions
2. Pneumonia
3. Pleuritis
4. Classic adult rheumatoid plumonary nodules are rare in children

Cardiovascular

1. Pericarditis is found by ECHO in almost half the children with JRA.
2. The conduction system of the heart may be involved.
3. Cardiac valves may reflect inflammatory changes.

Renal

1. Impaired creatinine clearance is common.
2. Renal failure is rare.

TABLE 14-2. Dysplastic disease of bone and cartilage
This group of skeletal diseases usually is diagnosed at birth and is united by several common features, most notably airway problems and multiple organ involvement.

Type	Clinical manifestations	Physiologic considerations	Anesthetic considerations
Achondroplasia	Proximal limb shortening Frontal bossing Large head, long trunk Prominent mandible	**CNS** Dilated ventricles Small foramen magnum Hydrocephalus Spinal cord compression **Bone** Narrow spinal canal Lumbar lordosis and kyphoscoliosis	Difficult intubation Neck instability May have increased risk of neurologic deficit after regional techniques Technical difficulties of regional techniques caused by spine and bone deformities
Asphyxiating thoracic dystrophy (Jeune syndrome)	Stiff, small thorax with short ribs Short, broad hands and feet Postaxial polydactyly	Respiratory dysfunction (may improve with age) Pulmonary hypertension Cardiac defects Renal disease	Small larynx May need invasive monitors for cardiopulmonary disease Baseline pulmonary and renal function tests needed May have decreased excretion of anesthetic drugs

Ellis van Creveld	Polydactyly Mesomelic dwarfism Long, narrow thorax Nail/teeth abnormalities	Absence of tracheal cartilage causes airway collapse and tension lobar emphysema Cardiac defects (usual septal)	Abnormalities of dentition and upper/lower airway High airway pressures may cause barotrauma Nitrous oxide should be avoided with emphysema May need invasive monitors for cardiopulmonary disease
Chondrodysplasia punctata (stippled epiphyses)	Frontal bossing Hypertelorism High palate/saddle nose Short neck and stature Tracheal stenosis	Atlantoaxial instability Cardiac defects Hydrocephalus or other CNS abnormalities Associated renal anomalies	Difficult intubation (facial and neck abnormalities) Renal, cardiac function need to be assessed Possible elevated intracranial pressure
Osteogenesis imperfecta	Brittle bones with multiple fractures Blue sclera	Scoliosis Deafness Intracranial hemorrhages Impaired platelet function	Difficult intubation (short neck, teeth easily broken) Extra padding and careful positioning required Respiratory dysfunction caused by scoliosis Succinylcholine fasciculations may cause fractures Propensity for temperature increase during anesthesia (responds to cooling unlike malignant hyperthermia)
Osteopetrosis (Albers-Schonberg disease)	Failure to thrive Ecchymoses Megalocephaly Hepatosplenomegaly	Pancytopenia Low serum calcium Brittle bones	Careful positioning required May have coagulopathy and platelet dysfunction Serum calcium deficit may cause arrhythmias, seizures, or prolonged neuromuscular blockade

Hematologic Manifestations

1. Anemia is typically microcytic, hypochromic, and refractory to iron therapy.
2. Bleeding secondary to platelet dysfunction is caused by chronic use of antiinflammatory agents.
3. Neutrophilia may be associated with a high fever.
4. Splenomegaly may be associated with thrombocytopenia.

Anesthetic Management

Preoperative Evaluation

1. Airway assessment
   a. Consider indirect laryngoscopy to evaluate glottis.
   b. Cervical spine x-rays should include flexion and extension films for evaluation of atlantoaxial joint stability.
2. Cardiac examination
   a. Include auscultation for murmurs.
   b. A chest x-ray should be obtained if clinically indicated.
   c. Electrocardiogram should be examined for conduction delays.
   d. An echocardiogram can provide information on the extent of pericardial effusions and cardiac valve involvement.
3. Laboratory tests
   a. A CBC with platelet count and differential
   b. Coagulation/bleeding parameters
   c. Electrolytes, BUN, creatinine
   d. Urinalysis
4. Medications/treatments:
   a. Perioperative stress steroid coverage is indicated if the patient is on chronic steroid therapy or if a recent history of steroid use is present (hydrocortisone 4 to 8 mg/kg/day in 3 divided doses).
   b. Premedication should be conservative because the airway may be difficult to secure.
   c. Preoperative transfusion may be required depending on the degree of anemia and cardiorespiratory function.

Intraoperative Management

Airway. Inhalation induction with face mask followed by nasal or oral intubation, awake fiberoptic intubation, or any combination of the above is advisable when a difficult airway is anticipated. Muscle relaxants should be used only after securing the airway.

Vascular access. Chronic illness and chronic steroid use can lead to difficult access. Alternative plans (cutdown or indwelling central catheter) should be considered preoperatively.

Positioning. All pressure points should be padded carefully. The degree of cervical spine involvement determines head positioning.

Anesthetic agent. A marginal airway necessitates an awake, alert patient before tracheal extubation. Cardiac and respiratory involvement may limit dosages. Infusion of short-acting agents may provide the most titratability without prolonged effects.

SLIPPED CAPITAL FEMORAL EPIPHYSIS

This condition occurs when the proximal femoral plate weakens, permitting the femoral head to slip off, usually posteriorly and medially.

Patient Characteristics

- Adolescents
- More common in males than in females
- Bilateral involvement occurs in 25% to 30% of patients
- Most patients fall into one of two body types:
  1. Short, obese, prepubescent
  2. Tall and thin

Anesthetic Considerations in Obese Children

The primary anesthetic considerations are those that apply to obese children. The airway should be assessed; inhalation induction is often disastrous in the obese child with redundant soft tissue. An obstructed airway results in rapid desaturation because of marginal pulmonary reserve. It is unwise to rely on the ability to place an intravenous catheter in the obese child rapidly during a difficult induction. Furthermore, details surrounding gastric emptying in obese children are limited, but it is anticipated that the risks of acid aspiration are increased. For these reasons, a rapid-sequence induction with preoperative placement of the intravenous catheter is recommended. The IV also permits premedication with an H_2 antagonist and metoclopramide. The judicious use of narcotics is recommended, especially if any history of obstructive sleep apnea or snoring is present. The trachea should not be extubated until the child is fully awake and alert.

NEUROMUSCULAR DISORDERS

Von Recklinghausen Disease (Neurofibromatosis)

Von Recklinghausen Disease (VRD) is an autosomal dominant trait with new mutations being common. The hallmark of the disease is cafe-au-lait spots (more than 6 that are greater than 1.5 cm in diameter) and neurofibromas.

Associated Conditions

1. Laryngeal and tracheal compression secondary to tumor
2. High incidence of kyphosis and progressive scoliosis
3. Increased incidence of neural tumors such as glioma, meningioma, acoustic neuroma, and pheochromocytoma (which may present as sustained hypertension)
4. Compression of spinal roots, cerebello-pontine angle, medulla oblongata, and other nonneural structures
5. Impaired mental function (usually mild)
6. Megaloencephaly
7. Malformations of the greater wing of the sphenoid bone with pulsating exophthalmos
8. Congenital pseudoarthrosis (commonly tibia and radius)
9. Increased incidence of cancer

Anesthetic Considerations

1. Airway abnormalities may lead to difficulties with intubation and ventilation.
2. Patients may have a prolonged response to nondepolarizing muscle relaxants.
3. Hypertension, tachycardia, or arrhythmias may indicate pheochromocytoma.
4. Increased intracranial pressure may require appropriate treatment.

Cerebral Palsy

The term cerebral palsy is attached to a group of disorders characterized by damage to upper motor neurons of the brain or spinal cord. Clinical manifestations include mental retardation and skeletal muscle spasticity, convulsions, and balance problems. Surgery frequently is required to mobilize joints, decrease contracture, and correct deformities.

Anesthetic Considerations

1. Patients are prone to GE reflux and aspiration caused by upper motor neuron damage. Full-stomach precautions are usually appropriate.
2. Spasticity and limited neck motion may complicate intubation and airway management.
3. Postoperative pulmonary complications are common.
4. Succinylcholine use has not been shown to cause abnormal potassium release.
5. A susceptibility to hypothermia necessitates careful monitoring of temperature and particular efforts to maintain normothermia.
6. Hypothermia combined with abnormal cerebral function can lead to delayed awakening from anesthesia.

Poliomyelitis

Associated Problems

Scoliosis secondary to polio can occur about 2 years after the acute illness. Although polio is now rare secondary to immunization, when scoliosis is present, the site of the curvature, age of the child, muscle function, and severity of curve influence prognosis.

Anesthetic Considerations

1. Significant respiratory compromise depends on the presence of scoliosis and extent of disease.
2. Sensitivity to nondepolarizing neuromuscular blocking agents may be present.
3. Succinylcholine use may cause hyperkalemia.

Friedreich Ataxia

This group includes hereditary disorders with onset in late childhood or adolescence resulting in progressive dysfunction of the spinocerebellar pathways and pyramidal tracts with peripheral neuropathy and impaired position and vibration senses. Muscle weakness affecting respiratory muscles can be significant.

Myotonic Dystrophy (See Table 14-3 for less common myotonic dystrophies)

Myotonic dystrophy is an autosomal dominant trait affecting primarily the limb muscles but also with extraocular and facial involvement. Clinical features can include poor sucking/swallowing, muscle atrophy, facial weakness, ptosis, cataracts, frontal baldness, gonadal atrophy, endocrine failure, and mental retardation.

TABLE 14-3. Less common myotonias

Type	Features	Anesthetic considerations
Myotonic chondrodystrophy (Schwartz-Jampel syndrome)	Progressive Autosomal recessive Dwarfism Muscle stiffness Skeletal abnormalities	Same as myotonic dystrophy Predisposed to malignant hyperthermia
Myotonia congenita (Thomsen disease)	Not progressive Autosomal dominant Myotonia and hypertrophy of voluntary muscle (decrease with exercise) No cardiac involvement No dystrophic changes	Same as myotonic dystrophy
Paramyotonia	Similar to myotonia congenita	Myotonia develops with exposure to cold

Anesthetic Considerations

1. Poor sucking/swallowing predisposes these patients to aspiration. Full-stomach premedications (antacids, H_2 antagonists, gastric motility stimulants), and induction techniques apply.
2. Patients may have a poor cough and gag reflex, resulting in an increased incidence of atelectasis, pneumonia, and aspiration.
3. Bradycardia and intraventricular conduction delays with death occurring secondary to arrhythmias are common. The extent of cardiac involvement does not correlate with the extent of muscle involvement.
4. A depressed respiratory response to CO_2 with pulmonary hypertension and weakened respiratory muscles can cause serious hypoxemia and hypercapnia. Respiratory dysfunction dictates the judicious use of preoperative medications, narcotics, benzodiazepines, barbiturates, and inhalation agents.
5. Myotonia worsens with hypothermia. Maintenance of normothermia is essential.
6. Muscle spasms may complicate airway management.
7. Succinylcholine may precipitate a myotonic crisis. General and spinal anesthesia cannot break a myotonic contracture. Nondepolarizing neuromuscular agents do not elicit contractures and can be used safely.

8. Reversal with neostigmine and an antimuscarinic can precipitate myotonic contracture. The use of newer short-acting nondepolarizing agents and close monitoring of twitch response with a neuromuscular blockade (NMB) monitor is recommended.
9. Patients frequently require postoperative mechanical ventilation. The trachea should not be extubated until the patient is recovered from anesthesia completely.

MUSCULAR DYSTROPHY

See also Table 14-4 for less common dystrophies.

Duchenne (Pseudohypertrophic)

An X-linked recessive trait that usually presents with a waddling gait, appearing in a child between the ages of 3 and 5 years. The hallmark of the disease is muscle degeneration, a process of atrophy that confines the patient to a wheelchair by their early teens. Death is usually secondary to congestive heart failure, cardiomyopathy, or pneumonia, and usually occurs by 20 years of age.

Anesthetic Considerations

1. Succinylcholine may cause hyperkalemia, myoglobinemia, cardiac arrest, and rhabdomyolysis and should therefore be avoided. These effects can be seen in the absence of clinical disease and in relatives of affected patients.
2. Sensitivity to nondepolarizing neuromuscular blockers is common.
3. As the disease progresses, patients are unable to protect their airways from secretions, resulting in frequent pneumonia.
4. Worsening kyphoscoliosis with advancing disease seriously affects pulmonary function. Spinal fusion can reduce the rate of advancement of pulmonary disease. Surgical risk is related to vital capacity (VC). For VC greater than 45% of that predicted, postoperative ventilation normally is not necessary. For VC less than 30% serious postoperative complications are more common, even with supportive postoperative ventilation.
5. Cardiac muscle degeneration can lead to decreased contractility, right ventricular outflow obstruction, and mitral regurgitation. Anesthetics with the potential for myocardial depression should be used judiciously.
6. A nasogastric tube may prevent the acute gastric dilatation that has been associated with cardiovascular compromise.
7. Muscular dystrophy may be associated with malignant hyperthermia so that triggering agents should be avoided. Dantrolene may cause significant muscle weakness in these patients.
8. Use of atropine and scopolamine should be avoided if possible.
9. Hypomotility and delayed gastric emptying increase the risk of aspiration. Administration of H_2 antagonists, neutralization of gastric acidity, agents to increase gastric emptying, possible rapid-sequence induction with a nondepolarizing agent, and/or awake intubation should be considered.

TABLE 14-4. Less common muscular dystrophies

Type	Features	Anesthetic considerations
Limb-girdle (Erb's, Leyden-Mobius)	Autosomal recessive Involves hips and shoulders Presents in second decade with severe involvement by third decade Rare cardiac involvement	As in Duchenne's Variable extent of disease
Late onset X-linked	Onset occurs after age 10 Slower onset severity	As in Duchenne's
Facioscapulo	Autosomal dominant Onset after age 10 Normal life expectancy Affects arms, shoulders, face; later may involve back and hips Atria may lack electrical activity and not respond to pacing	As in Duchenne's, depending on extent of disease Severe bradycardia may require ventricular pacing Weak accessory muscles may increase pulmonary complications
Distal	Autosomal dominant Seen only in people of Swedish descent	As in Duchenne's, depending on extent of disease
Ocular	Begins with ptosis and extraocular muscle weakness Onset before age 30 Slow progression with limited muscular involvement	Special care to eyes and facial pressure points Extreme sensitivity to curare (paralysis can occur with 10% of usual dose)

Multiple Sclerosis (MS)

Characteristics

Multiple sclerosis is a disease of the CNS occurring between 15 and 40 years of age. Demyelination occurs in the brain and spinal cord, resulting in a variety of symptoms related to the site of involvement. Symptoms include visual changes, limb weakness, paresthesia, urinary incontinence, and constipation. Brainstem involvement can affect ventilation.

MS improves with pregnancy but new symptoms may develop postpartum. High risk geographic areas include the United States, Europe, Scandinavia, Great Britain, and New Zealand.

Drug Therapy

Remission has been induced with corticosteroids, ACTH, azathioprine, and cyclophosphamide. Drugs for treatment of symptoms include muscle relaxants and carbamazepine for seizures, ataxias, and dysarthrias.

Anesthetic Considerations

1. Preoperative
   a. Neurologic deficits should be documented before and after surgery.
   b. The possibility of disease progression should be discussed with the patient and family in detail, and all questions should be answered. Anesthesia and surgery have been reported to exacerbate MS.
   c. Spinal anesthesia can cause exacerbations of MS and should be used only if conditions warrant.
   d. Appropriate laboratory values should be checked, including CBC with differential (if on carbamazepine), hematologic and hepatic functions, electrolytes, and glucose (especially if on steroid therapy).
2. Intraoperative
   a. Because minimal temperature increases (less than 1° C) can block conduction in demyelinated fibers, temperature should be monitored closely and elevations treated aggressively.
   b. Preoperative medications can affect anesthetic management. Steroid use may necessitate stress coverage (hydrocortisone 4 to 8 mg/kg/day in three divided doses). Some anticonvulsants (e.g., carbamazepine and phenytoin) can increase the requirement for nondepolarizing muscle relaxants.
   c. Autonomic dysfunction may cause marked hypotension with inhalation agents.
   d. Succinylcholine potentially can cause hyperkalemia, although this has not been reported.

Myasthenia Gravis

Characteristics

Myasthenia gravis is an autoimmune disorder that results in a decrease in the number of acetylcholine receptors at the neuromuscular junction. Antibodies to the receptors may be present.

Symptoms include weakness and fatiguability of voluntary muscles. Such symptoms worsen with exercise. Ptosis, diplopia, and dysphagia are common, and a significant decrease in respiratory function may occur.

Three forms of the disease occur in children:

1. Neonatal transient myasthenia seen in infants born to mothers with the disease. Symptoms are usually transient.
2. Congenital myasthenia has symptoms first noticeable in infancy that persist throughout life and are usually mild.
3. Juvenile myasthenia occurs after age 10 and closely resembles the adult form of the disease. It has a female predominance.

Treatment

Drug therapy. Oral neostigmine and pyridostigmine are used to elevate levels of acetylcholine by inhibiting cholinesterase. Side effects include increased secretions, sensitivity to narcotics, and prolongation of succinylcholine and ester local anesthesia.
Operative. In up to 25% of patients, thymectomy eliminates the need for further drug therapy.

Anesthetic Management

1. Preoperative
   a. Anticholinesterase therapy should be continued if generalized symptoms are present.
   b. Discontinuation of therapy with 24 hours of bed rest may be appropriate for patients with only ocular symptoms.
   c. Premedication should be avoided.
2. Intraoperative
   a. Mask induction with spontaneous ventilation obviates the need for muscle relaxation for intubation. The use of halothane will have less effect on muscle relaxation than enflurane or isoflurane.
   b. If absolutely necessary, nondepolarizing relaxants should be used in $\frac{1}{20}$ of the usual dose and titrated to effect. Reversal of neuromuscular blockade may be ineffective.
   c. Hypothermia and hypokalemia can further decrease respiratory function and reserve.
   d. Narcotics should be titrated carefully in the postoperative period.
   e. Patients should meet the following criteria prior to extubation:
      - Awake and alert
      - Adequate head lift
      - Vital capacity >15 ml/kg
      - Negative inspiratory force > -30 cm H_2O
      - Ability to swallow and handle secretions

Myasthenic Syndrome (Eaton-Lambert)

Involvement primarily of proximal limb muscles, not ocular or bulbar muscles, caused by a decrease of acetylcholine at the end plate. Impaired acetylcholine esterase activity is probably responsible. Associated diseases include leukemia, neuroblastoma, systemic lupus erythematosis, rheumatoid arthritis, hypothyroidism, and hyperthyroidism. Anesthetic management should parallel that for myasthenia gravis.

BIBLIOGRAPHY

Bernstein, RL: Anesthetic management of patients with scoliosis. In ASA refresher courses, Vol 16, 1988.

Duncan PG: Neuromuscular diseases. In Katz J and Steward DJ: Anesthesia and uncommon pediatric diseases, Philadelphia, 1987, WB Saunders Co.

Ellis FR: Neuromuscular disease and anaesthesia, Br J Anaesth 46:603, 1974.

Gershwin ME and Robbins DL, editors: Musculoskeletal diseases of children, New York, 1983, Grune & Stratton.

Goldstein LA and Waugh TR: Classification and terminology of scoliosis, Clin Orthop 92:10, 1973.

Huttenlocher PR: Neuromuscular diseases. In Behrman RE, Vaugham VC III, and Nelson WE, editors: Nelson's textbook of pediatrics, ed 13, Philadelphia, 1987, WB Saunders Co.

Kafer ER: Respiratory and cardiovascular functions in scoliosis and the principles of anesthetic management, Anesthesiology 52:339-51, 1980.

Libman RH: Anesthetic consideration for the patient with osteogenesis imperfecta, Clin Orthop 159:123, 1981.

Norman ME: The bones and joints. In Behrman RE, Vaugham VC III, and Nelson WE, editors: Nelson's textbook of pediatrics, ed 13, Philadelphia, 1987, WB Saunders Co.

Salem MR and Klowden AJ: Anesthesia for pediatric orthopedic surgery. In Gregory GA, editor: Pediatric anesthesia, ed 2, New York, 1989, Churchill Livingstone.

Sumner E, Hatch DJ, and Lynn A: Unusual conditions in pediatric anaesthesia, Clinics in Anaesthesiology—Pediatric Anaesthesia 3:3, Philadelphia, 1985, WB Saunders Co.

Walts LF, Finerman G, and Wyatt GM: Anaesthesia for dwarfs and other patients of pathological small stature, Canad Anaesth Soc J 22:703, 1975.

15

ANESTHESIA FOR PEDIATRIC OPHTHALMOLOGIC SURGERY

Kathryn E. McGoldrick

Sally Ann saw twice as much as any girl her age
Twice as many suns and moons and words upon the page.
But everyone thought Sally Ann saw nothing much at all
She couldn't read or write her name or catch a basketball.

Twice as sad was Sally Ann who figured not a whit
Why what she saw and how things looked
were not a perfect fit.
RIVIAN BELL

PREOPERATIVE PREPARATION

Preoperative preparation of the patient begins with the establishment of rapport and communication among the anesthesiologist, the surgeon, the patient, and the patient's parents. Most parents realize that surgery and anesthesia involve risks, and often they appreciate a candid discussion of potential complications, balanced with information describing probability, or frequency, of serious adverse sequelae.

1. As always, a thorough history and physical examination with a complete list of medications and appropriate laboratory data is necessary. Any history of allergies to drugs, foods, or adhesive tape should be elicited.
2. A personal or family history of adverse reactions to anesthesia is very important before eye surgery because of the relatively high incidence of masseter spasm and malignant hyperthermia associated with strabismus.
3. It is important to counsel the child that one or both eyes may be patched postoperatively. Not surprisingly, occluded vision from either patches or ointments may terrify children as they emerge from anesthesia.

Coexisting Problems

The presence of an ocular abnormality always should alert the anesthesiologist to the presence of other associated anomalies, genetic aberrations, or systemic disease (see box below). Premature infants or neonates are not uncommonly pediatric ophthalmic patients. Special age-related differences in physiology and pharmacology apply.

OCULAR ANOMALIES AND COEXISTING DISEASE

Anomalies frequently associated with coexisting problems

Aniridia
Colobomata
Optic nerve hypoplasia
Cataracts
Ectopia lentis

Partial listing of genetic, metabolic, and systemic diseases with ocular pathology

Apert
Down
Marfan
Wagner-Stickler
Zellweger
Trisomy 18
Gangliosidoses
Mucopolysaccharidoses
Hypercalcemia
Homocystinuria
Cystomegalovirus
Sickle cell disease
Congenital myotonic dystrophies
Crouzon
Lowe
Sturge-Weber
Riley-Day
Trisomy 13
Lipidoses
Galactosemia
Kartagener syndrome
Diabetes mellitus
Rubella
Herpes
Neurofibromatosis

Induction Techniques

A broad spectrum of induction techniques exists. In the appropriate settings, methohexital per rectum, thiopental (or another barbiturate) intravenously, or an inhalation induction (usually with halothane because it is relatively nonirritating) are all acceptable methods. Intravenous alfentanil may be particularly useful in outpatient settings. Flexibility is essential because the induction plan may have to be modified based upon circumstances.

Oculocardiac Reflex

Underlying Pathology

1. The oculocardiac reflex has trigeminal afferent (V) and vagal efferent (X) pathways.
2. It is triggered by pressure on the globe or traction of the extraocular muscles, the conjunctiva, or orbital structures. It can be elicited by performance of a retrobulbar block, by ocular trauma, or by direct pressure on remaining tissue in the orbital apex following an enucleation.

3. The most common manifestation is sinus bradycardia. However, a vast array of dysrhythmias may occur including junctional rhythm, ectopic atrial rhythm, atrioventricular block, ventricular bigeminy, multifocal premature ventricular contractions, wandering pacemaker, idioventricular rhythm, asystole, and ventricular tachycardia.
4. Hypercarbia, hypoxemia, or inappropriate depth of anesthesia can augment the severity of the problem.

Incidence

The incidence ranges from 16% to 82%.[1,2] Strabismus patients can have an incidence as high as 90%, if not pretreated with atropine.

Prophylaxis

1. For strabismus surgery, most anesthesiologists favor routine prophylaxis with atropine 0.02 mg/kg IV before the commencement of surgery.
2. Because nearly complete vagolytic blockade requires 0.03 to 0.05 mg/kg of atropine, and because the peak action of intramuscular atropine occurs approximately 30 minutes following administration, it is not surprising that the usual, much smaller doses of atropine routinely given intramuscularly more than 1 hour before surgery have afforded inconsistent protection.
3. Oral atropine 0.04 mg/kg given 60 to 90 minutes before surgery with a sip of water is an alternative method, although the drug is absorbed slowly and efficacy is erratic.

Treatment

1. Treatment of the oculocardiac reflex depends upon its nature and severity. Small decrements in cardiac rate are acceptable if unaccompanied by hypotension. Severe bradycardia or hypotension is treated by asking the surgeon to stop ocular manipulation. Once the heart rate has returned to normal, a small dose of atropine (0.01 mg/kg IV) should be given.
2. Ventricular dysrhythmias triggered by the reflex may require the administration of 1 to 2 mg/kg of IV lidocaine. Atropine should never be administered during a dysrhythmia or during surgical manipulation because an extremely dangerous rhythm can follow.

Ophthalmic Effects of Anesthetic Agents

Anesthetic Agents

1. Inhalation agents cause dose-related decreases in intraocular pressure (IOP). The precise mechanism(s) remains unclear. However, postulated etiologies are: depression of a central nervous system control center in the diencephalic region; reduced aqueous humor production; enhancement of aqueous humor outflow; or relaxation of extraocular muscle tension.
2. Narcotics, barbiturates, and etomidate all lower IOP, provided that normocapnia is maintained.
3. Ketamine has minimal, if any, effect on IOP, as indicated by recent studies.[3]

4. In general, asphyxia, hypoventilation, or administration of carbon dioxide will raise IOP while hypothermia, nondepolarizing muscle relaxants, ganglionic blockers, and hypertonic solutions such as dextran, urea, mannitol, or sorbitol will reduce IOP.

Muscle Relaxants

1. Succinylcholine raises IOP as much as 8 mm Hg and extrusion of vitreous humor following the administration of succinylcholine has been reported.[4] Postulated mechanisms for this phenomenon are: tonic contraction of the extraocular muscles; choroidal vascular dilation; and relaxation of orbital smooth muscle.
2. The efficacy of pretreatment with nondepolarizing muscle relaxants to prevent increases in IOP caused by succinylcholine is still questionable. Suggested regimens include:
   a. pretreatment with small amounts of curare or gallamine[5,6]
   b. premedication with sufentanil (0.05 μg/kg) plus pretreatment with a nondepolarizing relaxant followed by a high-dose thiopental induction (7 mg/kg)[7]
   c. alfentanil (150 μg/kg) induction following the pretreatment mentioned above
3. Lidocaine is unreliable in preventing the ocular hypertensive response from either succinylcholine or intubation.[8]
4. Nondepolarizing agents will lower IOP.

Anesthetic Implications of Topical Ocular Drugs

See Table 15-1 for ocular drugs and dosages in pediatrics.

Absorption of Topical Drugs

1. Systemic absorption occurs from either the conjunctiva or nasal mucosa (following drainage through the nasolacrimal duct). Absorption is more rapid and extensive from nasal mucosal surfaces and can be reduced by application of digital pressure to the inner canthus of the eye for 3 to 5 minutes.
2. The lacrimal apparatus is dependent upon an active blink reflex and muscle action. Systemic absorption therefore is decreased significantly under general anesthesia. Nasolacrimal duct occlusion is still advisable, even in the anesthetized state, as small children are more vulnerable to the toxic side effects of certain ocular drugs.
3. Potentially toxic drugs include atropine, cocaine, cyclopentolate, echothiophate, epinephrine, phenylephrine, scopolamine, and timolol.

Mydriatics

Atropine. Atropine is an anticholinergic agent that produces mydriasis and cycloplegia. Topical application in children and the elderly has a proclivity to result in systemic reactions, including flushing, thirst, tachycardia, dry skin, temperature elevation, and agitation.

Scopolamine. Scopolamine is also an anticholinergic agent. It is a potent mydriatic and cycloplegic. Toxicity is common, indicated by CNS excitation

TABLE 15-1. Topical ocular medication

Drug	Concentration (%)	Amount per drop (mg)	Pediatric dose	Indication(s)
Atropine	1	0.5	one drop	Mydriasis Cycloplegia
Cocaine	4	2	<1.5 mg/kg	Vasoconstriction during dacryocystorhinostomy
Cyclopentolate	0.5-1	0.25-0.5	one drop	Mydriasis Cycloplegia
Echothiophate	0.03-0.125	0.015-0.0625	one drop bid	Antiglaucoma
Epinephrine	0.25-1	0.125-0.5	one drop bid	Antiglaucoma
Phenylephrine	2.5	1.25	one drop	Mydriasis Vasoconstriction Decongestion
Scopolamine	0.5	0.25	one drop	Mydriasis Cycloplegia
Timolol	0.25-0.5	0.125-0.25	one drop bid	Antiglaucoma
Betaxolol	0.5	0.25	one drop bid	Antiglaucoma

and disorientation. The usual dose is 0.25 mg, or one drop of a 0.5% solution. Toxicity can be treated with physostigmine 0.01 mg/kg IV, repeated once or twice over a 20-minute period.

Cyclopentolate. This is a popular short-acting mydriatic that is a synthetic antimuscarinic agent. CNS toxicity is a problem and manifests as dysarthria, disorientation, seizures, and frank psychosis. Concentrations of 1% or less (available in 0.5%, 1%, and 2% solutions) are advised for pediatric usage.

Antiglaucoma Agents

Echothiophate iodide. Echothiophate is a long-acting anticholinesterase that is associated with cholinergic side effects such as vomiting, hypotension, and abdominal pain. Preoperative intravenous therapy with atropine is indicated to prevent severe bradydysrhythmias. Drugs that are metabolized by plasma pseudocholinesterase such as succinylcholine, procaine, cocaine, and chloroprocaine should be reduced in dosage or entirely avoided if the patient has received echothiophate iodide within the last 5 weeks.

Epinephrine. This β-agonist is used in individuals with open-angle glaucoma. Available concentrations range from 0.25% to 2%. The higher concentrations are associated with a higher incidence of systemic side effects such as hypertension, tachycardia, and dysrhythmias.

Timolol. Timolol maleate is a nonselective β-blocker commonly used as a 0.25% or 0.5% solution. It should be used with extreme caution in patients with known contraindications to systemic β-blockers (i.e., asthma, congestive heart failure, and first- or second-degree heart block). Timolol also has been implicated in the exacerbation of myasthenia gravis and postoperative apnea in neonates.

Betaxolol hydrochloride. Betoptic is a β-blocker. Systemic side effects are rare. However, its use is contraindicated in patients where cardiac β-blockade is potentially dangerous.

Vasoconstrictors

Cocaine. Cocaine is an ester-linked local anesthetic that has sympathomimetic properties secondary to its ability to block the reuptake of catecholamines. Cocaine has limited topical ocular use because of its corneal toxicity. It is, however, used in nasal packing during dacryocystorhinostomy for vasoconstriction and shrinkage of nasal mucosa. One drop of 4% cocaine solution contains 2 mg of cocaine. The maximum safe dosage is 3 mg/kg, but 1.5 mg/kg is recommended if a volatile anesthetic is being used. Furthermore, it must be appreciated that systemic reactions may transpire with as little as 20 mg of cocaine; there is, unfortunately, a narrow range from safety to toxicity to death with cocaine usage. Cocaine should not be administered in combination with epinephrine because of the facilitation of dysrhythmias, especially during halothane anesthesia. Cocaine is contraindicated in patients with hypertension or those receiving adrenergic modifying drugs. The CNS symptoms caused by cocaine toxicity may be treated with intravenous barbiturates. If serious cardiovascular complications ensue, intravenous labetalol should be given to counteract them. To avoid cocaine toxicity the physician should search out possible contraindications and then administer meticulously calculated doses of dilute solutions.

Phenylephrine. Phenylephrine (neosynephrine) is an alpha agonist used for pupillary dilation and capillary decongestion. Children are especially vulnerable to overdose and manifest severe bradycardia, hypertension, and ST-segment depression. Asystole also has been noted to occur. Only the 2.5% solution is recommended for pediatric use, with one drop (1.25 mg)/eye/hr.

Specific Surgical Procedures

Strabismus

1. Strabismus surgery is the most common pediatric ocular operation. Approximately 5% of the population have malalignment of the visual axes.
2. Strabismus is associated with an increased incidence of malignant hyperthermia (MH), and some studies show a three times–higher incidence of masseter spasm in children undergoing strabismus repair than in the general population.
3. The forced duction test (FDT) that is used to determine whether the muscle is paretic, as opposed to restricted in motion, will not be possible if succinylcholine has been used within 20 minutes of the test.
4. Intubation of the trachea can be achieved under deep inhalational anesthesia or with the use of a nondepolarizing agent. Such problems as succinylcholine-induced masseter spasm and FDT invalidation can be circumvented with these techniques.
5. Oculocardiac reflex prophylaxis is advised before intubation of the trachea and surgical manipulation. Intravenous atropine 0.02 mg/kg or glycopyrrolate 0.01 mg/kg can be used (see pp. 308-309, Oculocardiac Reflex).
6. Postoperative nausea and vomiting are very common. Droperidol 0.075 mg/kg given at the start of the procedure, before surgical manipulation, has been found to be most effective.[10] The antiemetic effects of lidocaine 1.5 to 2 mg/kg IV are variable.

Congenital Cataracts

1. Fifty percent of the cases of congenital cataracts are idiopathic. The remainder are associated with chromosomal disorders, inborn errors of metabolism such as galactosemia, intrauterine infections, trauma, and drugs such as corticosteroids.
2. Surgical removal is indicated as early as possible because the clouded lens will impede retinal stimulation and proper visual development. Visual outcome is compromised severely if surgery is delayed beyond 6 months of age.
3. Optimal surgical conditions include an immobile eye and a maximally dilated pupil that permits adequate observation of the red reflex to assure complete removal of the affected lens. Additionally, once the eye is open a uniform intraocular pressure should be maintained. Any coughing or "bucking" on the endotracheal tube could produce loss of the intraocular contents.

4. Mydriasis can be achieved with preoperative topical 2.5% phenylephrine and 1% cyclopentolate. Additional intraoperative mydriasis is induced by continuous infusion of epinephrine 1:200,000 in a balanced salt solution into the anterior chamber. The drug is simultaneously removed from the chamber by aspiration. The intense vasoconstriction of the iris and ciliary body are felt to limit any uptake of epinephrine. Certainly systemic uptake of epinephrine is always of concern. Nonetheless, under halothane anesthesia, in both children and adults, no increased incidence of dysrhythmias has been reported following direct instillation of epinephrine into the anterior chamber.
5. Paralysis with a nondepolarizing muscle relaxant is advocated strongly to maintain a motionless eye with stable IOP. A sufficiently deep level of anesthesia is indicated for similar reasons until the wound has been closed completely. If the patient should move unexpectedly when the eye is open, intravenous thiopental should be given immediately. Succinylcholine is contraindicated when the eye is surgically open.
6. Any inhalation agent or a balanced technique may be appropriate. Hypercarbia-associated elevations in IOP should be avoided by means of adequate ventilation. Many patients are neonates; an unnecessarily high F_IO_2 should be avoided because of the potential for retinopathy of prematurity (ROP).
7. The goal is safe extubation of the trachea without coughing. Intravenous lidocaine and extubation in the lateral position while the patient is still deeply anesthetized are current recommendations.
8. An IV-emetic therapy using a drug such as droperidol 0.075 mg/kg is urged strongly to prevent any increases in IOP from vomiting. (This should be administered at the start of the case, before ocular manipulation.)

Corneal Transplant

The anesthetic considerations for a penetrating keratoplasty are similar to those for cataract surgery. Both are exquisitely delicate intraocular procedures that demand meticulous attention to appropriate anesthetic depth.

Retinoblastoma

1. Retinoblastoma is the most common pediatric ocular malignancy. It usually is diagnosed during the first 3 years of life. Even so, these aggressive tumors account for 1% of all cancer-related pediatric deaths, despite relative rarity.
2. Common presenting symptoms include white pupillary reflex, strabismus, ocular inflammation, and glaucoma.
3. Treatment varies depending upon the grade and involvement of the tumor. Cryotherapy, photocoagulation, enucleation, chemotherapy, or radiation are current therapies. If enucleation is required, it is advised to administer intravenous atropine prophylactically because of the relatively high incidence of oculocardiac reflex.
4. Daily irradiation for a period of weeks is common therapy for these children. Providing anesthesia can be very challenging, because the pa-

tient must be motionless, but only briefly, and they must be left unattended because of the high-dose radiation exposure (see Chapter 20).

Sufficiently deep and short-lived anesthesia can be accomplished by a variety of techniques. Rectal or intramuscular methohexital, intravenous or intramuscular ketamine administered after an atropine premedication, or a brief inhalational anesthetic administered by either insufflation or intubation are several satisfactory techniques.

Open Eye and Full Stomach Situations

1. This clinical situation has become a frequent conundrum for the anesthesiologist. Methods and agents useful in protecting against aspiration of gastric contents must be balanced against their potential to increase IOP.
2. Trauma is the typical cause of the open globe. Other injuries such as intracranial trauma producing subdural or epidural hematoma, skull or orbital fractures, and thoracic or abdominal trauma need to be excluded before operation.
3. Any unnecessary stimulation should be avoided because coughing or vomiting can raise IOP as much as 40 mm Hg. The stomach should not be emptied by a nasogastric tube. Additionally, any external pressure on the globe by aggressive placement of an anesthetic mask or increases in venous pressure (as may result from narcotic-induced vomiting, coughing, or struggling) must be avoided.
4. Aspiration prophylaxis is advised with an H_2-receptor antagonist. Metoclopramide (0.15 mg/kg IV) is also useful to help stimulate peristalsis.
5. After pretreatment with a nondepolarizing agent, rapid-sequence induction is generally the method of choice for an open-globe injury in a patient with a full stomach (see Table 15-2 on the next page for induction techniques).[11] It is recommended that the patient be extubated in the lateral position when the patient is fully awake. Suction of the gastric contents while the child is still deeply anesthetized is advised before reversal of muscle relaxation.

Postoperative Problems

Nausea and Vomiting

The high incidence of nausea and vomiting associated with pediatric strabismus surgery has been reduced dramatically by the periinduction use of droperidol (0.075 mg/kg IV). Further postoperative nausea and vomiting can be treated with low dosages of droperidol (0.010 mg/kg IV), or with dimenhydrinate (Dramamine) in doses of 1 mg/kg IM or 2 mg/kg per rectum. If the patient appears excessively drowsy, metoclopramide 0.15 mg/kg may be administered instead.

Pain

Strabismus surgery, cryotherapy, and retinal detachment surgery frequently are associated with considerable postoperative pain. Analgesics such as codeine or morphine are helpful, if rectal tylenol does not provide adequate analgesia (see Chapter 22 for analgesic doses).

TABLE 15-2. Induction techniques for open globe/full stomach

Technique	Advantages	Disadvantages
Technique I		
1. Barbiturate (thiopental) 7 mg/kg 2. Pancuronium 0.15 mg/kg	Pancuronium lowers IOP	1. Possible aspiration and death during 75-150 sec of unprotected airway 2. Dramatic increase in IOP if intubation attempts produce coughing or straining 3. Prolonged muscle relaxation beyond length of procedure
Technique II		
1. Barbiturate 2. Atracurium 0.6 mg/kg or vecuronium 0.15 mg/kg	1. Shorter duration 2. Minimal cardiac effects 3. Minimal accumulation	Onset of action is the same as pancuronium (problems 1 and 2 above)
Technique III		
1. Priming dose (1/10 of intubating dose of nondepolarizer) 2. Barbiturate 3. Intubating dose of nondepolarizer 4 min after priming dose	1. May be able to intubate within 90 sec	1. Wide variability in onset of relaxation 2. Aspiration and respiratory dysfunction can occur with priming dose
Technique IV		
1. Pretreatment with nondepolarizing relaxant 2. Barbiturate (thiopental) 7 mg/kg 3. Succinylcholine 1-2 mg/kg	1. Rapid onset 2. Excellent intubating conditions 3. Short duration 4. No reports of extruded intraocular contents with this technique	1. Slight elevations in IOP may occur 2. Bradycardia associated with succinylcholine necessitates pretreatment with atropine

REFERENCES

1. Berler DK: Oculocardiac reflex, Am J Ophthalmol 12:56, 954, 1963.
2. Taylor C and others: Prevention of the oculocardiac reflex in children: comparison of retrobulbar block and intravenous atropine, Anesthesiology 24:646, 1963.
3. Ausinisch B and others: Ketamine and intraocular pressure in children, Anesth Analg 55:773-75, 1976.
4. Lincoff HA and others: Effect of succinylcholine on intraocular pressure, Am J Ophthalmol 40:501, 1955.
5. Miller RD, Way WL, and Hickey RF: Inhibition of succinylcholine-induced increased intraocular pressure by nondepolarizing muscle relaxants, Anesthesiology 29:123-26, 1968.
6. Meyers EF and others: Failure of nondepolarizing neuromuscular blockers to inhibit succinylcholine-induced increased intraocular pressure: a controlled study, Anesthesiology 48:149-51, 1978.
7. Badrinath SK, Braverman B, and Ivankovich AD: Alfentanil and sufentanil prevent the increase in IOP from succinylcholine, Anesth Analg 67:S5, 1988.
8. Smith RB, Babinski M, and Leano N: Effect of lidocaine on succinylcholine-induced rise in IOP, Can Anaesth Soc J 26:482, 1979.
9. Carroll JB: Increased incidence of masseter spasm in children anesthetized with halothane and succinylcholine, Anesthesiology 67:559-61, 1987.
10. Lerman J, Eustis S, and Smith DR: Effect of droperidol pretreatment on post-anesthetic vomiting in children undergoing strabismus surgery, Anesthesiology 65:322-25, 1986.
11. Libonati MM, Leahy JJ, and Ellison N: Use of succinylcholine in open eye surgery, Anesthesiology 62:637, 1985.

SUGGESTED READINGS

Abramowitz MD, Oh TH, and Epstein BS: Antiemetic effect of droperidol following outpatient strabismus surgery in children, Anesthesiology 59:579-83, 1983.

France NK: Ophthalmological disease. In: Katz J and Steward DJ, editors: Anesthesia and uncommon pediatric diseases, Philadelphia, 1987, WB Saunders Co.

McGoldrick KE: Anesthetic implications of congenital and metabolic diseases. In: Bruce RA, McGoldrick KE, and Oppenheimer P, editors: Anesthesia for Ophthalmology, Birmingham, 1982, Aesculapius.

16

ANESTHETIC MANAGEMENT OF CHILDREN WITH RENAL AND ENDOCRINE DYSFUNCTION

Francis X. McGowan
Susan M. Chlebowski

Roses are red,
Violets are blue,
Sugar is sweet
And so are you.
ANON

PEDIATRIC RENAL DISORDERS

Developmental Considerations

Renal function is depressed in the neonate, especially in the preterm infant under 34 weeks gestation. Replacement fluids should therefore approximate as closely as possible the content of the fluid being lost, while serum and urinary electrolyte values are monitored.

Glomerular Filtration Rate (GFR)

- Under 34 weeks gestation, GFR averages as little as 1 to 3 ml/min.
- A rapid increase to a value of 30 to 35 ml/min/1.73 M^2 occurs at term.
- During the first year of life, GFR increases linearly to mature values (about 100 to 125 ml/min/1.73 M^2).
- The GFR of the newborn is sufficient to meet the demands of growth and homeostasis, but there is little margin in the event of conditions that cause renal ischemia (e.g., perinatal asphyxia, hypotension, respiratory distress

syndrome (RDS), renal vein thrombosis, surgical procedures, vasodilating anesthetics).

Renal Tubular Maturation

- Tubular immaturity, when present, is seen at birth, particularly in premature infants.
- At any given gestational age, glomerular maturation probably exceeds that of the tubules, leading to glomerulotubular imbalance. As a result, the ability to reabsorb the filtered solute load is exceeded, leading to proteinuria, glycosuria, and bicarbonate wastage (renal tubular acidosis of prematurity).
- Negative sodium balance is also prominent.

Water Conservation and Excretion

- The neonate is relatively isosthenuric, unable to either maximally concentrate or dilute the urine.
- Newborns can only concentrate urine between 100 and 600 mOsm/L, which restricts their ability to respond to dehydration or to excrete a water load. The premature infant's concentrating ability may be even less than that of a full-term infant.
- Adult concentrating and dilutional ability ranges from 50 to 1,300 mOsm/L.

Renal Endocrine Functions

- The renin-angiotensin system functions at near normal levels in the infant, although the magnitude of response may be somewhat depressed.
- Aldosterone secretion, which causes sodium retention, increases slightly.
- An increase in atrial natriuretic peptide (ANP) occurs, particularly in preterm infants with respiratory disease. ANP increases excretion of sodium and water.

Acid-Base Functions

- The neonate has a decreased renal bicarbonate (HCO_3) resorptive capacity and a lower renal threshold for bicarbonate, which leads to increased filtration. Plasma bicarbonate levels are consequently lower than those of the adult (18 to 22 mEq/L).
- Acid excretion and the ability to acidify the urine are limited.
- The acid-base functions mature during the first several months of life.

Assessment of Renal Function

Urine Output

1. Normal urine output for infants and children ranges from 0.5 to 1.5 ml/kg/hr.
2. Causes of decreased urine output include the following:
   - Hypoperfusion
   - Acute tubular necrosis (ATN)
   - Inhalation anesthetics
   - Inferior vena cava (IVC) or renal vein obstruction

- Obstructed/kinked urinary catheter
- Hemolytic transfusion reaction
- Malignant hyperthermia
- Use of vasopressors

Serum Creatinine and BUN

- Creatinine crosses the placenta. Levels are therefore identical in both mother and fetus and do not reflect GFR.
- The level of creatinine will decrease by 50% within the first week of life for infants greater than 34 weeks gestation, reaching a normal infant value of 0.25 to 0.40 mg.
- Because there is little net loss of creatinine in preterm infants, values do not decrease until 34 weeks gestation, at which time GFR increases.
- The level of creatinine increases during the first 10 to 15 years of life in healthy children, ranging from 0.4 to 0.9 mg.
- BUN averages 8 to 12 mg in children aged 1 to 16 years. In newborns, 25 to 31 mg is the usual level for the first few days of life. Premature infants average 16 to 22 mg.

Urine Specific Gravity (SG) and Osmolality

- Interpretation of urine specific gravity is often confounded by the presence of substances such as glucose, protein, radiographic contrast agents, and mannitol, all of which artificially elevate the value. Nonosmotic diuretics typically produce dilute urine.
- Newborn values are 1.004 to 1.020 mOsm/L for SG and 100 to 600 mOsm/L for urine osmolality.

Proteinuria

- Small plasma proteins, such as albumin, are filtered and reabsorbed. The resorptive process is limited in newborns, leading to mild proteinuria.
- Normal protein excretion is 240 mg/M^2/day in infants and 100 mg/day in children. Urine dipstick values greater than 10 to 20 mg necessitate further investigation.
- Other causes of proteinuria not associated with renal disease include exercise, fever, dehydration, and orthostatic proteinuria.
- Disease states associated with proteinuria include nephrotic syndrome, glomerulonephritis, interstitial nephritis, urinary tract infection, renal vein thrombosis, significant hypertension, diabetes, and collagen vascular diseases.

Creatinine Clearance

- When interpreting measurements of creatinine clearance, certain factors must be taken into account, such as patient age, muscle mass, and age-related differences in GFR and serum creatinine.
- Infants over age 6 months have creatinine clearance values similar to those of older children and adults.

Oliguria and Acute Renal Failure

Prerenal. A prerenal cause must be excluded in all children with oliguria.

Etiology

- Renal hypoperfusion as a result of hemorrhage, dehydration, sepsis, hypotension, or intravascular volume depletion
- Renal vein thrombosis, associated most often with birth asphyxia, cyanotic heart disease, maternal diabetes, and polycythemia

Diagnosis

- Clinical history and physical evidence of heart failure, cardiac tamponade, shock, sepsis, bleeding, dehydration, or third-space losses may be present
- Blood pressure and central venous pressure are usually decreased; heart rate is increased.
- Bladder catheterization yields urine output less than 0.5 ml/kg/hr with elevated urine specific gravity and osmolarity.
- Electrolytes and creatinine may be initially normal. BUN may be elevated. Metabolic acidosis is present if systemic perfusion is compromised (see box below for complications of acute renal failure).
- Rarely are invasive monitors necessary for diagnostic purposes. Arterial and/or central venous pressure (CVP) catheters may be needed to guide therapy.

COMPLICATIONS OF ACUTE RENAL FAILURE

Hypovolemia

- Usually seen in prerenal azotemia
- May also be present as a result of fluid restriction in renal or postrenal state or after hemodialysis

Hypervolemia

- More common in renal or postrenal ARF
- May aggravate hypertension and heart failure

Hypertension

- Seen with volume overload and activation of renin-angiotensin system
- Treated with fluid and salt restrictions and antihypertensive agents
- Dialysis may be necessary

Hyperkalemia

- K^+ >5.5 mEq/L necessitates monitoring
- K^+ >6.5 mEq/L requires urgent treatment with close ECG monitoring

Metabolic Acidosis

- Perioperative concerns are worsening of acidosis by hypothermia, dehydration, bleeding, and poor perfusion.
- Intraoperative use of hyperventilation will increase pH.
- Administration of HCO_3, citrate, or lactate will also increase pH (last two require liver metabolism to HCO_3).

Treatment

- Intravascular volume is immediately restored with saline or lactated Ringer's, followed by replacement of estimated deficits. Appropriate rehydration should be accompanied by improved perfusion and hemodynamics and restoration of urine flow. (See Tables 16-1 and 16-2 for guides to fluid replacement in renal failure.)
- If no improvement in urine output is seen after appropriate restoration of the intravascular volume, a diuretic trial may be employed with mannitol (0.5 g/kg) IV or furosemide (1 to 2 mg/kg) IV.
- If there is no improvement in the oliguria/anuria, cessation of further diuretic or aggressive fluid management should be considered, and the patient evaluated for renal and postrenal causes of the oliguria.

TABLE 16-1. Guide to fluid replacement in renal failure

Type of defect	Replacement of fluid
Oliguria or anuria	Insensible losses (1/3 maintenance) + 1:1 replacement for bleeding, nasogastric suction, diarrhea, etc.
Na^+/H_2O losing	Insensible losses (1/3 maintenance) + 1:1 replacement of urine + 1:1 replacement for bleeding, nasogastric suction, etc.
Na^+/H_2O overload	Insensible losses (1/3 maintenance) + 1/3 to 1/2 urine output + additional losses if indicated

TABLE 16-2. Type of fluids used in renal failure

Replacement	Type of fluid
Insensible loss	5% or 10% dextrose
Urine output	Electrolyte content of urine guides choice of solution
Additional losses*	Lactated Ringer's Plasmacyte Normosol

*Solutions containing potassium are generally withheld if anuric or oliguric.

Renal

Etiology

- The most common cause of renal failure in children is renal ischemia caused by hypoperfusion and resulting in parenchymal damage
- Cyanotic children with shunting are thought to be at special risk.

- Other causes include nephrotoxins, acute tubular necrosis, nephritis, hemolytic-uremic syndrome, immunologic causes, hemoglobinuria, myoglobinuria, heart failure, and cyanosis.

Diagnosis

- The diagnosis of renal failure *must* exclude prerenal or postrenal causes.
- Creatinine clearance is markedly diminished, and serum creatinine is elevated.
- Frequently present are hyponatremia, hyperkalemia, hypervolemia, metabolic acidosis, and uremia (see box on p. 321 for complications of acute renal failure).
- A renal ultrasound helps to exclude obstruction. Radionuclide renal scanning helps to evaluate renal perfusion.
- The clinical history may provide clues about cause (e.g., severe trauma and shock, drug ingestion, crush injury with rhabdomyolysis, vasculitis).

Treatment

- Initial treatment should be as for prerenal azotemia to ensure adequate intravascular volume and renal perfusion. Urinary and serum electrolytes should be closely followed and potassium omitted from replacement regimens. Any predisposing causes should be vigorously treated.
- Attempting to alkalinize the urine and promote diuresis may be useful if myoglobin, hemoglobin, or tumor lysis are causative factors.
- Dopamine infused at 3 to 5 μg/kg/min to augment renal perfusion may be appropriate in states thought to have a low cardiac output component (e.g., congestive heart failure, shock, sepsis, postbypass, postanoxic insult).
- Urgent hemodialysis or peritoneal dialysis is indicated for the following:
  1. Volume overload leading to congestive heart failure or malignant hypertension
  2. Severe hyperkalemia (see Table 16-3 on the next page for treatment of hyperkalemia)

Postrenal

Etiology

- Obstruction as a result of congenital anomalies is the most common cause of postrenal failure.
- Posterior urethral valves are the most frequently occurring anomaly in male infants.
- Other causes include tumor, trauma, and retroperitoneal fibrosis.

Diagnosis

- Examination may reveal abdominal, flank, or bladder masses.
- Abdominal ultrasound is often diagnostic.

Treatment

- Therapy consists primarily of repair or bypass of the obstructed area.
- In cases of bilateral obstruction, the phenomenon of postobstructive diuresis may result.
  1. This is characterized by a transient (12 to 48 hour) diuresis that is the consequence of excretion of the salt, water, urea, and other products that accumulated during the obstruction.

TABLE 16-3. Emergency treatment of hyperkalemia

Drugs	Dosage and route of administration	Comments
Sodium polystyrene sulfonate (Kayexalate) in sorbitol (cation exchange resin)	1 gm/kg PO or PR The enema form must be retained for 50 min; may repeat q 4 hr.	• Each gram of resin exchanges 1-2 mEq Na^+ for 1 mEq K^+ • May cause Ca^{++} loss • Only method other than dialysis that removes K^+ from body
Calcium gluconate	50-100 mg/kg IV slowly	• Immediate but transient effect • Stabilizes myocardial transmembrane potential
Calcium chloride	10 mg/kg IV slowly (Preferred route is through a central vein)	• As for calcium gluconate
Sodium bicarbonate	1-2 mEq/kg IV (Should be diluted 1:2 for infants)	• Rapid, brief • Promotes intracellular movement of K^+ • Hypernatremia, volume overload, and intraventricular hemorrhage may occur in premature infant
Insulin (regular) + glucose	0.1-0.2 units/kg + 1 ml/kg of D50 IV	• To avoid hypoglycemia, follow serial blood glucose
Dialysis	Hemodialysis	• Hemodynamic instability, anticoagulation, access difficulties in small children • Time delay is needed to complete dialysis
	Peritoneal dialysis	• More rapidly initiated • Respiratory compromise may occur from abdominal fluid • Risk of infection (peritonitis)
	Ultrafiltration	• Requires vascular access and adequate perfusion pressure • More rapidly initiated and less cumbersome than hemodialysis

2. A natriuretic factor and damage to the tubules and collecting duct may also play a role.
3. Treatment initially involves replacement of electrolyte and water losses, according to plasma and urine electrolyte values.
4. Gradually restricting water and electrolyte replacement will progressively encourage the kidney to resume tubular and concentrating duties.

Chronic Renal Failure (CRF)

See box on the next page for manifestations of CRF.

Etiology

- Over half the cases of CRF in children are due to congenital anomalies, including obstructive uropathy, renal dysplasia, or polycystic kidney disease.
- Other causes include glomerulonephritis of various types, hemolytic-uremic syndrome, nephritis, and malignancy.

Pathophysiology

Knowledge of the type of defect can help guide fluid and drug therapy, because these patients are very sensitive to inappropriate fluid and electrolyte administration.

- Glomerulonephritis is a glomerulotubular imbalance leading to sodium and water retention, hypertension, edema, and occasionally congestive heart failure.
- Renal dysplastic and obstructive lesions cause defective concentrating mechanisms, resulting in obligate free water loss.
- Medullary cystic disease, sickle cell nephropathy, and hydronephrosis exhibit defective distal sodium resorption resulting in obligate sodium and free water requirements.
- End-stage renal disease (ESRD) exhibits severely limited GFR, which disables the filtering of sodium, water, potassium, acid, and other products of matabolism. Calcium and vitamin D metabolism are also impaired.

Anesthetic Considerations in Renal Failure

A wide variety of anesthetic techniques and agents have been used successfully in patients with renal failure. Primary consideration must be given to the specific manifestations of disease in each individual.

Pharmacokinetics and Pharmacodynamics

Renal disease has been shown to have the following effects:

- Decrease drug binding and volume of distribution
- Decrease excretion of renal drugs and metabolites
- Render the blood:brain barrier more permeable

Muscle Relaxants

- Succinylcholine may induce hyperkalemia when renal failure is present.
- Reduced requirements of nondepolarizing muscle relaxants are due to

MANIFESTATIONS OF CHRONIC RENAL FAILURE

Neurologic

- Fatigue and lethargy
- Somnolence
- Peripheral neuropathy
- Muscle weakness
- Uremic or hypertensive encephalopathy
- Autonomic nervous system dysfunction

Pulmonary

- Pulmonary edema
- Pleural effusions

Cardiac

- Hypertension
- CHF
- Peripheral edema
- Uremic pericarditis
- Pericardial effusion and tamponade

Metabolic

- Acidosis
- Hyperkalemia
- Hypocalcemia
- Hyperphosphatemia
- Hyperuricemia
- Secondary hyperparathyroidism

Hematologic

- Anemia
- Platelet dysfunction
- Coagulopathy
- Decreased immune function

Bone

- Rickets
- Osteomalacia
- Osteitis fibrosa

Growth

- Somatic growth retardation

decreased muscle mass and to muscle weakness. Increased sensitivity may be due to hypocalcemia, acidosis, hypermagnesemia, and hypokalemia.

- Renal elimination of muscle relaxants is as follows:

Muscle relaxant	Percentage of renal excretion
Gallamine	100%
Pancuronium and metocurine (biliary elimination may increase in the setting of renal failure)	70%
Tubocurare	60%

- Atracurium and vecuronium elimination are not significantly altered by CRF.

Inhalation Agents

- The pulmonary route of uptake and elimination removes the need to rely on the kidneys for drug excretion.
- All inhalation agents depress GFR by decreasing cardiac output from vasodilatation.
- Fluoride ion may accumulate during enflurane or halothane use; fluoride will accumulate when GFR is less than 16.

Narcotics

- The presence of oliguria or anuria may lengthen the duration of narcotic effects and potentiate respiratory depression.
- Meperidine's metabolite normeperidine (which causes CNS excitability) may accumulate in the presence of renal dysfunction.
- Adverse consequences have not been found to occur with the use of fentanyl or fentanyl/droperidol combinations.
- The effects of narcotics may also be potentiated by changes in underlying mental status and in the blood:brain barrier in uremic patients.

Thiopental

Since protein binding is significantly reduced, induction doses should be reduced by 50% to 75%. The duration of the drug will be prolonged.

Complications of Dialysis

- Complications of hemodialysis include anticoagulation, intravascular volume depletion, infection, hepatitis, and electrolyte imbalance.
- Complications of peritoneal dialysis include less rapid removal of potassium and toxins than with hemodialysis; infection; and respiratory compromise secondary to the presence of increased abdominal fluid. All patients should have dialysate drained before arrival in the operating room.

Cardiopulmonary Disease

- An increased respiratory rate may compensate for metabolic acidosis. The increased rate aggravates the work of breathing, which may hasten respiratory failure and actually worsen acidosis.

- In addition, patients may have the following conditions:
  - Pulmonary edema, pleural effusions, and pleuritis
  - Pericardial effusion and tamponade
  - Decreased myocardial contractility secondary to uremia
  - CHF caused by acidosis, volume overload, and diminished contractility
  - Hypertension (may be severe)
- Choice of anesthetic agents and use of invasive monitoring are based on severity of disease.

Anemia

- A normochromic, normocytic anemia is a common finding once creatinine is greater than 3 to 4 mg%.
- Increased cardiac output and rightward shift of the Hgb-O_2 dissociation curve (caused by metabolic acidosis and increased 2,3-DPG levels) help compensate for the anemia.
- Prophylactic transfusion is not indicated unless blood loss, severe infection, or significant cardiopulmonary disease is present. Hgb greater than 6 to 7 g/100 ml is acceptable in CRF.
- If transfusion is necessary, frozen washed RBCs have the lowest volume of fluid and level of potassium.

Platelet Dysfunction

- Unusual if creatinine is less than 6 to 7.
- Largely reversible by dialysis.
- May be corrected by desmopressin acetate (DDAVP) 0.3 μg/kg IV over 30 minutes with a peak effect in 60 to 90 minutes and a duration of 4 to 6 hours. Repeated doses may be less effective than the initial dose.

Hypertension

Etiology

- Unlike adult hypertension, most hypertension in infants and children is not primary (essential) but is related to renovascular or other renal diseases.
- Causes include renal artery stenosis, polycystic kidney disease, glomerulonephritis, renal vein thrombosis, umbilical artery catheter complications, Wilm's tumor, neuroblastoma, aortic coarctation, congenital adrenal hyperplasia, and medications such as steroids and cyclosporine A.

Diagnosis

- Knowledge of appropriate blood pressure for age is crucial (see Chapter 3).
- Misdiagnosis of hypertension is most frequently caused by the use of the wrong size blood pressure cuff. The correct size should cover two-thirds the length of the upper forearm, with the cuff bladder encircling more than half the upper arm over the brachial artery.
- Doppler techniques provide the most reliable noninvasive means of measuring systolic pressure in infants. The most accurate measurement provided by oscillometric methods is that of mean arterial pressure (e.g., Dinamapp), although measurement of systolic pressure is also fairly accurate by these methods.

- Hypertension is present at a blood pressure (BP) greater than 2 standard deviations above the mean for age, or above the 95th percentile for age.
- A hypertensive crisis exists under the following conditions:
  1. Values are significantly greater than 2 standard deviations above the mean.
  2. Diastolic BP is greater than 95 mm Hg in an infant or small child and greater than 110 mm Hg in an older child.
  3. Any cardiac (e.g., CHF, angina) or neurologic symptoms (headache, visual changes) are present.

Treatment

- Because of the higher incidence of organic causes in children, diagnostic investigation for treatable processes should be pursued.
- In the presence of acute or chronic renal failure, fluid and salt intake should be restricted and antihypertensive medications administered.
- Dialysis may be necessary.
- Diuretics, β-blockers, vasodilators, and angiotensin converting enzyme inhibitors form the mainstays of antihypertensive therapy in children.
- Weight reduction and sodium restriction are also important for the purpose of decreasing blood pressure.
- Causes of intraoperative hypertension in an otherwise healthy child include hypoxia, hypercarbia, a cuff that is too small, light anesthesia, or autonomic activity (e.g., tourniquet use).
- Postoperative hypertension is most often caused by pain, relative volume overload, or bladder distention, although hypoxia and hypercarbia must always be considered.

TABLE 16-4. Treatment of hypertensive crises in children

Drug	Dose (IV)	Comments
Vasodilators		
Sodium nitroprusside	0.5-10 mcg/kg/min	• Rapid onset. • Tachyphylaxis may develop if use is prolonged.
Hydralazine	0.1-0.3 mg/kg	• Onset: 20 min • IV duration relatively brief.
Diazoxide	2-6 mg/kg bolus	• Should be given rapidly with furosemide (1-2 mg/kg) IV to limit fluid retention. • Hyperglycemia may occur.
α, β-blocker		
Labetolol	1-3 mg/kg/hr	• Peak onset: 10 min • Duration: 5 hr • Should discontinue infusion when BP controlled and allow to self-taper.

TABLE 16-5. Common antihypertensive drugs in children

Drug	Dose (mg/kg)	Comments/side effects
β-blockers		
Propranolol	0.5-1.0 mg/kg/day divided q6-12h PO	• Contraindicated in asthma, CHF. • Use heart rate as guide to degree of β-blockade. Rebound BP if stopped acutely.
Metoprolol	1-2 mg/kg/day divided q12h PO	• More β_1-specific; otherwise as above.
Vasodilator		
Hydralazine	0.75-3 mg/kg/day divided q6-12h PO	• May cause lupuslike syndrome, tachycardia, volume retention.
Diuretics		
Hydrochlorothiazide	2-3 mg/kg/day divided q12h PO	• May cause hyperuricemia, photosensitivity, hypokalemia.
Chlorothiazide	20-30 mg/kg/day divided q12h PO	• May cause hypokalemia.
Furosemide	2 mg/kg/dose q6-12h PO	• May cause hypokalemia.
Spironolactone	1-3 mg/kg/day divided q6-12h PO	• K^+-sparing; avoid in hyperkalemia.
Converting enzyme inhibitor		
Captopril	Neonate: 0.1-0.4 mg/kg/dose q6-24h PO Infant: 0.5-0.6 mg/kg/day divided q6-12h PO Child: 25 mg/day divided q12h PO	• May precipitate renal failure with renal artery stenosis; may cause neutropenia.

ANESTHETIC MANAGEMENT OF SPECIFIC PEDIATRIC RENAL SYNDROMES

Hemolytic-Uremic Syndrome (HUS)

Etiology

Infectious agents such as viruses, shigella, and salmonella have all been implicated.

Manifestations

- Occurs most often in infants and young children.
- Usually preceded by a prodromal illness: diarrhea, vomiting, and upper respiratory infections.
- Acute renal failure, thrombocytopenia, and hemolytic anemia are due to microangiopathic disruption. Severe hypertension, hypovolemia, electrolyte imbalance, anemia, congestive heart failure, seizures, lethargy, and coma may accompany renal failure.
- Renal involvement can range from mild, transient depression of function to development of renal necrosis and chronic renal failure in approximately 20% to 30% of cases.

Treatment

- Causes of infection must be identified and treated.
- Early aggressive supportive therapy with red cell and platelet transfusions is necessary. Blood cells may have decreased survival because of ongoing consumptive and microangiopathic processes.
- Dialysis is required for the treatment of hyperkalemia, volume overload, acidosis, congestive heart failure, and hypertension.

Anesthetic Management

- Treatment of a child with renal failure complicated by coagulopathy and anemia includes preoperative dialysis, blood pressure control, and blood component therapy as indicated.
- Large-bore venous catheters and arterial and central venous access may help to assess the status of intraoperative fluids and electrolytes.

Nephrotic Syndrome

Etiology

- Nephrotic syndrome is defined as proteinuria, hypoalbuminemia, hyperlipidemia, and edema.
- Its most common causes in children are idiopathic or primary glomerular lesions.
- Lupus, the glomerulonephritides, diabetes, sickle cell disease, and amyloidosis are additional causes.

Manifestations

- Increased glomerular permeability to plasma proteins leads to significant proteinuria.
- Intravascular volume depletion is often associated with ascites and GI mucosal edema, resulting in nausea and vomiting.
- Decreased drug protein binding is present.
- Respiration is compromised by ascites and pleural effusions.

- There is a decrease in total serum calcium, although ionized calcium is usually normal because of decreased albumin.
- A hypocoagulable state is present.

Anesthetic Management

- Intravascular volume status must be assessed. It is usually contracted and must be reexpanded to preserve GFR. Placement of a CVP is indicated if a major surgical procedure is planned.
- Sodium-poor albumin (10 to 20 ml/kg infused slowly) helps to mobilize ascites and edema fluid and restore intravascular volume. Furosemide (1 to 2 mg/kg) PO or IV may be used in sequence with albumin to promote diuresis.
- Patients already receiving immunosuppressants and steroids should continue to do so perioperatively and should also receive stress dose steroids.
- A reduction in thiopental dosage is warranted because of decreased protein binding and tenuous volume status.

Renal Tubular Acidosis

Two major types of renal tubular acidosis (RTA) exist: proximal and distal.

Proximal RTA

- Bicarbonate normally appears in the urine when the proximal resorptive threshold is exceeded. In adults and older children, this occurs at 24 to 26 mEq/L; in infants at 20 to 22 mEq/L. In proximal RTA, the threshold is usually 16 to 18 mEq/L. Distal hydrogen ion secretion and urine acidification are not impaired.
- Major manifestations are metabolic; that is, hyperchloremic acidosis, hypocalcemia, and a urine pH that may or may not be alkaline. Salt and water wastage is usually associated with proximal RTA. Rickets and osteomalacia are late findings.
- A transient form occurs in preterm or term infants that may cause vomiting and growth retardation.
- Therapy includes bicarbonate replacement and potassium supplementation. Hydrochlorothiazide has been used to increase the bicarbonate threshold in proximal RTA.
- Volume expansion by means of sodium chloride may paradoxically worsen the acidosis by further promoting bicarbonate diuresis. Nevertheless, gradual volume replacement may be necessary in the perioperative period.

Distal RTA

- Distal RTA results from the distal tubules' inability to secrete hydrogen ions. Failure to acidify the urine renders the urine alkaline (pH usually greater than 6), potentiating the occurrence of nephrocalcinosis, osteomalacia, growth retardation, and progressive renal insufficiency.
- Acidosis, hypocalcemia and polyuria may also be found.
- Treatment consists of bicarbonate replacement.
- Responsiveness is generally greater in distal RTA patients than in those with proximal RTA.

Sickle Cell Nephropathy

Etiology

Sickle cell nephropathy can occur in both sickle cell trait (AS) and homozygous (SS) patients. The cause is believed to be increased sickling as a result of the normal hypertonicity and hypoxia found in the renal medulla.

Major Manifestations

- Hematuria.
- A progressive decline in the ability to concentrate urine. While initially reversible by means of red blood cell transfusions, it progresses to a fixed status with obligate dilute urine output so that the patient is unable to concentrate urine when dehydrated.
- Urine specific gravity and osmolarity do not reflect the patient's volume status.

Management

- Aggressive fluid management is usually advised.
- The basic principles underlying the treatment of sickle cell disease are observed. Essential are adequate oxygenation, avoidance of hypothermia or acidosis, and careful monitoring of hemodynamics.

Diabetic Nephropathy

- Diabetic nephropathy rarely occurs in children, usually requiring a minimum of 10 to 15 years to develop. The pathognomic lesion is that of nodular intercapillary glomerulosclerosis (Kimmelstiel-Wilson lesions).
- The initial indication of diabetic nephropathy is proteinuria, followed by a declining GFR and a rising serum creatinine. Patients may also become nephrotic.
- Hypertension is a frequently associated finding.
- In diabetics with renal failure, myocardial infarction is a major cause of morbidity and mortality.
- Anesthetic management includes routine care of the diabetic patient and monitoring fluids and electrolytes.

Wilm's Tumor (Nephroblastoma)

Manifestations

- Wilm's tumor is the most common abdominal tumor of childhood, usually appearing between 1 and 5 years of age. It is occasionally bilateral and sometimes associated with hemihypertrophy and aniridia.
- Symptoms of Wilm's tumor are usually a large abdominal mass, with hematuria, fever, and weight loss. Hypertension from increased renin secretion may be present. Anemia and fever often occur as a result of hemorrhage into the tumor.
- The tumor may be massive and involve the IVC, renal vein, or aorta.
- Wilm's tumor may metastasize to the lymph nodes, to the liver, and to the lungs.

Treatment

In conjunction with certain drugs, Wilm's tumor patients may be undergoing chemotherapy. The following side effects should be noted (see also Chapter 12):

Drug	Side Effect
Vincristine	Neuropathy, vomiting
Actinomycin D	Vomiting and thrombocytopenia
Cyclophosphamide	Bone marrow suppression and hemorrhagic cystitis
Adriamycin	Dose-related cardiotoxicity beginning at 300 to 400 mg/m^2 (may be detected by echocardiography).

Anesthetic Management

- The large tumor mass predisposes to reflux and regurgitation. Ranitidine (1 mg/kg) IV may be useful to decrease acidity. Metoclopramide must be used with caution in young children because of the high incidence of dystonic reactions. Rapid sequence induction is probably indicated for large abdominal masses. By impinging on diaphragmatic excursion, the mass may also compromise ventilation.
- Life-threatening hemorrhage may occur, particularly in the case of an extensive tumor with IVC extension or encasement of the aorta. IVC cross-clamping may be required during surgery. All of these factors can acutely compromise cardiac output intraoperatively.
- The use of multiple, large-bore IV catheters (preferably above the diaphragm), arterial, and CVP catheters should be considered for hemodynamic monitoring and blood sampling.
- Extensive third space losses are likely to occur because of prolonged and extensive dissection. Prolonged exposure of the abdominal contents may result in hypothermia.
- Young children often require postoperative intensive care unit management and mechanical ventilation after undergoing extensive surgery.

Anesthesia for Miscellaneous Urologic Procedures

Cystoscopy and Urodynamic Studies

- For cystoscopy and urodynamic studies, infants and children usually receive general anesthesia, often administered by face mask if the planned procedure is to be brief.
- Thiopental, deep inhalation anesthesia, narcotics, and atropine may inhibit bladder and sphincter tone and thereby interfere with urodynamic studies.

Hypospadias, Chordee, and Undescended Testicles

- Procedures for hypospadias, chordee, and undescended testicles are usually performed using general anesthesia. The major anesthetic concerns relate to the status of any coexisting disease.

- The manipulation of the testicles and the peritoneum that occurs during undescended testicle repair can produce prominent vagal stimulation. Atropine or glycopyrrolate are effective in ablating this response. Regional anesthetic techniques (caudal anesthesia) are effective in preventing vagal symptoms and are useful for postoperative analgesia.
- An undescended, unlocated testicle may require an intraabdominal approach, necessitating muscle relaxation and intubation. Spinal anesthesia has been advocated for infants at higher risk from coexisting pulmonary disease.

ENDOCRINE DISEASES

Diabetes Mellitus

General Characteristics

1. Diabetes mellitus is the most common childhood endocrine disorder.
2. A chronic metabolic disease, it is frequently genetic in origin and results in deranged metabolism of carbohydrates, protein, and fat.
3. Most common in children is insulin-dependent diabetes mellitus (IDDM), sometimes referred to as juvenile-onset, or type I, diabetes.
   - IDDM is a result of pancreatic β cell destruction, which ablates the ability to synthesize and release insulin. This may result from virus-induced autoimmune mechanisms.
   - IDDM is found in approximately 1 in every 500 school-age children.
   - IDDM shows no sexual predilection.
4. Noninsulin-dependent diabetes mellitus (NIDDM), formerly referred to as maturity-onset, or type II, diabetes, is commonly diagnosed in the adult. These patients have normal or high insulin levels and do not usually manifest ketoacidosis.

Clinical Manifestations

1. Children commonly have a history of the following:
   - Lethargy
   - Weakness
   - Weight loss
   - Polyuria
   - Polyphagia
   - Polydipsia
2. Diabetic ketoacidosis (DKA) is the initial presentation in 10% to 20% of children with diabetes mellitus.
   - DKA is a catabolic state often precipitated by trauma, infection, vomiting, or psychological stress.
   - Abdominal pain with leukocytosis may accompany DKA.
   - Metabolic alterations include hyperglycemia (serum glucose greater than 300 mg/100 ml), dehydration, ketonemia, metabolic acidosis, hypokalemia, and hyperlipidemia.
3. Renal insufficiency or failure may be present.
4. Insulin replacement in children approximates 0.5 to 1 units/kg/day initially and often declines after initial therapy to 0.3 units/kg/day or less.

- Hypoglycemia is a frequent complication of insulin therapy, manifested by trembling, diaphoresis, tachycardia, and nervousness. Symptoms may progress to a change in mental status, seizures, or coma.
- Treatment of hypoglycemia is oral or intravenous dextrose or glucagon (0.5 mg to 1 mg) IM.

Anesthetic Management

Preoperative assessment

1. The preoperative assessment of a diabetic requires the following information:
   - Age of onset of diabetes
   - Type and dosage of insulin
   - Dietary habits
   - Frequency of DKA and/or hypoglycemic episodes
2. Unstable diabetic patients should be admitted to the hospital before surgery so that their insulin therapy can be optimized and their serum glucose controlled. Children with stable diabetes undergoing surgical procedures of less than 1 hour's duration may be admitted on the day of surgery. Surgery should be scheduled as early as possible on the day of admittance.
3. Preoperative laboratory measurements include:
   - Serum glucose, electrolytes, creatinine, and blood urea nitrogen (BUN)
   - Urinary glucose and ketones
   - Glycosylated hemoglobin (Hgb A1c): may be helpful in evaluating blood sugar control for the preceding 3-month period.
4. The preoperative visit provides an opportunity to allay concerns and develop a rapport with the patient. Anxiety associated with surgery may heighten sympathetic or neuroendocrine activity, which will result in an elevated serum glucose level.
5. Preoperative sedatives should be prescribed in their usual dosages. Delayed gastric emptying is often present; maintenance of usual NPO times and use of H_2 antagonists and metoclopramide preoperatively are recommended.

Intraoperative management

- One of the following three protocols may be employed for the management of insulin therapy in the perioperative period.
  1. The most common method is a D_5.45 NS intravenous infusion begun early in the morning on the day of surgery at a maintenance rate. One-half the usual NPH insulin dosage is given after the dextrose infusion is begun. Blood glucose levels are measured before induction and frequently during the operative procedure. Plasma glucose is maintained between 100 and 250 mg/dl. Regular insulin doses of 0.1 mg/kg are given when plasma glucose exceeds 250 mg/dl.
  2. An alternative method is to begin simultaneous insulin and glucose infusions on the morning of surgery. The insulin infusion rate allows for 0.2 to 0.4 units of regular insulin per gram of glucose. This infusion results in 1 to 2 units of insulin per 100 ml of D_5W. Once again, blood glucose levels are maintained between 100 and 200 mg/dl by adjusting the insulin infusion rate.

3. The third method of preoperative diabetes management is to withhold both insulin and glucose infusions. This technique may be used for short procedures that occur early in the morning and permit oral intake in the recovery room. After oral intake is resumed, 40% to 50% of the usual insulin dose is given. Serum glucose should be monitored intraoperatively and postoperatively.

- Anesthesia and sedation may mask the occurrence of hypoglycemia. Regional anesthesia, if tolerated, may be used, with the advantage of allowing for assessment of the child's mental status if hypoglycemia should occur.

Postoperative management. The blood glucose should be measured every 4 to 6 hours beginning in the recovery room and continuing postoperatively. A sliding scale for insulin administration is frequently used until the usual oral intake is resumed.

Hypoparathyroidism

General Characteristics

- Primary hypoparathyroidism is caused by a decrease in hormone production. It may result from surgical excision of the glands during thyroid surgery.
- The pseudoform is an inherited disorder resulting from decreased end-organ responsiveness despite elevated hormone levels. Physical characteristics are shortness of stature, thick neck, short metacarpals and metatarsals, and mental retardation.

Clinical Manifestations

- Serum calcium is low, and a positive Chvostek or Trousseau sign is seen.
- Inspiratory stridor may be heard.
- The ECG shows a prolonged PR interval.
- Chronic diarrhea, skin infections, and cataracts may be present in older children.

Anesthetic Management

Preoperative assessment

- Surgery should be delayed until the serum calcium level becomes approximately normal.
- If emergent surgery is required, calcium gluconate (30 mg/kg) or calcium chloride (10 mg/kg) should be given with ECG monitoring, and pH should be measured frequently to avoid alkalosis.

Intraoperative management

- Serum ionized calcium should be monitored intraoperatively and treated when necessary.
- Ionized calcium concentrations can be decreased by rapid blood transfusions.
- Intraoperative hypotension may occur as a result of myocardial depression from anesthetic agents coupled with low serum ionized calcium.
- Responses to nondepolarizing muscle relaxants may be potentiated in the presence of decreased serum ionized calcium levels.

Postoperative management. An acute decrease in ionized calcium can result in laryngospasm.

Hyperparathyroidism

General Characteristics

- Hyperparathyroidism is classified as primary, secondary, or pseudoform.
- Primary hyperparathyroidism is usually due to a parathyroid adenoma during childhood. The infant has poor muscle tone, dehydration, and poor feeding habits with resultant weight loss. Poor rib development causes respiratory dysfunction.
- Secondary hyperparathyroidism results from renal or gastrointestinal disease.
- Pseudohyperparathyroidism is due to an ectopic release of parathyroid hormones or a parathyroid hormone–like substance.

Clinical Manifestations

In primary hyperparathyroidism, ionized serum calcium elevation with increased parathyroid hormone is diagnostic and a metabolic acidosis with hyperchloremia and hyperphosphatemia is present.

Anesthetic Management

Preoperative management

- The preoperative evaluation of hyperparathyroidism must include an ECG because the PR interval may be longer and the QT interval inversely proportional to the serum calcium. T waves are longer when serum calcium is sharply elevated.
- Blood pressure and electrolytes should be evaluated.
- Preoperative hydration is necessary.
- Serum calcium is lowered by normal saline infusions and furosemide.
- Mithramycin and calcitonin are also used.

Intraoperative management

- Thiopental or inhalation agents can be used for induction.
- Hypercalcemic crisis can occur intraoperatively and requires blood pressure support, hyperventilation, hydration, and urine output monitoring.

Postoperative management

- After parathyroid resection, airway obstruction secondary to hematoma, edema, or recurrent laryngeal nerve injury may occur.
- Hypocalcemia may be present, with cramps, paresthesias, and a widened QT interval. Therapy is calcium gluconate (30 mg/kg) or calcium chloride (10 mg/kg).

Hyperthyroidism

General Characteristics

Hyperthyroidism in children is most commonly congenital or is a result of Graves' disease.

1. Congenital hyperthyroidism is caused by the transfer of maternal thyroid-stimulating immunoglobulins in utero.
    - The birth is premature and the infant has a goiter.

- Tachycardia, respiratory distress, and congestive heart failure may be present.

2. Graves' disease occurs more frequently among adolescents than children and 4 to 5 times more frequently among females.

Clinical Manifestations

- Signs and symptoms of hyperthyroidism in children include goiter, exophthalmos, hypertension, tachycardia, widened pulse pressure, and tremor.
- The levels of serum thyroxine (T_4) and triiodothyronine (T_3) are elevated. Age adjusted normal values are needed because thyroid hormone levels are higher in children.
- Treatment of hyperthyroidism in children includes propylthiouracil and saturated solution of potassium iodide (SSKI). Although symptoms will resolve in 1 to 2 weeks, laboratory values may not normalize for 4 to 6 weeks. Propranolol is useful for cardiovascular symptomatology.

Preoperative Management

- Preoperatively, the child should have received 6 to 8 weeks of thiouracil therapy to assure a euthyroid state.
- One week before surgery, administration of Lugol's solution should be initiated.
- A larger goiter requires a computerized axial tomography (CAT) scan to determine if tracheal compression exists.
- Propranolol may be used preoperatively to control tachycardia.

Intraoperative Management

- Anticholinergics are to be avoided because they can interfere with heat dissipation by blocking the ability to perspire.
- Thiopental is used for induction because it may possess antithyroid effects. Increased cardiac output prolongs induction time with inhalation agents.
- In the presence of exophthalmus, special attention should be given to eye care.
- For muscle relaxation, atracurium or vecuronium are used because of their minimal cardiovascular effects.
- The use of ketamine is not recommended, because it usually further increases heart rate and blood pressure.
- Isoflurane is the inhalational agent used for maintenance because it does not sensitize the myocardium to catecholamines. Halothane should be avoided both because of its ability to precipitate arrhythmias in the presence of catecholamines and because of the altered metabolic rate in hyperthyroid patients.
- Surgical complications include bradycardia resulting from carotid sinus stimulation; thyroid storm; thoracic air dissection; unilateral or bilateral recurrent laryngeal nerve injury; and hypoparathyroidism.
- Airway obstruction may occur from edema, hematoma, tracheomalacia, or laryngeal nerve injury.
- Thyroid storm can mimic malignant hyperthermia, with hyperthermia, tachycardia, congestive heart failure, dehydration, and shock. It results

from the acute release of thyroid hormones. Treatment includes sodium iodide, cortisol, propranolol, and propylthiouracil.

Hypothyroidism

General Characteristics

1. Hypothyroidism is among the most common of endocrine disorders in children.
2. Congenital hypothyroidism occurs in 1:4000 to 1:7000 live births and is usually a result of thyroid dysgenesis. Females are affected twice as often as males.
3. Clinical features of hypothyroidism in infants include the following:
   - Puffy face, wide fontanelle and sutures, flat nasal bridge, large tongue, and a hoarse cry
   - Protuberant abdomen with umbilical hernia
   - Cold, mottled, or jaundiced skin
   - Sluggish reflexes
4. Acquired hypothyroidism is twice as common as the congenital form.
5. Causes of acquired hypothyroidism include chronic lymphocytic thyroiditis, radioactive iodine therapy, infiltrative diseases, hypopituitarism, surgical excision, and sick euthyroid syndrome.

Clinical Manifestations

- Hypothyroidism is often manifested during childhood by reduced growth velocity.
- The child may also appear lethargic and have a goiter or myxedema.
- Precocious sexual development may be in evidence.
- Possible intolerance to cold, a low pulse pressure, and bradycardia are often present.
- An elevated thyroid stimulating hormone (TSH) is the most sensitive index of primary hypothyroidism.
- Serum thyroxine (T_4) is low and the T_3 resin uptake (T_{3RU}) is low or normal.

Anesthetic Management

Preoperative assessment and medications

- The degree of hypothyroidism must be determined preoperatively.
- A minimal period of 2 weeks of thyroxine therapy is necessary to establish a euthyroid state.
- If there is cardiac involvement, treatment should begin gradually because of the risk of sudden death.
- Hypothyroid children are more sensitive to the depressant effects of medications on the respiratory and cardiovascular systems. Reductions in heart rate and stroke volume may result in a significant reduction in cardiac output.
- Preoperative sedation should be avoided.
- Thyroid medications should be continued preoperatively.
- Hydrocortisone should be given (2 mg/kg every 6 hours) because of the increased incidence of adrenocortical insufficiency and impaired response to adrenocorticotropic hormone (ACTH).

Intraoperative management

- Before induction, atropine may be used.
- Doses of medication should be reduced intraoperatively because of heightened sensitivity, which is attributed to decreased cardiac output, reduced intravascular volume, and altered baroreceptor function. There may also be a reduction in hepatic metabolism and renal excretion.
- Decreased intravascular volume may result in hypotension when vasodilating agents are used. Ketamine may prove beneficial in these situations.
- Use of arterial and central venous pressure catheters is recommended for hemodynamic monitoring.
- The risk of hypothermia is great. Operating room temperatures should be maintained at a minimum of 25° C. All fluids should be warmed and a heating mattress used.
- Prevention of hyponatremia and hypoglycemia is effected by the use of intravenous solutions containing sodium and dextrose and by frequent monitoring of sodium and glucose levels.

Postoperative management

- Compromised pulmonary function should be anticipated. The child's ventilatory response to hypercarbia and hypoxia may be impaired. Ventilatory assistance may be required postoperatively.
- Emergence from anesthesia may be prolonged.
- Cardiovascular and respiratory support may be required.
- Body temperature and serum glucose should be monitored into the postoperative period.
- The administration of corticosteroids and thyroid medications should be resumed as soon as the patient begins accepting oral fluids.

Hypopituitarism

General Characteristics

1. Hypopituitarism in children is often secondary to compression by a craniopharyngioma.
2. In children less than 14 years of age, 10% of all brain tumors are craniopharyngiomas.
   - Peak incidence is 7 years of age.
   - There is a higher incidence in males than in females.
   - This tumor results in failure to grow, elevated intracranial pressure, and visual losses.

Clinical Manifestations

- Physical characteristics of hypopituitarism include short stature, lack of sexual development, and obesity.
- Hypothyroidism, adrenal insufficiency, and diabetes insipidus may also be present.
- Hyperpituitarism may involve excesses of growth hormone, resulting in gigantism associated with glucose intolerance and hyperinsulinemia.
- Excessive secretion of ACTH results in Cushing's disease, which is characterized by obesity, reduced growth, and osteoporosis.
- The posterior pituitary may produce excessive antidiuretic hormone se-

cretion (SIADH), with hyponatremia, reduced serum osmolality, elevated urine osmolality, and decreased urine output.
- Children with pituitary pathology may have elevated intracranial pressures (ICP) evidenced by headache, vomiting, tense fontanelles, and behavioral changes.

Preoperative Management

- Preoperative sedation should be avoided in patients with elevated ICP.
- Corticosteroids and thyroid hormones should be given when indicated.

Intraoperative Management

- Surgical removal of pituitary tumors includes three approaches: stereotactic, transsphenoidal, and frontal craniotomy.
- Involvement of the cavernous sinus implies a significant risk of air embolism and bleeding.
- An induction designed to lower ICP with hyperventilation and thiopental is advocated, with intravenous lidocaine or fentanyl to blunt the cardiovascular response to laryngoscopy.
- Mannitol is used to reduce cerebral edema.
- Insertion of an arterial catheter permits continuous blood pressure monitoring and blood sampling.
- Nasogastric tubes are contraindicated in patients with pituitary tumors.
- Venous air embolism is a potential complication, particularly if the sitting position is used.
- Anesthesia is maintained with nitrous oxide, oxygen, and isoflurane.

Postoperative Management

1. Postoperative complications include diabetes insipidus (DI) in about 20% of patients, thyroid and ACTH deficiency, hyperthermia, and seizures.
2. Serum sodium, osmolality, glucose, and urine output and osmolality must be measured frequently for possible diabetes insipidus.
3. Signs of DI include the following:
   - Urine output greater than 3 ml/kg/hr
   - Elevated serum sodium
   - Decreased urine osmolality
   - Ratio of urine to serum osmolality greater than 1:1
4. DI is treated with vasopressin, hypotonic fluids, and potassium.

Neuroblastoma

General Characteristics

- Neuroblastoma is a malignant tumor originating in the adrenal medulla or paravertebral ganglia. It may be found in the abdomen, mediastinum, or spinal cord.
- Metastasis to the bone marrow, liver, and brain is common.
- Incidence is approximately 1 in every 10,000 live births.

- The tumor most often manifests itself in children who are less than 1 year of age.

Anesthetic Management

Preoperative management

- The extent of the tumor and metastasis should be determined preoperatively.
- There is potential for bone marrow depression and cardiac toxicity if chemotherapy has been given.
- Anemia should be corrected if necessary to increase oxygen carrying capacity.
- Children should be well hydrated in anticipation of substantial intraoperative blood loss and the occurrence of third space sequestrations.
- Vomiting and diarrhea (causing electrolyte abnormalities) may occur as a result of the tumor's release of vasoactive peptide.

Intraoperative management

- Intravenous catheters should be placed in the upper extremities or the external jugular vein in anticipation of inferior vena cava involvement.
- Placement of arterial and central venous pressure catheters is warranted in the presence of a large abdominal or thoracic tumor.
- Monitoring of room temperature, a heating mattress, and warm fluids are necessary to prevent hypothermia caused by evaporative losses from a large operative site.
- An intravenous or inhalation induction is acceptable. A rapid-sequence induction is indicated in the event of intestinal obstruction.
- It is possible for neuroblastomas to secrete catecholamines and cause hypertension, so the use of isoflurane is preferred.
- Atracurium and vecuronium are used for muscle relaxation because they produce minimal cardiovascular side effects.
- Manipulation of the inferior vena cava can result in tumor embolism. Symptoms of a pulmonary embolism, including hypotension, cardiac arrhythmia, and cardiac arrest, can be seen.

Pheochromocytoma

General Characteristics

- Pheochromocytoma is a catecholamine-secreting tumor that originates in the adrenal medulla (90%) but may also be found wherever chromaffin tissue is present, as in the sympathetic chain, which extends from the base of the skull to the pelvis.
- Approximately 10% of tumors are bilateral.
- In nearly 20% of patients, functional tumors occur in numerous sites.
- The tumor may be one of the diseases in multiple endocrine neoplasia type IIa or IIb.
- Malignant pheochromocytomas rarely occur in children.
- There is a greater incidence of pheochromocytoma in puberty than childhood.

Clinical Manifestations

- The elevation in plasma norepinephrine or epinephrine associated with pheochromocytoma usually causes headaches, nausea, vomiting, diaphoresis, visual complaints, and weight loss.
- The child looks pale, has cool extremities, and appears anxious.
- Hypertension may be intermittent or persistent.
- Sustained hypertension is associated with large tumors that secrete norepinephrine.
- Orthostatic hypotension reflects the reduction in intravascular fluid volume resulting from sustained hypertension.

Anesthetic Management

Preoperative management

- Serum electrolytes, creatinine, fasting blood sugar, and possibly a glucose tolerance test should be obtained preoperatively. Hyperglycemia results from adrenergic inhibition of insulin release and glycogenolysis.
- Chronically elevated plasma catecholamines may result in a cardiomyopathy, necessitating an ECG and echocardiogram.
- α-adrenergic blockade should be instituted several days before surgery. Phenoxybenzamine, an α-1 and α-2 receptor antagonist, or prazosin, an α-1 receptor antagonist, is used. α blockade prevents vasoconstriction in response to catecholamines and facilitates insulin release. Since the child's blood volume is contracted, a reduction in hematocrit indicates a return to normal blood volume.
- Although cardiac arrhythmias and tachycardia are rare in the pediatric population, the use of β-adrenergic blockade may be necessary. β-adrenergic blocking drugs should not be used in the absence of α-adrenergic blockade. Unopposed α-adrenergic vasoconstriction increases systemic vascular resistance (afterload) and prevents the β-blocked heart from maintaining adequate cardiac output.
- Alphamethyltyrosine reduces catecholamine synthesis and is an alternative therapy for children.
- Preoperative sedation serves to reduce anxiety and the associated catecholamine release.

Intraoperative management

1. Medications that stimulate the sympathetic nervous system should be avoided.
2. α-adrenergic blockade should be continued until the day of surgery.
3. An arterial catheter should be placed before induction.
4. Anesthesia may be induced with thiopental, diazepam, or inhalation agents. Halothane is avoided because of the likelihood of arrhythmias in the presence of excess circulating catecholamines.
5. Theoretically, succinylcholine-induced fasiculations could increase catecholamine release by the tumor, but this effect is not visible clinically.

6. Atracurium and vecuronium are the recommended muscle relaxants because they produce minimal cardiovascular side effects.
7. Lidocaine or fentanyl given intravenously 1 minute before laryngoscopy may diminish an increase in blood pressure and prevent cardiac arrhythmias.
8. Anesthesia can be maintained with nitrous oxide, oxygen, enflurane, or isoflurane.
9. Hypertension is controlled by the use of sodium nitroprusside (1 to 4 μg/kg/min) or phentolamine (30 μg/kg).
10. As the veins draining the pheochromocytoma are ligated, a decline in blood pressure may result from the decrease in plasma catecholamines.
11. An infusion of norepinephrine is necessary if hypotension persists.
12. Intravascular volume is evaluated by means of a central venous pressure catheter.
13. Serial arterial blood gases should be obtained and frequent measurements of electrolytes taken.
14. Hyperglycemia is common before surgery. Hypoglycemia is evident after the tumor has been removed.

Postoperative management

- Invasive monitoring should be maintained until the child's cardiovascular and pulmonary status stabilize.
- Between 24 and 48 hours postoperatively, blood pressure returns to normal values if the entire tumor has been excised.
- Plasma catecholamine concentrations should normalize in 7 to 10 days.

BIBLIOGRAPHY

Berry FA: The renal system. In Gregory GA, editor: Pediatric anesthesia, ed 2, vol 1, New York, 1989, Churchill Livingstone.

Cramolini GM: Diseases of the renal system. In Katz J and Steward DJ, editors: Anesthesia and uncommon pediatric diseases, Philadelphia, 1987, WB Saunders Co.

Dogramaci I, Drash AL, and Finberg L: Disorders of metabolism. In Ziai M, editor: Pediatrics, ed 3, Boston, 1984, Little, Brown & Co.

Kern T and Templeton J: Diseases of the endocrine system. In Katz J and Steward D, editors: Anesthesia and uncommon pediatric diseases, Philadelphia, 1987, WB Saunders Co.

Loughran PG and Gieseche AH: Diabetes mellitus: anesthetic considerations, Semin Anesth 3:207, 1984.

Roizen M: Endocrine abnormalities and anesthesia: implications for the anesthesiologist. In Hershey SG, editor: ASA Refresher Courses, vol 12, Philadelphia, 1984, JB Lippincott Co.

Rosenbaum S: Anesthetic management of the diabetic patient. In Hershey SG, editor: ASA Refresher Courses, vol 9, Philadelphia, 1981, JB Lippincott Co.

Spear RM, Deshpande JK, and Davis PJ: Systemic disorders in pediatric anesthesia. In Motoyama EK, editor: Smith's anesthesia for infants and children, ed 5, St Louis, 1990, The CV Mosby Co.

Travis LB: Kidney and urinary tract. In Rudolph AM, editor: Textbook of pediatrics, ed 18, Norwalk, 1987, Appleton and Lange.
Ziai M and Mosier HD, Jr: The endocrine glands. In Ziai M, editor: Pediatrics, ed 3, Boston, 1984, Little, Brown & Co.

17

PEDIATRIC SYNDROMES AND ANESTHETIC IMPLICATIONS

Gail E. Rasmussen
Charlotte Bell

Oh, wouldn't it be nice to be a hammer or a horn,
And know that you are perfect from the moment that you're born?
RIVIAN BELL

The following is a list of abbreviations used in this chapter:

ALL	acute lymphoblastic leukemia
ASA	acetylsalicylic acid
ATN	acute tubular necrosis
AV	atrioventricular, arteriovenous
AVM	arteriovenous malformation
C-spine	cervical spine
CAD	coronary artery disease
CHD	congenital heart disease
CHF	congestive heart failure
CN	cranial nerve
CNS	central nervous system
CV	cardiovascular
DDAVP	desmopressin acetate
DIC	disseminated intravascular coagulation
DTR	deep tendon reflexes
EACA	epsilon-amino-caproic acid
ETT	endotracheal tube
FFP	fresh frozen plasma
GE	gastroesophageal
GI	gastrointestinal
HDL	high-density lipoprotein
HTN	hypertension
ICP	intracranial pressure
Ig	immunoglobulins
INH	isoniazid
IUGR	intrauterine growth retardation
IV	intravenous
IVH	intraventricular hemorrhage
LFTs	liver function tests
MAC	minimum alveolar concentration
MH	malignant hyperthermia

MVP	mitral valve prolapse
N_2O	nitrous oxide
NSAID	nonsteroidal antiinflammatory drugs
PDA	patent ductus arteriosis
PFTs	pulmonary function tests
PS	pulmonic stenosis
SVT	supraventricular tachycardia
TEF	tracheoesophageal fistula
TMJ	temporomandibular joint
TPL	thiopentothal
URI	upper respiratory infection
VF	ventricular fibrillation
VSD	ventriculoseptal defect

CARDIOTHORACIC SYNDROMES (See also Chapter 11)

Congenital cardiac lesions are responsible for more than 90% of all cases of heart disease in children. The incidence of congenital heart disease (CHD) is 2 to 3 times higher in preterm than full-term infants. A thorough understanding of the anatomy and physiology of a specific lesion, by either echocardiography or cardiac catheterization, is essential when developing an anesthetic plan. It is also important to appreciate that the same lesion in two different children may present varying degrees of disability depending on the amount of stenosis, magnitude of shunt, severity of failure, and previous corrective procedures. Children with CHD often have associated noncardiac defects, usually of the genitourinary system.

Syndromes and Diseases

Ebstein's anomaly
Eisenmenger's syndrome
Holt-Oram syndrome (heart-hand syndrome)
Ivemark syndrome
Jervell and Lange-Nielsen syndrome
Kartagener's syndrome
Kawasaki disease (mucocutaneous lymph node syndrome)
Progeria (Hutchinson-Gilford syndrome)
Romano-Ward syndrome
Rubinstein-Taybi syndrome
Shone syndrome
Tuberous sclerosis
VATER syndrome
Weber-Christian disease (chronic nonsuppurative panniculitis)
Werner syndrome
Williams syndrome
Wilson-Mikity syndrome
Wolff-Parkinson-White syndrome

CHROMOSOMAL SYNDROMES

This category includes syndromes involving specific chromosomal aberrations present in every cell and therefore every organ system. Often the gene has variable penetrance, which affects the severity of the syndrome and the degree of organ involvement. Most of the chromosomal syndromes are associated with mental retardation, which may limit patient cooperation, even in the older child or adolescent. Intramuscular ketamine (4 to 5 mg/kg) is often useful in the large uncooperative or hyperactive child because of its ease of use, rapid and predictable onset, and preservation of spontaneous ventilation.

Syndromes

Cri-du-chat syndrome
Down's syndrome (trisomy 21)
Edward's syndrome (trisomy 18)
Klinefelter's syndrome (XXY)
Noonan's syndrome (male Turner's)
Patau syndrome (trisomy 13)
Turner's syndrome (XO)

CONNECTIVE TISSUE DISORDERS

This category of syndromes primarily affects collagen synthesis, resulting in defective tensile strength properties. Multiple organ systems are usually affected.

These patients are often seen for hernia repair because of increased tissue laxity. Joint hyperflexibility requires extra care in positioning during operative procedures. Involvement of the cervical spine may increase the patient's susceptibility to injury during intubation. Airway management can be affected by arytenoid laxity or dislocation and preexisting tracheomalacia. Generalized alterations of vascular endothelium lead to an increased incidence of accelerated cardiovascular disease. Altered collagen structure may compromise cardiac valvular function.

These patients often have long histories of salicylate, nonsteroidal antiinflammatory drug, and steroid use. Stress dose steroid coverage and a coagulation profile should be considered preoperatively.

Syndromes and Diseases

Arthrogryposis multiplex congenita
Christ-Siemens-Touraine syndrome (anhidrotic ectodermal dysplasia)
Conradi's syndrome
CREST syndrome
Cutis laxa
Ehlers-Danlos syndrome
Juvenile rheumatoid arthritis (Still's disease)
Klippel-Feil syndrome
Klippel-Trenaunay-Weber syndrome
Larsen's syndrome
Marfan's syndrome
Pseudoxanthoma elasticum (Groenblad-Strandberg syndrome)
Scleroderma

CRANIOFACIAL DISORDERS

Children with craniofacial deformities often require many corrective operations, with the problem of airway management at issue on each occasion. Preoperative airway assessment becomes more difficult in the nonverbal or preverbal child or if psychomotor retardation is present. Some techniques commonly used for the difficult intubation (awake or fiberoptic intubation) become more difficult in the uncooperative child. Mask induction of anesthesia in spontaneously breathing patients before endotracheal intubation is often a successful option. The endotracheal tube must be adequately secured because it may be present in the operative field and not accessible to the anesthesiologist. Postoperatively, even minimal airway trauma or edema may necessitate prolonged ventilation.

Associated problems in these patients include elevated intracranial pressure, seizure disorders, and congenital heart disease. The extent of neurologic or cardiovascular involvement should be considered when devising anesthetic plans.

Syndromes and Diseases

Anderson's syndrome
Apert's syndrome
Beckwith-Wiedemann syndrome (infantile gigantism)
Carpenter's syndrome
Cherubism
Cornelia de Lange syndrome
Crouzon syndrome
Freeman-Sheldon syndrome (whistling face syndrome)
Goldenhar syndrome (oculoauriculovertebral syndrome)
Goltz's syndrome (focal dermal hypoplasia)
Gorlin-Chaudhry-Moss syndrome
Hallerman-Streif syndrome (oculomandibulofacial syndrome)
Leopard syndrome
Meckel syndrome
Mobius syndrome (congenital facial disease)
Oro-facial-digital syndrome
Pfeiffer syndrome
Pierre-Robin syndrome
Pyle's disease (metaphyseal dysplasia)
Saerthre-Chotzen syndrome
Smith-Lemli-Opitz syndrome
Sotos syndrome (cerebral gigantism)
Treacher-Collins syndrome (mandibulofacial dysostosis)

DERMATOLOGIC DISORDERS

Children affected by syndromes of primarily dermatologic origin often require repeated surgical intervention. Skin disruption results in increased vulnerability to mechanical trauma and necessitates meticulous care in positioning for surgery. Simple securing of intravenous catheters and endotracheal tubes, placement of ECG pads, and routine eye care should be accomplished without adhesives. Skin injury can be minimized by use of circumferential gauze bandages, padding under blood pressure cuffs, use of needle electrodes, avoidance of tape, suturing of intravenous catheters into place, and wiring of endotracheal tubes to teeth.

Disruption of the normal integument causes an inability to maintain body temperature, making temperature monitoring essential and maintenance of normothermia difficult. Standard practices of warming intravenous fluids, warming and humidifying inhaled gases, using warming lights and blankets, and elevation of room temperature should be used.

Intraoperative fluid losses are increased with loss of skin integrity and may be worsened by excessive bleeding from vascular malformations. Fluid and electrolyte balance should be monitored during lengthy procedures.

Syndromes and Diseases

Bloch-Sulzberger syndrome (incontinentia pigmenti)
Cockayne-Touraine syndrome (dystrophic epidermolysis bullae)
Epidermolysis bullosum (Herlitz's syndrome)
Erythema multiforme
Erythema multiforme major (Stevens-Johnson syndrome)
Ichthyosiform erythrodermia (congenital ichthyosis) (harlequin fetus)
Kohlmeier-Degos disease
Lyell disease (toxic epidermal necrolysis)
Rothmund-Thomson syndrome (poikiloderma atrophicans vasculare)
Seip-Lawrence syndrome
Staphylococcal scalded skin syndrome (Ritter disease)
Xeroderma pigmentosum

HEMATOLOGIC DISORDERS (See also Chapter 12)

Patients with congenital hematologic disorders often have anemia and decreased oxygen carrying capacity. The decision to transfuse the patient for elective surgery should be made preoperatively depending on the patient's overall condition. Also, the presence of dyshemoglobins (particularly Hemoglobin S [HgS]) may interfere with the accuracy of SpO_2 (oximetry) and thereby influence the decision to transfuse preoperatively. Coagulopathy diathesis, increased susceptibility to thrombosis, or both may also be present. These patients require specific identification of the clotting defect and delineation of the proposed treatment before the time of operation. Large-bore intravenous access and invasive monitoring should be considered if significant volume losses are anticipated.

Syndromes and Diseases

Blackfan-Diamond syndrome
Hemolytic uremic syndrome
Henoch-Schonlein purpura
Letterer-Siwe disease (acute disseminated histiocytosis)
Moschkowitz disease (thrombotic thrombocytopenic purpura)

Osler-Weber-Rendu syndrome (hereditary hemorrhagic telangiectasia)
TAR syndrome (thrombocytopenia and absent radius)
von Willebrand's disease

IMMUNOLOGIC DISORDERS

These syndromes impair the body's defense mechanism by affecting the T cells, B cells, immunoglobulins, or the complement cascade. Chronic pulmonary infections often occur, compromising pulmonary function and reserve. These patients require meticulous aseptic technique in the operating room for all invasive procedures including endotracheal intubation, intravenous (IV) catheter placement, and injection of any drugs into IV tubing.

Also included in this category are syndromes of probable autoimmune etiology involving multiple organ systems (granulomatous disease, systemic lupus). These patients usually require stress dose steroids in the perioperative period.

Syndromes and Diseases

Ataxia telangiectasia (Louis Bar syndrome)
Behcet's syndrome
DiGeorge syndrome (thymic hypoplasia)
Hand-Schuller-Christian disease
Hereditary angioneurotic edema
Systemic lupus erythematosis
Urbach-Wiethe disease
Wegener's granulomatosis
Wiskott-Aldrich syndrome

HEMATOLOGIC AND IMMUNOLOGIC DISORDERS
Syndromes and Diseases

Chediak-Higashi syndrome
Hereditary angioneurotic edema
Kasabach-Merritt syndrome

METABOLIC/OBESITY DISORDERS

Children with these syndromes share the primary clinical manifestations of obesity, whether from a known metabolic derangement or an unknown specific defect. The degree of obesity can be determined from standard growth charts and from calculation of the body mass index (BMI):

$$\text{BMI} = \frac{\text{Wt (kg)}}{\text{Ht}^2\ (\text{m}^2)}$$

$$\text{Normal} = 20 \text{ to } 30$$

$$\text{Obese} = \text{over } 30$$

Multiorgan system dysfunction should be anticipated in the obese pediatric patient including the cardiovascular, endocrine, musculoskeletal, and autonomic nervous systems. There is an increased incidence of respiratory disease and decreased respiratory reserve.

Specific anesthetic difficulties include airway obstruction from redundant soft tissue, delayed gastric emptying, increased aspiration risk, poor vascular access, and blood pressure lability. A loss of functional residual capacity impairs pulmonary reserve. Decreased sympathetic and parasympathetic function and an increased susceptibility to cardiac failure and pulmonary edema have been described. An increased production of serum fluoride may occur with halothane use.

Preoperative placement of an intravenous catheter and rapid sequence induction are recommended. Mask induction with spontaneous ventilation often results in acute airway obstruction and rapid oxygen desaturation.

Syndromes

Alstrom syndrome
Bandet-Biedle syndrome
Lawrence-Moon-Biedle syndrome
Noack's syndrome
Prader-Willi syndrome

INBORN ERRORS OF METABOLISM

In these diseases, a simple genetically determined biochemical defect results in the blockage of a specific metabolic process. As a result, precursors to the defective reaction accumulate and anticipated products are not made.

Since errors can occur in any biochemical pathway, a broad range of clinical symptoms and pathophysiology should be anticipated. However, most of these diseases produce some common attributes, most notably mental and motor retardation, neurologic abnormalities, and developmental disability. Multisystem involvement is common, particularly hepatorenal dysfunction and cardiomyopathy. Musculoskeletal defects and myotonia may result in respiratory compromise.

Anesthetic management of these patients requires specific delineation of the metabolic defect and thorough evaluation of the organ systems involved and the degree of involvement. Intra- and perioperative monitoring of biochemical functions (fluid, electrolyte, and glucose metabolism) is essential. Cardiopulmonary dysfunction and musculoskeletal abnormalities may result in an exaggerated response to inhalation anesthetics, sedatives, narcotics, and muscle relaxants. Prolonged drug action and impaired drug elimination may necessitate postoperative ventilation.

Syndromes and Diseases

Albright-Butler syndrome (primary distal renal tubular acidosis)
Bartter's syndrome
Bassen-Kornzweig syndrome (abetalipoproteinemia)
Cerebrohepatorenal syndrome (Zellweger syndrome)
Cretinism (congenital hypothyroidism)
Cystinosis
Fabry's disease (lysosomal storage disease)
Fanconi syndrome
Farber's disease

Favism (G-6-PD deficiency)
Gardner's syndrome
Gaucher disease
Glycogen storage disease:
- Type I—von Gierke's disease
- Type II—Pompe disease
- Type III—Cori disease
- Type IV—Andersen's disease
- Type V—McArdle disease
- Type VI—Hers disease
- Type VII—Tauri disease

Hartnup disease
Hemochromatosis
Homocystinuria
Lesch-Nyhan syndrome
Maple syrup urine disease
Mucopolysaccharidoses:
- Type I—Hurler's syndrome (Gargoylism)
- Type II—Hunter's syndrome
- Type III—Sanfilippo syndrome
- Type IV—Morquio syndrome
- Type V—Scheie disease
- Type VI—Maroteaux-Lamy syndrome

Niemann-Pick disease
Phenylketonuria (PKU)
Porphyria
Prune belly syndrome (urethral obstruction malformation complex)
Refsum's syndrome
Sipple syndrome (multiple endocrine neoplasia—type II)
Tangier disease (analpha lipoproteinemia)
Tay-Sachs disease
Wermer's syndrome (multiple endocrine neoplasia—type I)
Wilson's disease (hepatolenticular degeneration)
Wolman's disease (familial xanthomatosis)

MUSCULAR DISORDERS

Progressive weakness is the hallmark of most pediatric syndromes that primarily affect muscle. These myopathies result in atrophy of skeletal muscle and contractures necessitating careful padding and positioning in the operating room. Cardiac muscle involvement may cause cardiomyopathy with arrhythmias, conduction disturbances, or congestive heart failure.

Weakness of respiratory muscles may impair the patient's ability to ventilate. Exaggerated responses to muscle relaxants or sedatives may further decrease ventilatory response. Absent cough or gag may result in recurrent aspiration, with chronic infections and pneumonia. Prolonged airway protection and the need for mechanical ventilation are often necessary in the postoperative period.

Syndromes and Diseases

Amyotonia congenita (infantile muscular atrophy)
Bowen's syndrome (cerebrohepatorenal syndrome)
Central core disease
Duchenne muscular dystrophy
Familial periodic paralysis:
  Type I—hypokalemic
  Type II—hyperkalemic
  Type III—normokalemic
Fazio-Londe syndrome
King-Denborough syndrome
Kugelberg-Welander disease
Lowe syndrome (oculocerebrorenal syndrome)
Myasthenia gravis
Myositis ossificans (fibrodysplasia ossificans)
Myotonia congenita (Thomsen's disease)
Myotonic dystrophy
Paramyotonia congenita (Eulenberg syndrome)
Rieger syndrome
Schwartz-Jampal syndrome
Werdnig-Hoffman disease (progressive infantile spinal muscle atrophy)

NEUROLOGIC DISORDERS (See Chapter 13)

Although this category encompasses a broad spectrum of clinical problems, the two most commonly encountered are elevation of intracranial pressure (ICP) and seizure disorders. Usual techniques for patients with increased ICP include a barbiturate induction, intraoperative hyperventilation, pharmacologic agents to decrease cerebral edema (osmotic diuretics and steroids), and avoiding narcotic premedications, which may raise $PaCO_2$. In general, it is best to avoid ketamine, which elevates ICP.

Barbiturates and benzodiazepines possess antiseizure properties that make them useful agents for patients with seizure disorders. Ketamine can raise seizure threshold. Conversely, enflurane may lower seizure threshold at 2.5 MAC in the presence of hypocarbia.

Syndromes and Diseases

Arnold-Chiari malformation
Charcot-Marie-Tooth disease
Dandy Walker syndrome
Encephalocele (cranium bifidum)
Friedrich's ataxia
Guillain-Barré syndrome
Hallervorden-Spatz disease
Leber's hereditary optic neuropathy
Leigh's syndrome
Krabbe's disease (globoid cell leukodystrophy)
Myelomeningocele (spina bifida)

Neurofibromatosis (von Recklinghausen syndrome)
Riley-Day syndrome (familial dysautonomia)
Shy-Drager syndrome
Sturge-Weber syndrome (encephalotrigeminal angiomatosis)
Sydenham's chorea
Syringomyelia
Von Hippel-Lindau syndrome

SKELETAL DISORDERS

Most congenital disorders of the skeletal system can be categorized under the multiple forms of osteochondrodysplasias (dwarfism). Although symptoms and organ system involvement can vary widely, several features commonly occur.

Short stature, joint laxity or fixed contractures, and brittle bones prone to pathologic fractures necessitate careful padding and positioning in the operating room. Odontoid hypoplasia or atlantoaxial instability may predispose the spinal cord to compression during intubation and positioning. Airway management is further compromised by limited neck mobility or the presence of associated anomalies (micrognathia, cleft palate, tracheal stenosis).

Kyphoscoliosis is a common feature and may result in significant restrictive pulmonary disease and decreased pulmonary reserve. It also increases the problem of positioning, particularly if spinal stenosis with neurologic deficits is present.

A significant association exists between many forms of osteochondrodysplasia and congenital cardiac defects, seizure disorders, hydrocephalus, and bone marrow dysfunction (coagulopathy). The full extent of organ system involvement needs to be elucidated during the preoperative evaluation.

Syndromes

Forms of dwarfism (osteochondrodystrophies)

1. Achondrogenesis
2. Thanatophenic dwarfism
3. Short rib-polydactyly syndromes type I and type II
4. Type I osteogenesis imperfecta
5. Camptomelic dwarfism (lethal form)
6. Cerebrocostomandibular syndrome
7. Hypophosphatasia

Jeune syndrome (asphyxiating thoracic dystrophy)
Osteopetrosis (Albers-Schonberg disease, or marble bone disease)
Seckel syndrome (bird headed dwarfism)
Stickler syndrome (arthroophthalmomyopathy)

TABLE 17-1. Pediatric syndromes and anesthetic implications

Syndrome or disease	Primary system affected	Clinical manifestations	Physiologic considerations	Anesthetic implications
Abetalipoproteinemia (see Bassen-Kornzweig syndrome)				
Acute disseminated histiocytosis (see Letterer-Siwe disease)				
Albers-Schonberg disease (see Osteopetrosis)				
Albright-Butler syndrome (primary distal renal tubular acidosis)	Metabolic	• Anorexia • Vomiting • Constipation • Polyuria • Dehydration • Growth retardation	• Nephrocalcinosis causing interstitial nephritis and renal failure • Potassium loss causing weakness and periodic paralysis (may be severe)	• Hypokalemia • Impaired renal drug excretion • Fluid and electrolyte imbalance

Alstrom syndrome	Metabolic/ Obesity	• Obesity
		• Diabetes mellitus
		• Blindness
		• Deafness
		• Medullary cystic kidney
			• Complications of obesity:
			  • Delayed gastric emptying
			  • Altered autonomic nervous system response
			  • Poor vascular access
				• Impaired renal drug excretion
				• Aspiration precautions required
				• Impaired glucose and electrolyte regulation secondary to diabetes

Continued.

TABLE 17-1. Pediatric syndrome and anesthetic implications—cont'd

Syndrome or disease	Primary system affected	Clinical manifestations	Physiologic considerations	Anesthetic implications
Analbuminemia	Metabolic	• Almost absent albumin (4-100 mg%)	• Altered drug binding and metabolism	• Very sensitive to protein-bound drugs including thiopental, curare, coumarin, and bupivacaine
Analpha lipoproteinemia (see Tangier disease)				
Andersen's disease (Glycogen storage disease—type IV)	Metabolic	• Hepatosplenomegaly • Failure to thrive • Muscle weakness	• Cirrhosis • Hypoglycemia	• Requires maintenance glucose infusion and monitoring of blood glucose • Impaired hepatic drug metabolism • Liver function tests and coagulation profile may be abnormal • Exaggerated response to muscle relaxants
Anderson's syndrome	Craniofacial	• Severe midface hypoplasia • Mandibular prognathism • Abnormal structure and angle of mandible (triangular facies) • Kyphoscoliosis	• Restrictive lung disease	• Potentially difficult airway • Decreased pulmonary function and reserve

Anhidrotic ectodermal dysplasia (see Christ-Siemens-Touraine syndrome)				
Apert's syndrome (acrocephalosyndactyly)	Craniofacial	• Craniosynostosis • Sphenoethmoidomaxillary hypoplasia • Hypoplastic midface and prominent mandible • Cleft palate • Hydrocephalus • Exophthalmos • Associated CHD	• Elevated ICP • Psychomotor retardation	• Potentially difficult airway • Management of elevated ICP • Preoperative assessment of congenital heart defects required
Arnold-Chiari malformation	Neurologic	• Dysphagia • Apnea • Stridor • Aspiration • Opisthotonos • Decreased gag reflex • Associated with meningomyelocele and syringomyelia	• Elongation of cerebellar vermis and choroid plexus through foramen magnum with kinking of medulla and upper cervical cord • Compression causes cranial nerve palsies	• Potentially difficult airway • Vocal cord paralysis • Postoperative ventilation or tracheostomy often required • Aspiration precautions required

Continued.

TABLE 17-1. Pediatric syndrome and anesthetic implications—cont'd

Syndrome or disease	Primary system affected	Clinical manifestations	Physiologic considerations	Anesthetic implications
Arthrogryposis multiplex congenita	Connective tissue	• CHD • Inguinal hernia • Cleft palate • Scoliosis • TMJ rigidity • Decreased muscle mass • Spinal cord involvement causes leg and arm contractures	• Restrictive pulmonary disease	• Care in positioning required • Potentially difficult airway • May have exaggerated response to muscle relaxants • Contractures worsen vascular access • Pulmonary dysfunction may necessitate postoperative ventilation
Arthroopthalmomyopathy (see Stickler syndrome)				
Asphyxiating thoracic dystrophy (see Jeune syndrome)				
Ataxia telangiectasia (Louis Bar syndrome)	Immunologic	• Progressive cerebellar ataxia • Pulmonary infections • Bronchiectasis • If survival to adolescence, may develop malignant lymphoma	• Decreased IgA and IgE	• Significant pulmonary dysfunction

Bandet-Biedl syndrome	Metabolic/ Obesity	• Obesity
		• Polydactyly
		• Hypogenitalism
		• CHD
			• Psychomotor retardation
			• Renal dysfunction
			• Complications of obesity:
			  • Delayed gastric emptying
			  • Altered autonomic nervous system response
			  • Poor vascular access
				• Impaired renal drug excretion
				• Preoperative cardiac evaluation required
				• Aspiration precautions necessary

Bartter's syndrome	Metabolic	• Hyperaldosteronism with normal blood pressure
		• In infancy:
		  • Anorexia
		  • Failure to thrive
		  • Polyuria
		  • Polydipsia
			• Decreased response to angiotensin and norepinephrine
			• Increased prostaglandins
			• Hypokalemic, hypochloremic metabolic alkalosis
				• Fluid and electrolyte imbalance
				• Decreased response to vasopressors, particularly norepinephrine
				• Impaired renal drug excretion

Bassen-Kornzweig syndrome (Abetalipoproteinemia)	Metabolic	• Retinal abnormalities • Strabismus • Ptosis • Spinocerebellar degeneration with ataxia • Steatorrhea	• Vitamin A deficiency	• Association with strabismus and MH • Exaggerated response to muscle relaxants

Continued.

TABLE 17-1. Pediatric syndrome and anesthetic implications—cont'd

Syndrome or disease	Primary system affected	Clinical manifestations	Physiologic considerations	Anesthetic implications
Beckwith-Wiedemann syndrome (infantile gigantism)	Craniofacial	• Birth weight greater than 4,000 g • Macroglossia • Visceromegaly • Exophthalmos • Omphalocele • CHD	• Persistent severe neonatal hypoglycemia secondary to islet cell hyperplasia, hyperinsulinemia (especially in response to glucose) • Medullary renal dysplasia	• Potentially difficult airway management • Requires constant glucose infusion, avoidance of IV glucose boluses, and close monitoring of blood glucose • Impaired renal drug excretion

Behcet's syndrome	Immunologic	• Triad:
		  • Recurrent uveitis
		  • Aphthous stomatitis
		  • Genital ulcerations
		• Conjunctivitis
		• Choroiditis
		• Optic atrophy
		• Dermatitis and abscesses
		• CNS signs (relapse and remit), spastic paresis, ataxia, seizures
		• Cardiovascular:
		  • Pericarditis
		  • Vasculitis
		  • Hemoptysis
			• Probable immunologic cause with multisystem involvement and chronic progressive course
			• Obstructive pulmonary disease
			• Caval obstruction
				• Oropharyngeal scarring causes potentially difficult airway
				• May require stress dose steroids
				• Preoperative assessment of pulmonary dysfunction needed
				• Cardiovascular involvement may necessitate invasive monitoring

Bird headed dwarfism (see Seckel syndrome)				
Blackfan-Diamond syndrome	Hematologic/Immunologic	• Hepatosplenomegaly • Recurrent pulmonary infections • Thrombocytopenia	• Congenital idiopathic red cell aplasia	• May require stress dose steroids • Anemia and abnormal coagulation profile often present
Bloch-Sulzberger syndrome (incontinentia pigmenti)	Dermatologic	• Skin lesions, erythematous streaks, verrucous lesions, hyperpigmentation • CNS manifestations leading to developmental retardation, cortical atrophy, spastic paresis, seizures, and hydrocephalus • Ocular manifestations: strabismus, cataracts, retinal detachment • Skeletal anomalies: spina bifida, cleft lip or palate, pegged teeth, microcephaly	• CNS manifestations may cause elevated ICP • Impaired thermoregulation	• Management of patient with elevated ICP • Succinylcholine should be avoided in presence of spastic paresis • Teeth are susceptible to injury during laryngoscopy

Continued.

TABLE 17-1. Pediatric syndrome and anesthetic implications—cont'd

Syndrome or disease	Primary system affected	Clinical manifestations	Physiologic considerations	Anesthetic implications
Bowen's syndrome (cerebrohepatorenal syndrome)	Muscular	• Neonatal jaundice/hepatomegaly • Polycystic kidneys • CHD • Muscular hypotonia	• Renal dysfunction • Hypoprothrombinemia	• Extremely exaggerated response to muscle relaxants • Impaired renal drug excretion • Electrolyte imbalance • Abnormal coagulation profile
Carpenter's syndrome (acrocephalopolysyndactyly)	Craniofacial	• Short neck • Hypoplastic mandible • Omphalocele • CHD • Hypogenitalism	• Premature closure of all cranial sutures and elevated ICP • Psychomotor retardation	• Potentially difficult airway • Requires preoperative assessment of CHD • Management of elevated ICP
Central core disease	Muscular	• Muscular dystrophy • Hypotonia with muscle wasting	• Increased risk of malignant hyperthermia	• Increased sensitivity to respiratory depressants • Exaggerated response to muscle relaxants • MH triggers should be avoided
Cerebral gigantism (see Sotos syndrome)				
Cerebrohepatorenal syndrome (see Bowen's syndrome)				

Cerebrohepatorenal syndrome (Zellweger syndrome)	Metabolic	• Flat facies • Growth retardation • Hepatomegaly • Polycystic kidneys • Hypotonia • Neonatal jaundice • Long bone calcific deposits • CHD	• Psychomotor retardation • Renal dysfunction • Hypoprothrombinemia	• Requires preoperative cardiac assessment • Impaired renal drug excretion • Abnormal coagulation profile • Exaggerated response to muscle relaxants
Charcot-Marie-Tooth disease	Neurologic	• Weakness of limbs	• Sympathetic postganglionic fibers impair autonomic function, particularly the control of temperature by sweating	• Impaired thermoregulation • Autonomic nervous system hypersensitivity
Chediak-Higashi syndrome	Hematologic/ Immunologic	• Albinism • Hepatosplenomegaly • Recurrent chest infections (streptococcus, staphylococcus) • Terminal lymphoreticular malignancy • Prolonged bleeding time • Bruising, GI bleeding	• Peroxidase and lysosomal granules in granulocytes of peripheral blood • Thrombocytopenia	• May require stress dose steroids • Abnormal coagulation profile

Continued.

TABLE 17-1. Pediatric syndrome and anesthetic implications—cont'd

Syndrome or disease	Primary system affected	Clinical manifestations	Physiologic considerations	Anesthetic implications
Cherubism	Craniofacial	• Intraoral vascular masses • Mandibular and maxillary tumors	• Chronic upper airway obstruction may cause pulmonary HTN, cor pulmonale	• Tracheostomy may be necessary for extremely difficult airway • Potential pulmonary and cardiac dysfunction

Christ-Siemens-Touraine syndrome (anhidrotic ectodermal dysplasia)	Connective tissue	• Triad:
		  • Absence of sweat glands
		  • Partial or complete absence of teeth
		  • Hypotrichosis
		• Hypoplastic mandible and maxilla
			• Heat intolerance and inability to control temperature by sweating
			• Persistent respiratory infection because of poor mucus production
				• Potentially difficult airway
				• Impaired thermoregulation
				• Risk of hyperpyrexia
				• Anticholinergics decrease sweat production and may further contribute to hyperthermia

Chronic nonsuppurative panniculitis (see Weber-Christian disease)				

Cockayne-Touraine syndrome (dystrophic epidermolysis bullae)	Dermatologic	• Subepidermal bullae primarily on hands, feet, sacral areas, mucous membranes • Recurrent respiratory infections • Scarring of skin leading to strictures and contractures, especially of oral aperture • Poor nutritional status	• Anemia • Growth retardation is common	• Potentially difficult airway • Friction on skin surfaces (adhesives) disrupt skin integrity • Fluid and electrolyte imbalance • Impaired thermoregulation
Congenital facial disease (see Mobius syndrome)				
Congenital hypothyroidism (see Cretinism)				
Congenital ichthyosis (see Ichthyosiform erythrodermia)				
Conradi syndrome	Connective tissue	• Chondrodystrophy with contractures • Saddle nose • CHD	• Psychomotor retardation • Renal dysfunction	• Impaired renal drug excretion • Requires preoperative cardiac assessment

Continued.

TABLE 17-1. Pediatric syndrome and anesthetic implications—cont'd

Syndrome or disease	Primary system affected	Clinical manifestations	Physiologic considerations	Anesthetic implications
Cori disease (glycogen storage disease—Type III)	Metabolic	• Splenomegaly • Hepatomegaly	• Amylo-1,6 glucosidase deficiency • Glycogen deposition in liver and muscle • Hypoglycemia, acidosis, and hyperuricemia	• Requires glucose infusion, frequent monitoring of blood glucose and acid-base status • Exaggerated response to muscle relaxants • Abnormal coagulation profile
Cornelia de Lange syndrome	Craniofacial	• High arched palate • Short stature • Strabismus • Microcephaly • Hirsutism • Weak cry • Hand and feet malformations • Micrognathia • Macroglossia • Cleft palate • CHD	• Upper airway obstruction	• Preoperative cardiac evaluation required • Potentially difficult airway • Strabismus associated with MH

Cranium bifidum (see Encephalocele)				
CREST syndrome	Connective tissue	• Calcinosis • Raynaud's phenomenon • Esophageal dysmotility • Scleroderma, syndactyly • Telangiectasias	• Renal dysfunction • Pulmonary hypertension	• Restriction of oral aperture and difficult intubation • Pulmonary dysfunction • May require stress steroids • Impaired renal drug excretion • Cardiac function may be impaired • Hands and feet must be kept warm to prevent vasoconstriction
Cretinism (congenital hypothyroidism)	Metabolic	• Goiter • Macroglossia • Hypotension with markedly decreased intravascular volume • Low cardiac output • Cold intolerance • Myxedema • Delayed gastric emptying	• If untreated can lead to neurologic deficits • Decreased metabolic rate • Respiratory depression and impaired ventilatory response to hypoxia and hypercarbia • Hypoglycemia • Hyponatremia • Adrenal insufficiency	• Increased sensitivity to cardiovascular and respiratory depressants • May need postoperative ventilatory support • Prolonged recovery from opioids • Exaggerated response to sedation and premedication • Fluid and electrolyte imbalance • Aspiration precautions • Stress dose steroids may be required

Continued.

TABLE 17-1. Pediatric syndrome and anesthetic implications—cont'd

Syndrome or disease	Primary system affected	Clinical manifestations	Physiologic considerations	Anesthetic implications
Cri-du-chat syndrome	Chromosomal	• Abnormal larynx leading to a catlike cry • Strabismus • Microcephaly • Micrognathia • CHD	• Deletion or translocation of chromosome 5 • Psychomotor retardation • Hypothermia	• Difficult intubation • Stridor caused by laryngomalacia may be worsened by anesthesia • Preoperative cardiac evaluation required • Difficulty maintaining normothermia
Crouzon syndrome (craniosynostosis)	Craniofacial	• Wide skull • Proptosis • Maxillary hypoplasia: sagittal and coronal suture synostosis • Exophthalmos • Strabismus • Nystagmus • High arched palate and cleft palate	• Elevated ICP	• Potentially difficult airway • Management of increased ICP • Strabismus associated with MH

Cutis laxa	Connective tissue	• Skin hangs on body in loose pendulous folds
		• Premature wrinkling
		• Hoarse cry secondary to vocal cord laxity
		• Propensity for hernias
		• Diaphragmatic atony
		• GI tract diverticula
		• Rectal prolapse
			• Disorder of elastin synthesis
			• In severe form:
			  • Emphysema
			  • Pulmonary artery stenosis
			  • Aortic aneurysmal dilation
				• Cardiopulmonary dysfunction
				• Vascular catheters are difficult to maintain
				• Soft tissue laxity around larynx may lead to airway obstruction

Cystinosis	Metabolic	• Fanconi syndrome • Epistaxis • Portal hypertension • Esophageal varices • Hypothyroidism • Diabetes	• Renal dysfunction • Anemia and coagulopathy	• Impaired renal drug excretion • Anemia and abnormal coagulation profile
Dandy Walker syndrome	Neurologic	• Hydrocephalus • Associated malformations (meningomyelocele)	• Elevated ICP	• Management of elevated ICP • See meningomyelocele

Continued.

TABLE 17-1. Pediatric syndrome and anesthetic implications—cont'd

Syndrome or disease	Primary system affected	Clinical manifestations	Physiologic considerations	Anesthetic implications
DiGeorge syndrome	Immunologic	• Parathyroid deficiency leading to hypocalcemia, tetany, and cardiac failure • Thymic hypoplasia • Tetanic seizures • CHD • Micrognathia • Tracheomalacia	• Defect of third and fourth branchial arches • Increased susceptibility to viral, fungal, and mycobacterial infections	• Potentially difficult airway • Requires frequent monitoring of serum calcium • Exaggerated response to nondepolarizing muscle relaxants • Requires preoperative cardiac evaluation • Blood transfusions must be irradiated with 3,000 rad to prevent graft-versus-host reaction
Down's syndrome (Trisomy 21)	Chromosomal	• Microcephaly • Hypotonia • CHD: VSD, tetralogy of Fallot, PDA, endocardial cushion defect, AV canal • Duodenal atresia • Atlantoaxial instability and other cervical spine abnormalities • Macroglossia • Congenital subglottic stenosis • Increased neoplastic disease (ALL, thyroid cancer)	• Airway obstruction • Polycythemia in neonates • Increased susceptibility to infections • Hypothyroidism	• Potentially difficult airway • Increased risk of laryngospasm • Prolonged duration of topical atropine (ophthalmic) • Decreased CNS catecholamine stores may decrease MAC • Exaggerated response to muscle relaxants • C-spine evaluation useful before intubation • Decreased functional residual capacity and pulmonary reserve

Duchenne muscular dystrophy	Muscular	• Progressive muscle weakness • Kyphoscoliosis, lumbar lordosis • Pharyngeal weakness, dysphagia, aspiration • Cardiac arrhythmias, impaired contractility • CPK elevation with myoglobinuria and rhabdomyolysis • CHF • Progressive respiratory dysfunction	• Proximal muscles affected first and distal muscles appear hypertrophied • Restrictive lung disease	• Postoperative ventilation may be required • Association with malignant hyperthermia • Succinylcholine causes increased serum K^+ and possible cardiac arrest • Exaggerated response to respiratory depressants, muscle relaxants, and inhalation agents
Dystrophic epidermolysis bullae (see Cockayne-Touraine)				
Ebstein's anomaly	Cardiothoracic	• Patent foramen ovale • Small right ventricle • Coexistent tricuspid stenosis and tricuspid insufficiency	• Cyanosis from intraatrial shunting • Congestive heart failure (primarily right sided) • Cardiac arrhythmia, usually paroxysmal, atrial tachycardia	• Management of CHF, cyanotic heart disease • Agents that precipitate tachycardia should be avoided
Edward's syndrome (Trisomy 18)	Chromosomal	• CHD • Micrognathia • Renal malformations • Rocker bottom feet	• Apneic spells and airway obstruction • Renal dysfunction	• Potentially difficult airway • Impaired renal drug excretion

Continued.

TABLE 17-1. Pediatric syndrome and anesthetic implications—cont'd

Syndrome or disease	Primary system affected	Clinical manifestations	Physiologic considerations	Anesthetic implications
Ehlers-Danlos syndrome	Connective tissue	• Joint hyperextensibility • Lens subluxation • Retinal detachment • Glaucoma • Cystic renal involvement • GI bleeding • Dissecting aortic aneurysm • Mitral valve prolapse and conduction defects • Kyphoscoliosis • Inguinal hernia	• Deficiency of protocollagen lysyl hydroxylase • Restrictive lung disease • Coagulopathy	• Increased risk of spontaneous pneumothorax • Skin integrity easily disrupted • Impaired renal drug excretion • Abnormal coagulation profile • Impaired cardiac function
Eisenmenger's syndrome	Cardiothoracic	• Pulmonary hypertension and increased pulmonary vascular resistance • Right to left shunt at both atrial and ventricular level • Cor pulmonale	• Abnormal PFTs: decreased total lung capacity, vital capacity, and compliance; increased residual and closing volumes • Cyanosis	• Abnormal ventricular function • Positive pressure ventilation may increase right to left shunt and worsen cyanosis • Prolonged postoperative ventilation may be necessary

Encephalocele (cranium bifidum)	Neurologic	• Anterior encephalocele appears as mass in nasopharynx • Basal encephalocele may cause feeding difficulties and respiratory obstruction • Posterior encephalocele associated with hydrocephalus, epilepsy, paraplegia, spasticity, and blindness	• Herniation of cerebral tissue and meninges through defect in skull • Abnormalities in thermoregulation	• Potentially difficult airway • Difficulty maintaining normothermia • Brain stem compromise may precipitate changes in heart rate and blood pressure
Encephalotrigeminal angiomatosis (see Sturge-Weber syndrome)				
Epidermolysis bullosum (Herlitz's syndrome)	Dermatologic	• Narrow scarred airway and restriction of oral aperture • Mucous membrane involvement • Feeding problems and poor nutrition • Mitten hand deformities	• Separation of epidermis and dermis following shear forces; leads to bullae formation after minor trauma to skin (Nikolsky sign) • Possible associated porphyria • Anemia	• Often requires fiberoptic intubation • Regional anesthetic techniques may also cause bullae • Meticulous avoidance of trauma with: 1. Routine airway manipulation 2. IV, ETT securement 3. Pressure point padding 4. Eye care • Need preoperative evaluation of nutritional status • May need stress dose steroids • Impaired thermoregulation

Continued.

TABLE 17-1. Pediatric syndrome and anesthetic implications—cont'd

Syndrome or disease	Primary system affected	Clinical manifestations	Physiologic considerations	Anesthetic implications
Erythema multiforme	Dermatologic	• Erythematous plaques, blisters, and target, or bull's eye, lesions of distal extremities and mucous membranes • Associated malignancies	• Spectrum of acute inflammatory diseases with IgM and complement deposition in tissues in response to vascular damage • Causes: viral, fungal, and bacterial infections, drugs, or unknown	• Loss of skin integrity • Sulfonamides, salicylates, penicillins, barbiturates, and hydantoins should be avoided
Erythema multiforme major (Stevens-Johnson syndrome)	Dermatologic	• Prodrome: fever, malaise, arthralgia, URI • Extensor surface bullae • Bullae of visceral pleura may cause pneumothoraces, pleural effusions, and pulmonary infections • GI ulceration and hemorrhage • Pericarditis • Atrial fibrillation • Corneal ulcerations, uveitis, and staphylococcal panophthalmitis	• Inflammatory process • Anemia • Dehydration • Poor nutritional status • Renal: ATN and nephritis	• Preoperative cardiac evaluation required • Fluid and electrolyte imbalance • Avoidance of skin trauma • Bullae may compromise upper airway, causing difficult intubation • May need stress dose steroids • Sulfonamides, salicylates, penicillins, barbiturates, and hydantoins should be avoided

Eulenberg syndrome (see Paramyotonia congenita)				
Fabry's disease (lysosomal storage disease)	Metabolic	• Angiokeratomas of skin • Corneal opacities • HTN • Myocardial ischemia • Renal disease: proteinuria, polyuria, tubular dysfunction, and progressive azotemia	• Galactosidase deficiency • Lipid deposition in blood vessels	• Preoperative cardiac evaluation required • Impaired renal drug excretion
Familial dysautonomia (see Riley-Day syndrome)				
Familial periodic paralysis: Type I—Hypokalemic Type II—Hyperkalemic Type III—Normokalemic	Muscular	• Severe muscle weakness, may spare respiratory muscles • Loss of cough reflex, dysphagia • Cardiac dysrhythmias	*Type I* • Paralysis (lasts 36 hr) exacerbated by high-carbohydrate meals, salt loading, exercise, or cold • Treatment: spironolactone, acetozolamide *Type II* • Paralysis (lasts 1-2 hr) related to exercise and cold • Treatment: calcium, insulin, and glucose *Type III* • Weakness may last several days • Recurrent respiratory infections	• May have exaggerated response to nondepolarizing muscle relaxants • Careful monitoring of fluids and electrolytes • Avoidance of hypothermia *Type I* • IV fluids should be free of sodium and dextrose *Type II* • IV fluids should contain dextrose and be free of potassium *Type III* • As for type I

Continued.

TABLE 17-1. Pediatric syndrome and anesthetic implications—cont'd

Syndrome or disease	Primary system affected	Clinical manifestations	Physiologic considerations	Anesthetic implications
Familial xanthomatosis (see Wolman's disease)				
Fanconi syndrome	Metabolic	• Metabolic acidosis • Hypokalemia • Hypophosphatemia • Hypercalciuria • Glucosuria • Aminoaciduria • Polyuria • Rickets, osteomalacia, and pathologic fractures • Slow progression to chronic renal failure	• Impaired tubular reabsorption of glucose, amino acids, phosphate, bicarbonate, uric acid, and K^+	• Requires careful preoperative evaluation and frequent intraoperative monitoring of fluids, electrolytes, and acid-base status • Impaired renal drug excretion
Farber's disease	Metabolic	• Triad: Subcutaneous nodules; Arthritis; Hoarseness • Dysphagia and respiratory difficulties due to epiglottis and larynx granuloma formation • Macroglossia • Hepatomegaly • Cardiomyopathy	• Deficiency of acid ceramidase leading to ceramide deposition in tissues • Airway obstruction	• Potentially difficult airway • Need preoperative assessment of cardiopulmonary function • Impaired hepatic metabolism

Favism (G-6-PD deficiency)	Metabolic	• Hemolytic anemia • Vitreous hemorrhage • Recurrent infections • Hepatitis • Bacterial pneumonia • Mononucleosis	• Hemolysis occurs with oxidant drugs: • Salicylates • Sulfa • Phenacetin • Vitamin K • Methylene blue • INH • Quinidine • Antimalarials • Nitrofurans	• Prilocaine may cause methemoglobinemia • Impaired hepatic drug metabolism • Liver function and coagulation need preoperative assessment
Fazio-Londe syndrome	Muscular	• Bulbar neuropathy impairs swallowing and gag reflexes	• Anterior horn cell degeneration of bulbar nuclei and cervical and upper thoracic cord	• Aspiration precautions needed • Succinylcholine may cause hyperkalemia • May have exaggerated response to muscle relaxants
Fibrodysplasia ossificans (see Myositis ossificans)				
Focal dermal hypoplasia (see Goltz's syndrome)				

Continued.

TABLE 17-1. Pediatric syndrome and anesthetic implications—cont'd

Syndrome or disease	Primary system affected	Clinical manifestations	Physiologic considerations	Anesthetic implications
Forms of dwarfism (osteochondrodystrophies) 1. Achondrogenesis 2. Thanatophenic dwarfism 3. Short rib-polydactyly syndromes—type I and type II 4. Type I osteogenesis imperfecta 5. Camptomelic dwarfism (lethal form) 6. Cerebrocosto-mandibular syndrome 7. Hypophosphatasia	Skeletal	• Odontoid hypoplasia and/or atlantoaxial instability • Micrognathia • Cleft palate • Tracheal stenosis and malacia • Small chest cavity • Kyphoscoliosis • CHD	• Restrictive lung disease • Airway obstruction	• Need preoperative C-spine and cardiac evaluation • Potentially difficult airway • Care in positioning

Freeman-Sheldon syndrome (whistling face syndrome)	Craniofacial	• Craniocarpotarsal dysplasia • Strabismus • Hypertelorism • Blepharophimosis • Bulging cheeks • Small mouth; pursed lips • V-shaped fibrous tissue band at the midchin	• Airway obstruction • Elevated ICP	• Potentially difficult airway • Association with strabismus and MH • Management of elevated ICP
Friedrich's ataxia	Neurologic	• Scoliosis • Myocardial necrosis, muscle degeneration • Arrhythmias • Ataxia due to degeneration of spinocerebellar tract and loss of large myelinated fibers of dorsal root ganglia	• Progressive degeneration throughout CNS, including mental deterioration • Restrictive lung disease	• Preoperative cardiopulmonary evaluation required • May have exaggerated response to muscle relaxants
G-6-PD deficiency (see Favism)				
Gardner's syndrome	Metabolic	• Multiple polyposis • Bony tumors • Sebaceous cysts • Fibromas	• Anemia from GI bleeding	• May have loss of skin integrity • Care in positioning required

Continued.

TABLE 17-1. Pediatric syndrome and anesthetic implications—cont'd

Syndrome or disease	Primary system affected	Clinical manifestations	Physiologic considerations	Anesthetic implications
Gaucher disease	Metabolic	• Triad of trismus, strabismus, and retroflexion of head • Hepatosplenomegaly • Aseptic necrosis of femoral head • Vertebral fractures • Joint swelling • Chronic aspiration • Spasticity • Hypersplenism	• Defect of glucocerebrosidase • Most common metabolic disorder of glycolipid metabolism • Thrombocytopenia, leukopenia, and anemia • Increased acid phosphatase	• Preoperative coagulation profile needed • Potentially difficult airway • Association with strabismus and MH • Aspiration precautions • May have impaired hepatic drug metabolism • May need careful padding or positioning
Globoid cell leukodystrophy (see Krabbe's disease)				
Glycogen storage disease Type I—von Gierke's disease Type II—Pompe disease Type III—Cori disease Type IV—Andersen's disease Type V—McArdle disease Type VI—Hers disease Type VII—Tauri disease				

Goldenhar syndrome (oculoauriculovertebral syndrome)	Craniofacial	• Unilateral facial hypoplasia • Congenital heart disease • Mandibular hypoplasia • Micrognathia • Macrostomia • Colobomas, epibulbar dermoids • Cleft or high arched palate • Hemivertebra or vertebral fusion; may involve upper neck and odontoid elongation • Spina bifida	• Decreased pulmonary reserve • Upper airway obstruction • Psychomotor retardation	• Potentially difficult airway and intubation • Requires preoperative assessment of cardiac status and cervical spine
Goltz's syndrome (focal dermal hypoplasia)	Craniofacial	• Hypoplasia and change in skin pigmentation • Papillomas of mucous membranes • Strabismus • Enamel hypoplasia • CHD • Head asymmetry • Propensity for hernias • Incomplete segmentation of cervical and thoracic vertebrae	• Mesenchymal and ectodermal defect • Renal dysfunction • Airway obstruction from laryngeal papillomas	• Potentially difficult airway • Impaired renal drug excretion • Association with strabismus and MH • Need preoperative cardiac and C-spine evaluation • Teeth may fracture easily

Continued.

TABLE 17-1. Pediatric syndrome and anesthetic implications—cont'd

Syndrome or disease	Primary system affected	Clinical manifestations	Physiologic considerations	Anesthetic implications
Gorlin-Chaudhry-Moss syndrome	Craniofacial	• Craniofacial dysostosis • Hypertrichosis • Dental and ocular anomalies • CHD (PDA common)	• Possible CHF	• Potentially difficult airway • Preoperative cardiac evaluation needed
Groenblad-Strandberg syndrome (see Pseudoxanthoma elasticum)				
Guillain-Barré syndrome	Neurologic	• Acute polyneuropathy • Peripheral neuritis involving cranial nerves • Bulbar palsy leading to hypoventilation and hypotension	• Autonomic dysfunction causes swings in blood pressure and heart rate	• Succinylcholine may cause hyperkalemia • Bulbar involvement may necessitate tracheostomy and mechanical ventilation • CV instability • Drugs potentiating catecholamine release should be avoided

Hallermann-Streif syndrome (oculomandibulofacial syndrome)	Craniofacial	• Dwarfism • Hypotrichosis • Macrocephaly • Microphthalmia • Nystagmus • Strabismus • Malar hypoplasia • Micrognathia • TMJ displacement • Lordosis, scoliosis, spina bifida	• Restrictive lung disease • Psychomotor retardation	• Potentially difficult airway • Evaluation of pulmonary function and reserve required • Association with strabismus and MH
Hallervorden-Spatz Disease	Neurologic	• Dystonia leading to scoliosis, trismus, torticollis	• Disorder of basal ganglia • Dementia • Restrictive lung disease	• Succinylcholine should be avoided • Potentially difficult airway • Preoperative pulmonary evaluation needed • Inhalation agents may relax torticollis
Hand-Schuller-Christian disease	Hematologic	• Histiocytic granuloma in bones and viscera including larynx, lungs, liver, and spleen • Laryngeal fibrosis • Hypersplenism • CNS: diabetes insipidus	• Respiratory failure • Cor pulmonale • Pancytopenia	• Preoperative assessment of pulmonary status needed • May need stress dose steroids • Coagulation profile may be abnormal

Continued.

TABLE 17-1. Pediatric syndrome and anesthetic implications—cont'd

Syndrome or disease	Primary system affected	Clinical manifestations	Physiologic considerations	Anesthetic implications
Harlequin fetus (see Ichthyosiform erythrodermia)				
Hartnup disease	Metabolic	• Scaly red skin • Cerebellar ataxia	• Defective intestinal absorption of tryptophan, leading to niacin deficiency and pellagra • Emotional instability and psychosis	• Potential for loss of skin integrity • Behavioral disturbances may have implications for induction techniques
Heart-Hand syndrome (see Holt-Oram syndrome)				
Hemochromatosis	Metabolic	• Hepatic fibrosis and cirrhosis • Diabetes mellitus • Abnormal skin pigmentation • CHF and cardiac arrhythmias	• Inherited disorder of iron metabolism with iron deposition in liver, pancreas, skin, heart	• Preoperative cardiac evaluation needed • May have abnormal coagulation status • Impaired hepatic drug metabolism

Hemolytic uremic syndrome	Hematologic	• Triad:
		  • Nephropathy
		  • Thrombocytopenia
		  • Microangiopathic hemolytic anemia
		• Seizures
		• Cardiac failure caused by HTN, volume overload, severe anemia, and progressive renal disease
			• Associated metabolic derangements:
			  • Hyperkalemia
			  • Metabolic acidosis
			  • Hypocalcemia
			  • Hyponatremia
				• May have abnormal coagulation profile
				• Fluid-electrolyte imbalance

Henoch-Schonlein purpura	Hematologic	• Purpuric skin rash • Arthritis • Abdominal pain • Nephritis can progress to renal failure • GI hemorrhage • Subcutaneous, scrotal, and periorbital edema	• Vasculitis of small blood vessels • Nonthrombocytopenic purpura • Often associated with recent URI	• Impaired renal drug excretion • May have abnormal coagulation profile • May need stress dose steroids

Continued.

TABLE 17-1. Pediatric syndrome and anesthetic implications—cont'd

Syndrome or disease	Primary system affected	Clinical manifestations	Physiologic considerations	Anesthetic implications
Hepatolenticular degeneration (see Wilson's disease)				
Hereditary angioneurotic edema	Hematologic/ Immunologic	• Episodic brauny edema of trunk, extremities, face, abdomen, and airway lasting (average) 24-92 hr • Mortality about 30%, mostly from laryngeal edema • Often induced by vibration or trauma, may have prodromal tingling or tightness	• Abnormal levels of C_1 and C_4 esterase inhibitors and accumulation of vasoactive substances, which increase vascular permeability	• Preoperative complement assay needed • Hoarseness or dysphagia may be present • Recommended prophylaxis: EACA for 2-3 days and/or FFP 1 day preoperatively • Acute attack is treated with epinephrine, antihistamines, and steroids • Extreme care should be exercised in airway manipulation because minor trauma may elicit response
Hereditary hemorrhagic telangiectasia (see Osler-Weber-Rendu syndrome)				

Herlitz's syndrome (see Epidermolysis bullosum)				
Hers Disease (Type VI—glycogen storage disease)	Metabolic	• Hepatomegaly • Poor muscle development	• Hypoglycemia	• Continuous glucose infusion • Need acid-base and glucose monitoring • May have coagulopathy • May have exaggerated response to muscle relaxants
Holt-Oram syndrome (Heart-hand syndrome)	Cardiothoracic	• Upper limb anomalies (e.g., radial dysgenesis) • CHD: septal defects, dextrocardia, tetralogy of Fallot	• Sudden death secondary to pulmonary embolus or coronary occlusion reported	• Preoperative cardiac evaluation required
Homocystinuria	Metabolic	• Ectopia lentis • Kyphoscoliosis • Hepatomegaly • Osteoporosis • Arterial and venous thrombosis secondary to hypercoagulability	• Deficiency of hepatic cystathionine synthase leading to increased plasma and urinary levels of methionine and homocystine • Growth retardation • Restrictive lung disease	• Increased incidence of cerebral, pulmonary, renal, mesenteric, and coronary thrombosis in perioperative period • May have abnormal coagulation profile • Preoperative assessment of pulmonary status and reserve needed

Continued.

TABLE 17-1. Pediatric syndrome and anesthetic implications—cont'd

Syndrome or disease	Primary system affected	Clinical manifestations	Physiologic considerations	Anesthetic implications
Hunter syndrome (Type II—mucopolysaccharidosis)	Metabolic	• Stiff joints • Dwarfism • Hepatosplenomegaly • Pectus excavatum • Prone to respiratory infections • Kyphoscoliosis • Valvular heart disease and cardiomyopathy • Retinitis pigmentosa • Nodular, ivory-colored skin lesions • Hydrocephaly • Tracheomalacia	• Airway obstruction • Restrictive lung disease • Elevated ICP • Psychomotor retardation	• Potentially difficult airway because of abnormal anatomy and tracheal collapse • Upper airway obstruction from infiltration of lymphoid tissue in larynx • Need preoperative cardiopulmonary evaluation • Management of elevated ICP

Hurler syndrome (Type I—mucopolysaccharidosis)	Metabolic	• Coarse facies (gargoylism) • Macroglossia • Large tonsils and adenoids • Short, thick neck • Narrowing of laryngeal inlet and tracheobronchial tree • Hydrocephalus • Hepatosplenomegaly • Odontoid hypoplasia and atlantoaxial subluxation • Decreased joint mobility • Thoracic kyphosis • Flexion contractures • Severe CAD and valvular disease • Cardiomyopathy	• Airway obstruction • Restrictive lung disease and recurrent pulmonary infection • Psychomotor retardation	• Preoperative evaluation of C-spine and cardiopulmonary status required • Potentially difficult airway • Coagulation profile may be abnormal • Postoperative subglottic edema (croup) common

Continued.

TABLE 17-1. Pediatric syndrome and anesthetic implications—cont'd

Syndrome or disease	Primary system affected	Clinical manifestations	Physiologic considerations	Anesthetic implications
Hutchinson-Gilford syndrome (see Progeria)				
Ichthyosiform erythrodermia (congenital ichthyosis or harlequin fetus)	Dermatologic	• Contraction and decreased thickness of skin • Strangulation of smaller appendages (i.e., ears, lips, nose, and digits)	• Impaired thermoregulation	• Maintenance of normothermia • Loss of skin integrity
Immotile cilia syndrome (see Kartagener's syndrome)				
Incontinentia pigmenti (see Bloch-Sulzberger syndrome)				

Infantile gigantism (see Beckwith-Wiedemann syndrome)				
Ivemark syndrome	Cardiothoracic	• Malposition of abdominal viscera • Complex cyanotic congenital heart disease (transposition of great vessels, tricuspid atresia)	• Splenic agenesis may cause immunocompromise	• Cardiac status should be evaluated preoperatively • Aseptic technique required
Jervell and Lange-Nielsen syndrome	Cardiothoracic	• Prolonged QT, RT intervals on ECG • Congenital deafness • Syncopal attacks due to paroxysmal ventricular fibrillation, torsade de pointes	• Extreme sensitivity to sympathetic stimulation	• Cardiac status needs preoperative evaluation • Halothane, lidocaine, catecholamines, phenothiazines, quinidine, and procainamide should be avoided • Failure of medical therapy may necessitate left stellate ganglion blockade or pacemaker

Continued.

TABLE 17-1. Pediatric syndrome and anesthetic implications—cont'd

Syndrome or disease	Primary system affected	Clinical manifestations	Physiologic considerations	Anesthetic implications
Jeune syndrome (asphyxiating thoracic dystrophy)	Skeletal	• Dwarfism • Stiff thorax • Short ribs, prominent rib rosary in midaxillary line • Small larynx • Hands and feet are short and broad • Pulmonary hypoplasia and cysts	• Respiratory dysfunction; may require ventilatory support at birth to allow growth but tends to improve with age • Renal disease with proteinuria, uremia • HTN is problem if child survives infancy	• May require surgical intervention to enlarge thorax, with substantial blood loss • High incidence of barotrauma, hypoxia, and hypercarbia • Minimal pulmonary reserve • Impaired renal drug excretion • Small larynx may necessitate smaller endotracheal tube
Juvenile rheumatoid arthritis (Still's disease)	Connective tissue	• Synovitis • Joint effusions and subluxation • Cervical spine arthritis; atlantoaxial subluxation • TMJ involvement and decreased oral aperture • Mandibular hypoplasia • Cricoarytenoid arthritis • Myocarditis and conduction abnormalities	• Anemia • Renal dysfunction	• Potentially difficult airway; may require fiberoptic intubation • C-spine and cardiac evaluation needed preoperatively • May need stress dose steroids • ASA, NSAIDs may cause coagulopathy

Kartagener's syndrome (immotile cilia syndrome)	Cardiothoracic	• Dextrocardia • Bronchiectasis • Chronic bronchitis • Sinusitis • Heart block	• Dysfunction of cilia, causes male sterility • Chronic pulmonary disease	• Preoperative cardiopulmonary evaluation needed • Nitrous oxide should be avoided with bronchiectasis
Kasabach-Merritt syndrome	Hematologic/Immunologic	• Giant hemangiomas of cavernous type (usually on face and scalp) • Thrombocytopenia • Hypofibrinogenemia	• Deficient immune response • Chronic consumptive coagulopathy (platelets trapped in cavities stimulate activation of clotting mechanism)	• May need stress dose steroids • Surgical excision of hemangiomas can precipitate DIC • Invasive monitoring and large bore IVs needed for volume resuscitation • Airway difficulties depend on hemangioma location
Kawasaki disease (mucocutaneous lymph node syndrome)	Cardiothoracic	• Desquamative conjunctivitis • Stomatitis • Nonsuppurative lymphadenitis • Myocarditis, coronary artery aneurysms, and ischemia	• Acute febrile erythematous disease • Pyelonephritis and renal failure • Heart failure and arrhythmias	• Preoperative cardiac evaluation needed

Continued.

TABLE 17-1. Pediatric syndrome and anesthetic implications—cont'd

Syndrome or disease	Primary system affected	Clinical manifestations	Physiologic considerations	Anesthetic implications
King-Denborough syndrome	Muscular	• Slow progressive myopathy with contractures • Low set ears • Malar hypoplasia • Micrognathia • Pectus carinatum • Kyphoscoliosis • Cryptorchidism • Growth retardation	• MH susceptible • Restrictive lung disease • May be subset of Noonan's syndrome	• Potentially difficult airway • MH precautions and treatment needed • Preoperative evaluation of pulmonary function needed • May have exaggerated response to muscle relaxants
Klinefelter's syndrome (XXY)	Chromosomal	• Tall stature • Vertebral collapse due to osteoporosis • Microcephaly • Prognathism • Strabismus, lens dislocation • Hypogenitalism	• Aggressive behavior	• Care in positioning • Potentially difficult airway • Management of disruptive and uncooperative patient
Klippel-Feil syndrome	Connective tissue	• Scoliosis • Congenital heart disease • Sprengel deformity • Congenital synostosis of cervical vertebrae	• Renal dysfunction	• Care in neck manipulation for intubation • Assessment of CHD • Impaired renal drug excretion

Klippel-Trenaunay-Weber syndrome	Connective tissue	• Vascular malformations: port wine nevus, venous varicosities, AV aneurysms (primarily in legs) • Poly- and syndactyly	• High-output cardiac failure with significant AV shunt	• Drugs that decrease myocardial contractility should be avoided
Kohlmeier-Degos disease (malignant atrophic papulosis)	Dermatologic	• Multiple infarcts of skin, GI tract, and CNS • Porcelain white papules that form atrophic scars • GI lesions may cause perforation and peritonitis • CNS infarcts • Pleural effusions • Pericarditis and pericardial effusions	• Occlusive vasculitis of unknown etiology • Restrictive pulmonary disease • Cerebral edema, increased ICP, and herniation	• Preoperative cardiorespiratory evaluation • Management of elevated ICP
Krabbe's disease (globoid cell leukodystrophy)	Neurologic	• Blindness • Deafness • Significant mortality by age 2	• Progressive CNS deterioration becomes apparent in infancy • Psychomotor retardation	• Supportive care
Kugelberg-Welander disease	Muscular	• Hypotonia • Cardiac arrhythmias • CHF • Kyphoscoliosis	• Juvenile proximal hereditary muscular atrophy • Anterior horn cell degeneration	• Succinylcholine may induce hyperkalemia • May have exaggerated response to muscle relaxants and respiratory depressants • Aspiration precautions needed

Continued.

TABLE 17-1. Pediatric syndrome and anesthetic implications—cont'd

Syndrome or disease	Primary system affected	Clinical manifestations	Physiologic considerations	Anesthetic implications
Larsen's syndrome	Connective tissue	• Congenital joint dislocations • Cartilage weakness in ribs, epiglottis, arytenoids • Cleft palate • Hydrocephalus	• Elevated ICP • Chronic respiratory dysfunction	• Potentially difficult intubation • Management of elevated ICP

Lawrence-Moon-Biedl syndrome	Metabolic/ Obesity	• Obesity
		• Retinitis pigmentosa
		• Polydactyly
		• CHD
		• Psychomotor retardation
			• Complications of obesity:
			  • Delayed gastric emptying
			  • Altered autonomic nervous system response
			  • Poor vascular access
			• Renal defects, diabetes insipidus, urinary concentrating defect
				• Impaired renal drug excretion
				• Preoperative cardiac evaluation needed
				• Aspiration precautions needed

Leber's hereditary optic neuropathy	Neurologic	• Bilateral loss of central vision from neuroretinal degeneration • Cardiac dysrhythmias	• Rhodanase deficiency • May have encephalopathy	• Inability to metabolize sodium nitroprusside leads to severe cyanide toxicity • Preoperative cardiac evaluation needed
Leigh's syndrome	Neurologic	• Encephalopathy • Optic atrophy • Lactic acidosis • Psychomotor retardation	• Lesions affecting basal ganglia and brain stem	• Acid-base status needs frequent monitoring • May have impaired ventilatory response

Leopard syndrome	Craniofacial	• Congenital pulmonary stenosis • Hypertelorism • Cardiac conduction defects • Large skin freckles • Ptosis • Kyphosis, pectus carinatum	• Restrictive lung disease	• Preoperative ECG and cardiopulmonary evaluation needed • Potentially difficult airway

Lesch-Nyhan syndrome	Metabolic	• Hyperuricemia, causing:
		  • Urolithiasis
		  • Urinary obstruction
		  • Acute oliguric renal failure
		  • Self-mutilation
		  • Hyperreflexia, sustained clonus
			• Absence of hypoxanthine-guanine phosphoribosyl transferase needed for purine metabolism
			• Severe psychomotor retardation and aggressive behavior
				• Careful hydration needed to maintain alkaline urine
				• Impaired renal drug excretion
				• Exaggerated response to muscle relaxants

Letterer-Siwe disease (acute disseminated histiocytosis)	Hematologic	• Lymphocytic infiltration of liver, spleen, lymph nodes, lung, and bone • Seborrhea, eczema • Mandibular hypoplasia • Diabetes insipidus if sella turcica involved • Fulminant and fatal in infancy	• Pulmonary fibrosis, respiratory failure, cor pulmonale • May have leukocytosis or pancytopenia • High serum uric acid leading to red cell damage and renal stones	• Potentially difficult airway; may have laryngeal fibrosis • Loss of skin integrity • May need stress steroids • May have had chemotherapeutic agents • Preoperative pulmonary evaluation and coagulation profile needed • Impaired renal drug excretion

Continued.

TABLE 17-1. Pediatric syndrome and anesthetic implications—cont'd

Syndrome or disease	Primary system affected	Clinical manifestations	Physiologic considerations	Anesthetic implications
Louis Bar syndrome (see Ataxia telangiectasia)				
Lowe syndrome (oculocerebrorenal syndrome)	Muscular	• Hypotonia • Cataracts • Glaucoma • Strabismus • Osteoporosis and rickets • Seizures	• Psychomotor retardation • Renal tubular dysfunction • Hyperchloremic metabolic acidosis	• Management of seizure disorder • Impaired renal drug excretion • Electrolyte and acid-base imbalance • Strabismus associated with MH susceptibility • Exaggerated response to muscle relaxants
Lyell disease (toxic epidermal necrolysis)	Dermatologic	• Acute bullous eruption of skin and mucous membranes, oropharynx, tongue, tracheobronchial tree • Pneumonia • GI hemorrhage • Septicemia, shock, hypovolemia • DIC	• Impaired thermoregulation	• Loss of skin integrity • Fluid and electrolyte imbalance • May have abnormal coagulation profile • May need stress dose steroids

Lysosomal storage disease (see Fabry's disease)				
Malignant atrophic papulosis (see Kohlmeier-Degos disease)				
Mandibulofacial dysostosis (see Treacher Collins syndrome)				
Maple syrup urine disease	Metabolic	• In early infancy: • Poor feeding • Vomiting • High-pitched cry • Hypotonicity or hypertonicity • Seizures, stupor, and/or coma	• Decreased activity of oxoacid dehydrogenase causes increased leucine, isoleucine, valine, and oxoacids • Severe acidosis, hyperammonemia, and hypoglycemia can occur	• Frequent monitoring of acid-base status, blood glucose, fluids, and electrolytes is needed

Continued.

TABLE 17-1. Pediatric syndrome and anesthetic implications—cont'd

Syndrome or disease	Primary system affected	Clinical manifestations	Physiologic considerations	Anesthetic implications
Marble bone disease (see Osteopetrosis)				
Marfan's syndrome	Connective tissue	• Joint instability and dislocation • Dilation of aortic root (aortic aneurysm) • Aortic valvular insufficiency and mitral valve prolapse • Kyphoscoliosis, pectus excavatum • Bullous emphysema • Lens subluxation • Strabismus • Prone to hernias • Arachnodactyly • Atlantoaxial instability	• Cystic medial necrosis leading to coronary artery disease, valvular disease • Restrictive pulmonary disease	• Preoperative cardiopulmonary evaluation needed • Requires care in positioning • Increased potential for pneumothorax • C-spine evaluation before laryngoscopy useful

Maroteaux-Lamy syndrome (Type VI—mucopolysaccharidosis)	Metabolic	• Short stature • Coarse facies • Joint stiffness • Corneal clouding • Hydrocephalus • CHD • Odontoid hypoplasia • Kyphosis	• Elevated ICP • Restrictive lung disease	• Management of elevated ICP • Requires care in positioning • Potentially difficult airway • Preoperative C-spine and cardiopulmonary evaluation needed
McArdle disease (Type V—glycogen storage disease)	Metabolic	• Muscle cramps • Myoglobinuria • Muscle wasting	• Deficiency of muscle phosphorylase	• Succinylcholine may cause hyperkalemia • IV regional technique (Bier block) may increase chance of muscle ischemia • Symptoms may be confused with malignant hyperthermia
Meckel syndrome	Craniofacial	• Occipital encephalocele • Microcephaly • Micrognathia • Cleft epiglottis, lip, and palate • Polycystic kidney • CHD • Polydactyly • Abnormal genitalia • Cataracts	• Renal dysfunction	• Potentially difficult airway • Preoperative assessment of CHD needed • Impaired renal drug excretion

Continued.

TABLE 17-1. Pediatric syndrome and anesthetic implications—cont'd

Syndrome or disease	Primary system affected	Clinical manifestations	Physiologic considerations	Anesthetic implications
Metaphyseal dysplasia (see Pyle's disease)				
Mobius syndrome (congenital facial disease)	Craniofacial	• Limb deformities • Micrognathia and upper airway obstruction • Feeding difficulties • Recurrent aspiration • Muscle weakness of tongue, neck, chest	• Nonprogressive deterioration of motor nuclei of CN VI and VII causing facial palsy	• Potentially difficult airway • Preoperative evaluation of pulmonary dysfunction because of chronic aspiration • Exaggerated response to muscle relaxants may occur in distribution of involved nerves
Morquio syndrome (Mucopolysaccharidosis—type IV)	Metabolic	• Coarse facies • Prominent maxilla • Severe skeletal abnormalities • Short neck • Pectus carinatum • Joint laxity • Kyphoscoliosis • Odontoid hypoplasia with atlantoaxial subluxation	• Defective degradation of keratin sulfate • Restrictive lung disease and recurrent pulmonary infections	• Potentially difficult intubation • Preoperative C-spine and pulmonary evaluation needed
Moschkowitz disease (thrombotic thrombocytopenic purpura)	Hematologic	• Hemolytic anemia • Thrombocytopenia • Neurologic damage • Renal disease	• Coagulopathy	• May need stress dose steroids • Impaired renal drug excretion • May have abnormal coagulation profile

Mucocutaneous lymph node syndrome (see Kawasaki disease)				
Mucopolysaccharidoses Type I—Hurler syndrome Type II—Hunter syndrome Type III—Sanfilippo syndrome Type IV—Morquio syndrome Type V—Scheie disease Type VI—Maroteaux-Lamy syndrome				
Multiple endocrine neoplasia Type I—see Wermer's syndrome Type II—see Sipple syndrome				
Myasthenia gravis	Muscular	• Weakness and easy fatiguability of voluntary muscles • Ocular muscles commonly involved (ptosis, diplopia) • Dysarthria and dysphagia	• Autoimmune disorder of the neuromuscular junction caused by a decreased number of acetylcholine receptors	• Increased sensitivity to nondepolarizing muscle relaxants (use $\frac{1}{20}$ of normal dose) • May be resistant to effects of succinylcholine for muscle relaxation • Potentiation of narcotics by anticholinesterase therapy • Hypothermia and hypokalemia may worsen respiratory function • Regional techniques may decrease need for postoperative ventilation

Continued.

TABLE 17-1. Pediatric syndrome and anesthetic implications—cont'd

Syndrome or disease	Primary system affected	Clinical manifestations	Physiologic considerations	Anesthetic implications
Myelomeningocele (spina bifida)	Neurologic	• Hydrocephalus • Risk of CNS infection • Thoracic lesions can cause progressive spinal deformity (kyphosis, scoliosis, lordosis), resulting in restrictive lung disease	• Failure of fusion of vertebral arches • Usually varying degrees of paralysis below level of lesion	• Care in positioning required • Large blood and fluid losses should be anticipated during repair • Lateral position should be used for intubation to avoid trauma to sac • May be difficult to maintain normothermia
Myositis ossificans (fibrodysplasia ossificans)	Muscular	• Bony infiltration of tendons, fascia aponeuroses, and muscle	• Decreased thoracic compliance • Recurrent aspiration	• Difficulty opening mouth and necessity for neck manipulation may hinder intubation • Decreased pulmonary reserve • Aspiration precautions needed
Myotonia congenita (Thomsen's disease)	Muscular	• Decreased ability to relax muscles after contraction • Muscle hypertrophy	• Nonprogressive • Absence of cardiac involvement	• See myotonic dystrophy

Myotonic dystrophy	Muscular	• Weakness primarily of limb muscles • Ptosis • Baldness • Cataracts • Gonadal atrophy • Cardiac conduction defects and arrhythmias • Impaired ventilation • Dysphagia, aspiration • Increased CPK • Mental retardation	• Myotonia made worse by exercise and cold • Endocrine failure	• Succinylcholine and neostigmine can precipitate myotonic crisis • Exaggerated response to nondepolarizing muscle relaxants • Extreme sensitivity to respiratory depressants • Aspiration precautions needed • Often requires prolonged postoperative ventilation
Neurofibromatosis (von Recklinghausen syndrome)	Neurologic	• CNS neurofibromas • Café-au-lait spots • Peripheral tumors in nerve trunk • Increased incidence of pheochromocytoma • Kyphoscoliosis • Honeycomb cystic lung changes • Renal artery dysplasia and HTN • Tumors may involve larynx and right ventricle outflow tract	• Restrictive lung disease	• Preoperative screening for pheochromocytoma and pulmonary function needed • Impaired renal drug excretion • Prolonged paralysis with depolarizing muscle relaxants • Difficult airway management if tumor involvement

Continued.

TABLE 17-1. Pediatric syndrome and anesthetic implications—cont'd

Syndrome or disease	Primary system affected	Clinical manifestations	Physiologic considerations	Anesthetic implications
Niemann-Pick disease	Metabolic	• Hepatosplenomegaly • Epilepsy • Psychomotor retardation	• Deficiency of sphingomyelinase leading to tissue (cerebral) deposition of sphingomyelin • Thrombocytopenia and anemia	• May have abnormal coagulation profile • Management of seizure disorder

Noack's syndrome	Metabolic/Obesity	• Craniosynostosis
		• Obesity
		• Digital anomalies
			• Complications of obesity:
			  • Decreased respiratory reserve
			  • Delayed gastric emptying
			  • Autonomic nervous system dysfunction
				• Potential elevation of ICP
				• Aspiration precautions needed
				• Preoperative pulmonary evaluation needed
				• Difficult vascular access
				• Potentially difficult airway

Noonan's syndrome (Male Turner)	Chromosomal	• Short stature • CHD • Micrognathia • Hydronephrosis or hypoplastic kidneys	• Psychomotor retardation	• Preoperative cardiac evaluation needed • Impaired renal drug excretion • Potentially difficult airway
Oculoauriculovertebral syndrome (see Goldenhar syndrome)				

Oculocerebrorenal syndrome (see Lowe syndrome)				
Oculomandibulofacial syndrome (see Hallerman-Streif syndrome)				
Oro-facial-digital syndrome	Craniofacial	• Cleft lip and palate • Lobed tongue • Hypoplasia of mandible and maxilla • Hydrocephalus • Polycystic kidney • Digital abnormalities	• Elevated ICP • Renal dysfunction	• Potentially difficult airway • Management of elevated ICP • Impaired renal drug excretion
Osler-Weber-Rendu syndrome (hereditary hemorrhagic telangiectasia)	Hematologic	• Ectatic vascular lesions in skin, mucosa, viscera • Initial sign may be repeated epistaxis • Pulmonary AV fistulas	• Normal clotting factors, but bleeding may be difficult to control and cause severe anemia • Recurrent chest infections, dyspnea, and cyanosis	• Traumatic intubation may cause severe bleeding from oral mucosal lesions • Nasal intubation is contraindicated • Large AVMs can cause significant shunts (Qs/Qt) • Preoperative pulmonary evaluation needed • Large-bore intravenous catheters may be needed for volume replacement

Continued.

TABLE 17-1. Pediatric syndrome and anesthetic implications—cont'd

Syndrome or disease	Primary system affected	Clinical manifestations	Physiologic considerations	Anesthetic implications
Osteochondrodystrophies (see Forms of dwarfism)				

Osteogenesis Imperfecta
Type I:
O.I. congenita (newborn, most severe)
Type II:
O.I. tarda gravis (birth-1 year)
Type III:
O.I. tarda levis (1 year onward)
	Skeletal	• Classic Triad:
		  • Blue sclera
		  • Multiple fractures
		  • Deafness
		• Poor dentition
		• Bleeding diathesis
		• IVH from fractures sustained at delivery
		• Kyphoscoliosis
		• Cardiac anomalies
			• Defect in synthesis of collagen and associated dysfunction of platelet aggregation
			• Increased metabolic rate
			• Thoracic involvement leading to respiratory failure or impaired pulmonary reserve
				• Requires careful positioning and padding
				• Hyperpyrexia under anesthesia not felt to be MH
				• Preoperative coagulation profile and pulmonary evaluation needed
				• Tourniquets and blood pressure cuffs may cause fractures

Osteopetrosis (Albers-Schonberg disease, or marble bone disease)	Skeletal	• Petechiae, ecchymoses • Megalocephaly or hydrocephalus • Optic atrophy and abnormal eye movements • Hepatosplenomegaly • Generalized skeletal density on x-ray with disturbed mineralization at the growth plates similar to rickets	• Failure to thrive • Brittle bones and high incidence of pathologic fractures • Anemia, neutropenia, thrombocytopenia • Hypocalcemia with propensity for cardiac arrhythmias and seizures	• Requires care in positioning and padding • Management of seizure disorder • Potential for cardiac arrhythmias • May have coagulopathy • May have exaggerated response to nondepolarizing muscle relaxants

Paramyotonia congenita (Eulenberg syndrome)	Muscular	• Myotonia on exposure to cold and stress • Paroxysmal weakness	• Serum K^+ fluctuations	• Close monitoring of serum K^+ required • Succinylcholine may induce hyperkalemia • Nondepolarizers do *not* relax myotonia • Halothane can cause shivering and induce myotonia • Extreme sensitivity to respiratory depressants
Patau syndrome (Trisomy 13)	Chromosomal	• Microcephaly • Micrognathia • Dextrocardia and CHD • Cleft lip and/or palate • Fatal by age 3	• Psychomotor retardation	• Potentially difficult airway • Preoperative cardiac evaluation needed
Pfeiffer syndrome (acrocephalopolysyndactyly)	Craniofacial	• Craniosynostosis • Wide towering skull • Hypoplastic maxilla and nasal bridge • Hypertelorism • Proptosis • Strabismus • Cleft palate • Congenital deafness	• Normal mental function	• Management of difficult airway • Association of strabismus with MH

Continued.

TABLE 17-1. Pediatric syndrome and anesthetic implications—cont'd

Syndrome or disease	Primary system affected	Clinical manifestations	Physiologic considerations	Anesthetic implications
Phenylketonuria (PKU)	Metabolic	• Seizures • Pyloric stenosis • Eczema • Hyperactivity	• Deficiency of phenylalanine hydroxylase • Progressive mental retardation as accumulation of phenylalanine interferes with brain maturation and myelination	• Management of seizure disorder • Loss of skin integrity
Pierre-Robin syndrome	Craniofacial	• Micrognathia • Glossoptosis • Cleft palate • CHD	• Chronic upper airway obstruction may cause hypoventilation, pulmonary HTN, and cor pulmonale	• Difficult intubation • In supine position the tongue may cause total airway occlusion, which may require nasal airway, tongue suture, or tracheostomy
Poikiloderma atrophicans vasculare (see Rothmund-Thomson syndrome)				
Pompe disease (Type II—glycogen storage disease)	Metabolic	• Hypotonia • Hepatomegaly • Cardiomegaly and CHF • Macroglossia • Glossoptosis	• Absence of acid maltase • Airway obstruction • Recurrent pneumonia	• Potentially difficult airway • Cardiac and pulmonary depressants should be avoided • May have exaggerated response to muscle relaxants • Coagulation profile may be abnormal

Porphyria	Metabolic	• Flaccid paralysis and skeletal muscle weakness • Autonomic nervous system imbalance leading to HTN and tachycardia • Diabetes mellitus • Severe abdominal pain	• Autosomal dominant inherited disorder of increased delta aminolevulinic acid synthetase and decreased uroporphyrinogen synthetase activity resulting in increased porphobilinogen • Demyelination of peripheral nerves and axonal degeneration • Psychiatric disorders	• Drugs that induce liver enzymes precipitating an attack include: 1. Barbiturates 2. Steroids 3. Etomidate 4. Enflurane 5. Ketamine • Safe anesthetics include: Narcotics; Local anesthetics; N_2O, O_2, isoflurane, halothane; Atropine • Exaggerated response to muscle relaxants • Careful preoperative documentation of neurologic deficits • Frequent monitoring of glucose, fluids, and electrolytes
Prader-Willi syndrome	Metabolic/ Obesity	• Neonate: 1. Hypotonia and absent reflexes 2. Poor feeding • Older child: 1. Uncontrollable polyphagia, obesity 2. Hypogonadism 3. Hyperactivity	• Psychomotor retardation • Prone to hypoglycemia • Complications of obesity: • Delayed gastric emptying • Altered autonomic nervous system response • Poor vascular access	• Propensity to cardiopulmonary failure requiring postoperative ventilation • Continuous glucose infusion needed • May have prolonged response to muscle relaxants • Aspiration precautions needed

Continued.

TABLE 17-1. Pediatric syndrome and anesthetic implications—cont'd

Syndrome or disease	Primary system affected	Clinical manifestations	Physiologic considerations	Anesthetic implications
Primary distal renal tubular acidosis (see Albright-Butler syndrome)				
Progeria (Hutchinson-Gilford syndrome)	Cardiothoracic	• Cardiac disease: HTN, ischemia, cardiomegaly • Alopecia • Micrognathia • Joint stiffness • Small stature • Thick, inelastic skin	• Premature aging (starts 6 mo-3 yr)	• Management as for adults with myocardial ischemia or coronary artery disease • Careful padding and positioning • Potentially difficult airway
Progressive infantile spinal muscle atrophy (see Werdnig-Hoffman disease)				
Prune belly syndrome (urethral obstruction malformation complex)	Metabolic	• Deficiency of abdominal wall musculature • Bladder distention • Renal dysplasia • Pulmonary hypoplasia • Cryptorchidism • Colonic malrotation	• Congenital urinary tract obstruction and renal dysfunction • Ineffective cough from lack of abdominal wall musculature • Recurrent respiratory infections	• Preoperative pulmonary evaluation required • Impaired renal drug excretion

Pseudoxanthoma elasticum (Groenblad-Strandberg syndrome)	Connective tissue	• Skin papules • Poor skin turgor • Decreased visual acuity, retinal detachment • GI hemorrhage • Angina, claudication	• Degenerative multisystem disorder of elastin tissue • Premature peripheral, cerebral and coronary vascular disease • Renal hypertension	• Loss of skin integrity • Need preoperative evaluation of cardiac and renal function
Pyle's disease (metaphyseal dysplasia)	Craniofacial	• Enlarged mandible • Cranial nerve palsies • Skeletal anomalies	• Not significant	• Potentially difficult airway
Refsum's syndrome	Metabolic	• Peripheral polyneuropathy • Ichthyosis • Cardiac arrhythmias and heart block • Optic nerve atrophy • Limb weakness • Cerebellar ataxia • Nerve deafness	• Deficiency of phytanic acid alpha hydroxylase	• Preoperative cardiac evaluation • Loss of skin integrity • Requires care in padding and positioning
Rieger syndrome	Muscular	• Hypoplastic maxilla • Abnormal dentition • Imperforate anus • Hypertelorism	• Psychomotor retardation • Subset of myotonic dystrophy	• Succinylcholine may cause hyperkalemia • Difficult airway management • Sensitivity to respiratory depressants and nondepolarizing muscle relaxants

Continued.

TABLE 17-1. Pediatric syndrome and anesthetic implications—cont'd

Syndrome or disease	Primary system affected	Clinical manifestations	Physiologic considerations	Anesthetic implications
Riley-Day syndrome (familial dysautonomia)	Neurologic	• Hypotonia • Deficient tear production • Absent corneal reflex and DTRs • Insensitivity to pain • Recurrent aspiration and pneumonia	• Focal demyelination of posterior columns of spinal cord and degeneration of dorsal root ganglia • Emotional lability • Deficiency of dopamine β-hydroxylase leads to hypo- and hypertensive attacks • Chronic lung disease • Respiratory insensitivity to CO_2	• Lack of compensatory cardiovascular reflexes, especially in presence of potent cardiovascular depressants • Difficult to assess anesthetic depth because of pain insensitivity and autonomic lability • Aspiration precautions needed • Phenothiazines and β-blockers recommended for adrenergic blockade • Exaggerated response to muscle relaxants • Impaired thermoregulation
Ritter disease (see Staphylococcal scalded skin syndrome)				
Romano-Ward syndrome	Cardiothoracic	• Familial ventricular tachycardia • Syncopal attacks secondary to paroxysmal VF	• Cardiac conduction defects (e.g., prolongation of QT interval)	• Halothane, lidocaine, procaine, quinidine, and phenothiazines may adversely affect cardiac conduction • Sympathetic stimulation may stimulate ventricular tachydysrhythmias

Rothmund-Thomson syndrome (poikiloderma atrophicans vasculare)	Dermatologic	• Atrophic telangiectatic dermatosis • Cataracts • Sparse hair • Defective dentition • Hypogenitalism	• Congenital bone defects including pathologic fractures	• Poor dentition requires caution with laryngoscopy • Loss of skin integrity • Care in positioning and padding required
Rubinstein-Taybi syndrome	Cardiothoracic	• CHD: ASD, PS • Microcephaly • Dysphagia, aspiration	• Psychomotor retardation • Recurrent pulmonary infections	• Aspiration precautions • Antibiotic prophylaxis for CHD needed • Preoperative cardiac evaluation required
Saerthre-Chotzen syndrome (acrocephalopolysyndactyly)	Craniofacial	• Craniosynostosis • Prominent mandible • Strabismus • High arched palate	• Renal dysfunction	• Potentially difficult airway • Impaired renal drug excretion • Association of strabismus with MH
Sanfilippo syndrome (Type III—mucopolysaccharidosis)	Metabolic	• Coarse facial features • Joint stiffness • Usually fatal by second decade	• Severe psychomotor retardation	• Induction technique should be appropriate for uncooperative child
Scheie disease (Type V—mucopolysaccharidosis)	Metabolic	• Corneal clouding • Hernias • Joint stiffness, especially in hands and feet • Aortic insufficiency	• Deposition of mucopolysaccharides in connective tissue • Normal intelligence	• Requires care in positioning • Need preoperative cardiac evaluation (echocardiogram)

Continued.

TABLE 17-1. Pediatric syndrome and anesthetic implications—cont'd

Syndrome or disease	Primary system affected	Clinical manifestations	Physiologic considerations	Anesthetic implications
Schwartz-Jampal syndrome	Muscular	• Dwarfism • Skeletal abnormalities • Muscle stiffness and abnormal contractions	• Progressive myotonic dystrophy	• Elevated temperature with anesthesia that resembles MH • Requires careful positioning • Management as for myotonic dystrophy
Scleroderma	Connective tissue	• Inflammatory polyarthritis • Joint contractures • Diffuse pulmonary fibrosis and cor pulmonale • Cardiac conduction defects • Esophageal dysmotility, increased GE reflux, and strictures • Telangiectasias may cause anemia	• Autoimmune process causing deposition of fibrous tissue in skin and internal organs • Renal dysfunction • Pulmonary hypertension	• Restriction of oral aperture causes difficult intubation • May need stress steroids • Impaired renal drug excretion • Need preoperative cardiopulmonary evaluation • Aspiration precautions needed

Seip-Lawrence syndrome	Dermatologic	• Generalized loss of subcutaneous fat • Prominent veins • Hirsutism • Skin pigmentation • Hepatomegaly • Cirrhosis	• Generalized lipodystrophy • Impaired thermoregulation • Development of insulin-resistant nonketotic diabetes mellitus • Propensity to hypoglycemia • Renal dysfunction leading to glomerulonephritis • Accelerated skeletal growth	• Renal and hepatic drug excretion may be impaired • Close monitoring of blood glucose required • May have coagulopathy • Requires care in positioning and padding • Maintain normothermia
Shone syndrome	Cardiothoracic	• Mitral stenosis • Associated aortic stenosis and mitral regurgitation • Coarctation of aorta	• Parachute mitral valve (all chordae tendinae insert into a single papillary muscle) • Increased susceptibility to pulmonary infections	• Need preoperative cardiopulmonary evaluation
Shy-Drager syndrome	Neurologic	• Orthostatic hypotension • Decreased sweating	• Defective baroreceptor response causes blood pressure and heart rate lability • Diffuse CNS degeneration and autonomic dysfunction	• Impaired thermoregulation • Neosynephrine used to treat hypotension • Anticholinergics that decrease sweating should be avoided
Sipple syndrome (multiple endocrine neoplasia—type II)	Metabolic	• Pheochromocytoma (75% bilateral) • Medullary carcinoma of thyroid • Parathyroid adenoma • CNS tumors • Cushing's disease	• Electrolyte imbalance • Altered calcium homeostasis	• Management of pheochromocytoma with adequate preoperative alpha and beta blockade • Preoperative thyroid function tests needed • Frequent monitoring of electrolytes and fluids

Continued.

TABLE 17-1. Pediatric syndrome and anesthetic implications—cont'd

Syndrome or disease	Primary system affected	Clinical manifestations	Physiologic considerations	Anesthetic implications
Smith-Lemli-Opitz syndrome	Craniofacial	• Microcephaly • Micrognathia • Hypotonia • Pyloric stenosis • Strabismus • Hypospadias • Cryptorchidism • Syndactyly	• Increased susceptibility to recurrent infections • Psychomotor retardation • Thymic hypoplasia	• Potentially difficult airway • Decreased pulmonary reserve from recurrent infections • Association of strabismus with MH • May have exaggerated response to muscle relaxants
Sotos syndrome (cerebral gigantism)	Craniofacial	• Acromegalic features (large mandible and maxilla)	• Normal ICP but dilated ventricles	• Potentially difficult airway
Spina bifida (see Myelomeningocele)				

Staphylococcal scalded skin syndrome (Ritter disease)	Dermatologic	• Prodrome of:
		  • Malaise
		  • Fever
		  • Conjunctivitis
		  • URI
		• Bullous impetigo
			• Epidermolysis and intraepidermal desquamation
			• Staphylococcal sepsis secondary to exotoxin
				• Loss of skin integrity
				• Fluid and electrolyte imbalance
				• Strict aseptic technique required
				• Impaired thermoregulation

Steven's-Johnson syndrome (see Erythema multiforme major)				
Stickler syndrome (arthroophthalmomyopathy)	Skeletal	• Cataracts • Retinal detachment • Glaucoma • Joint laxity and arthritis • Cleft palate • Kyphoscoliosis • Deafness • Micrognathia • Flat facies	• Restrictive lung disease	• Potentially difficult airway • Need preoperative pulmonary evaluation
Still's disease (see Juvenile rheumatoid arthritis)				

Sturge-Weber syndrome (encephalotrigeminal angiomatosis)	Neurologic	• Hemangiomas:
		  • Eyelid or conjunctiva
		  • Face (along distribution of CN V)
		  • Meninges
		• Intracranial calcifications cause seizure disorder
		• Hemiparesis
		• Congenital glaucoma
			• Impaired mental function	• Hemangioma may be present in airway
				• Significant intraoperative blood loss should be anticipated

Continued.

TABLE 17-1. Pediatric syndrome and anesthetic implications—cont'd

Syndrome or disease	Primary system affected	Clinical manifestations	Physiologic considerations	Anesthetic implications
Sydenham's chorea	Neurologic	• Involuntary choreoathetoid movements • Emotional lability	• Antistreptococcal antibodies to neurons of the subthalamic and caudate nuclei • Persistent dopaminergic supersensitivity	• Central stimulants and neuroleptics should be avoided
Syringomyelia	Neurologic	• Associated with Arnold Chiari malformation • Skeletal muscle wasting • Scoliosis • Bulbar involvement, dysphagia, aspiration	• Defect in intermedullary blood supply to cord • Restrictive lung disease • Impaired thermoregulation	• See Arnold-Chiari malformation • Aspiration precautions needed • Exaggerated response to muscle relaxants • Succinylcholine-induced hyperkalemia
Systemic lupus erythematosus	Immunologic	• Nephritis • HTN • Arthritis • Dermatitis (malar butterfly rash) • Photosensitivity • Alopecia • CNS involvement, seizures, chorea • Pericarditis • Pleuritis • Hepatosplenomegaly	• Immune complex vasculitis with inflammatory involvement of connective tissue • ANA antibodies • Anemia • Thrombocytopenia	• Preoperative cardiac evaluation needed • Impaired renal drug excretion and hepatic drug metabolism • ASA, NSAIDs may impair coagulation studies • May need stress dose steroids

Tangier disease (analpha lipoproteinemia)	Metabolic	• Orange tonsils and rectal mucosa • Splenomegaly • Peripheral neuropathy • Premature coronary artery disease • Muscle wasting	• Decreased HDL • Anemia, thrombocytopenia	• May have exaggerated response to muscle relaxants • May have coagulopathy • Need preoperative evaluation for cardiac ischemia
TAR syndrome (thrombocytopenia, and absent radius)	Hematologic	• Bilateral radial aplasia • High incidence of intracranial hemorrhage • CHD	• Profound thrombocytopenia (< 15,000)	• Coagulopathy • Preoperative cardiac evaluation needed • Elective surgery should be avoided in first year of life
Tauri disease (glycogen storage disease—type VII)	Metabolic	• Muscle cramps • Myoglobinuria	• Altered liver function	• Confusion with MH • May have abnormal coagulation profile
Tay-Sachs disease	Metabolic	• Motor weakness causing dysphagia • Deafness • Blindness • Seizures • Cherry red spot on macula	• Ganglioside storage disease • Psychomotor retardation • Recurrent respiratory infections	• Aspiration precautions needed • Management of seizure disorder • May have decreased pulmonary reserve

Continued.

TABLE 17-1. Pediatric syndrome and anesthetic implications—cont'd

Syndrome or disease	Primary system affected	Clinical manifestations	Physiologic considerations	Anesthetic implications
Thomsen's disease (see Myotonia congenita)				
Thrombocytopenia and absent radius (see TAR syndrome)				
Thrombotic thrombocytopenic purpura (see Moschkowitz disease)				
Toxic epidermal necrolysis (see Lyell disease)				
Treacher-Collins syndrome (mandibulofacial dysostosis)	Craniofacial	• Bilateral facial hypoplasia, aplastic zygomatic arches • Micrognathia • Eyelid coloboma • Microstomia • Choanal atresia • CHD • Pharyngeal hypoplasia	• Airway obstruction	• Marked narrowing of airway above larynx; extremely difficult intubation • Preoperative cardiac evaluation needed
Trisomy 13 (see Patau syndrome)				

Trisomy 18 (see Edward's syndrome)				
Trisomy 21 (see Down's syndrome)				
Tuberous sclerosis	Cardiothoracic	• Hamartomas in lungs, kidney, heart • Cardiac arrhythmias • Adenoma sebaceum of skin • Seizures • Intracranial calcification	• Psychomotor retardation	• Impaired renal drug excretion • Rupture of lung cysts can occur • Management of seizure disorder • Preoperative cardiac evaluation needed
Turner's syndrome (XO)	Chromosomal	• Short stature • Micrognathia • Web neck • Pectus excavatum • Dissecting aortic aneurysm • Aortic coarctation • Pulmonary stenosis	• Renal dysfunction	• Potentially difficult airway • Impaired renal drug excretion • Preoperative cardiac evaluation needed
Urbach-Wiethe disease	Immunologic	• Cutaneous-mucosal hyalinosis • Hyaline deposits in larynx and pharynx cause hoarseness and aphonia	• Histiocytosis • Similar to Hand-Schuller-Christian disease	• Potentially difficult airway

Continued.

TABLE 17-1. Pediatric syndrome and anesthetic implications—cont'd

Syndrome or disease	Primary system affected	Clinical manifestations	Physiologic considerations	Anesthetic implications
Urethral obstruction malformation complex (see Prune belly syndrome)				
VATER syndrome	Cardiothoracic	• Vertebral segmentation • Imperforate anus • TEF • Absent radius • CHD (VSD)	• Renal dysfunction • Recurrent pulmonary infections	• See management of TEF (Chapter 18) • Impaired renal drug excretion • Preoperative cardiac evaluation needed

von Gierke's disease (glycogen storage disease—type I)	Metabolic	• Poor muscle development
		• Hyperlipidemia
		• Severe hypoglycemia
		• Short stature
		• Increased bleeding time and platelet dysfunction
			• Deficiency of G-6-phosphatase
			• Glycogen accumulation leading to massive hepatomegaly
			• Fanconi-like syndrome:
			  • Acidosis
			  • Aminoaciduria
			  • Glycosuria
			  • Phosphaturia
			  • Hyperuricemia
				• Increased intraabdominal pressure from hepatomegaly
				• Preoperative coagulation profile needed
				• Impaired hepatic drug metabolism and renal drug excretion
				• May have exaggerated response to muscle relaxants

Von Hippel-Lindau syndrome	Neurologic	• Retinal or CNS hemangioblastomas (posterior fossa or spinal cord) • Renal, pancreatic, and hepatic cysts	• Neurologic changes resulting from compression or hemorrhage	• Associated with pheochromocytoma • Possible impaired hepatic drug metabolism and renal drug excretion

Von Recklinghausen's syndrome (see Neurofibromatosis)				
Von Willebrand's disease	Hematologic	• Prolonged bleeding time	• Decreased factor VIII activity causing defective platelet adhesiveness	• Preoperative coagulation profile needed • Salicylates should be avoided • May need cryoprecipitate or DDAVP preoperatively (see Chapter 12)
Weber-Christian disease (chronic nonsuppurative panniculitis)	Cardiothoracic	• Necrosis of fat, including pericardial, retroperitoneal, and meningeal • Pericardial involvement causing restrictive pericarditis • Seizures	• Retroperitoneal involvement may cause acute or chronic adrenal insufficiency	• Preoperative cardiac evaluation needed • Heat, cold, and pressure may increase fat necrosis • May need stress steroids • Management of seizure disorder
Wegener's granulomatosis	Immunologic	• Recurrent pulmonary infections • Upper respiratory tract bleeding and hemoptysis • Glomerulonephritis	• Necrotizing granulomatous angiitis	• May need stress dose steroids • Potentially difficult airway • Need preoperative pulmonary evaluation • May have impaired renal drug excretion

Continued.

TABLE 17-1. Pediatric syndrome and anesthetic implications—cont'd

Syndrome or disease	Primary system affected	Clinical manifestations	Physiologic considerations	Anesthetic implications
Werdnig-Hoffman disease (progressive infantile spinal muscle atrophy)	Muscular	• Generalized muscle weakness • Kyphoscoliosis • Pectus excavatum • Bulbar involvement leads to recurrent aspiration and pneumonia	• Degenerative disease of anterior horn cells and cranial nerve motor nuclei • Decreased respiratory reserve	• Succinylcholine may cause hyperkalemia • Increased sensitivity to nondepolarizing muscle relaxants • Aspiration precautions needed • May need postoperative ventilatory support
Wermer's syndrome (multiple endocrine neoplasia—type I)	Metabolic	• Hyperparathyroidism • Pituitary tumors • Pancreatic islet cell tumors • Gastric ulcers • May have carcinoid tumor of bronchial tree	• Altered calcium homeostasis • May have renal failure secondary to calculi • Glucose instability with propensity to hypoglycemia	• Frequent monitoring of blood glucose needed • Impaired renal drug excretion • Potential for carcinoid syndrome • Aspiration precautions needed • Fluid and electrolyte imbalance
Werner syndrome	Cardiothoracic	• Coronary artery disease, ischemia, CHF • Arrest of growth in puberty • Scleroderma-like changes • Alopecia • Hypogonadism	• Psychomotor retardation • Premature aging • Diabetes mellitus	• Preoperative cardiac evaluation and monitoring for ischemia and coronary artery disease needed • Management of diabetes (Chapter 16)

Whistling face syndrome (see Freeman-Sheldon syndrome)				
Williams syndrome	Cardiothoracic	• Elfin facies • Hypercalcemia • Supravalvular aortic stenosis: fixed cardiac output • Dental abnormalities • Joint contractures	• Psychomotor retardation • Left ventricular failure and ischemia	• Preoperative cardiac evaluation and monitoring for ischemia needed • May need stress dose steroids • Serum calcium should be monitored • Careful positioning and padding required
Wilson-Mikity syndrome	Cardiothoracic	• Prematurity $< 1,500$ g birth weight • Pulmonary fibrosis and cystic areas • Right heart failure	• Severe chronic lung disease • Recurrent chest infections and aspiration	• Decreased pulmonary reserve • Aspiration precautions needed • May need stress dose steroids • Cardiac depressants should be avoided
Wilson's disease (hepatolenticular degeneration)	Metabolic	• Kayser-Fleischer rings on cornea • Malabsorption syndrome • Hepatic failure: cirrhosis and jaundice	• Decreased plasma ceruloplasmin causing abnormal copper deposition in liver and CNS (degeneration of lenticular nucleus and basal ganglia) • Renal tubular acidosis and aminoaciduria	• Decreased pseudocholinesterases • Impaired renal and hepatic drug clearance • Abnormal coagulation profile

Continued.

TABLE 17-1. Pediatric syndrome and anesthetic implications—cont'd

Syndrome or disease	Primary system affected	Clinical manifestations	Physiologic considerations	Anesthetic implications
Wiskott-Aldrich syndrome	Immunologic	• Severe recurrent bacterial and opportunistic infections • Seborrheic dermatitis and eczema • Bloody diarrhea leading to severe anemia • Intracranial hemorrhage	• X-linked recessive immunodeficiency (T cell and IgM) • Thrombocytopenia • Propensity for hypothermia • Progressive renal dysfunction	• Chronic debilitation • Absolute aseptic technique required • Impaired renal drug clearance • May need preoperative transfusions of red cells and platelets (irradiated to prevent graft-versus-host disease) • Antibiotic prophylaxis preoperatively • Preoperative evaluation and optimization of pulmonary and renal status
Wolff-Parkinson-White syndrome	Cardiothoracic	• Arrhythmias; SVT • May be in heart failure or cardiogenic shock due to tachycardia • Associated CHF, most commonly with Ebstein anomaly	• Reentry pathway: accessory bundle of Kent	• Sympathetic stimulation or atropine may trigger tachyarrhythmias • Halothane may predispose to PACs and trigger reentry pathway • Digoxin often used to control arrhythmias, rarely causes VF in children • Countershock should be used for SVT • Consider antibiotic prophylaxis if associated CHD

Wolman's disease (familial xanthomatosis)	Metabolic	• Xanthomatous visceral changes • Adrenal calcification • Hepatomegaly • Hypersplenism • Death by 6 months of age	• Foam cell infiltration of tissue including myocardium	• May have abnormal coagulation profile and platelet function • Preoperative cardiac evaluation needed
Xeroderma pigmentosum	Dermatologic	• Excessive erythema and blistering following minimal sun exposure • Keratosis and skin cancer develop at an early age despite aggressive treatment	• Disorder of pyrimidine metabolism	• Loss of skin integrity • Potentially difficult airway if extensive head and neck involvement
Zellweger syndrome (see Cerebrohepatorenal syndrome)				

BIBLIOGRAPHY

Birkinshaw KJ: Anesthesia in a patient with an unstable neck (Morquio's syndrome), Anesthesia 30:46-49, 1975.

Divekar VM and Sircar BN: Anesthetic management in Treacher-Collins syndrome, Anesthesiology 26:692-93, 1965.

Feingold M and Baum J: Goldenhar's syndrome, Am J Dis Child 132:136-38, 1978.

Gurkowski MA and Rasch DK: Anesthetic considerations for Beckwith-Wiedemann syndrome, Anesthesiology 70:711-12, 1989.

Jones AEP and Pelton DA: An index of syndromes and their anesthetic implications, Canadian Journal of Anaesthesia 23:206-26, 1976.

Kaplan P and others: Contractures in patients with Williams syndrome, Pediatrics 84:895-99, 1989.

Katz J and Steward DJ: Anesthesia and uncommon pediatric diseases, Philadelphia, 1987, WB Saunders Co.

Kobel M, Creighton RE, and Steward DJ: Anaesthetic considerations in Down's syndrome: experience with 100 patients and a review of the literature, Canadian Journal of Anaesthesia 29:593-99, 1982.

Lawlor F: Progress of a harlequin fetus to nonbullous ichthyosiform erythroderma, Pediatrics 82:870-73, 1988.

Oski FA and others: Principles and practice of pediatrics, Philadelphia, 1990, JB Lippincott Co.

Parker WD, Oley CA, and Parks JK: A defect in mitochondrial electron-transport activity (NADH-coenzyme Q oxidoreductase) in Leber's hereditary optic neuropathy, N Engl J Med 320:1331-33, 1989.

Ravindran R and Stoops CM: Anesthetic management of a patient with Hallermann-Streif syndrome, Anesth Analg 58:254-55, 1979.

Ryan JF and others: A practice of anesthesia for infants and children, Orlando, FL 1986, Grune & Stratton, Inc.

Singh G, Lott MT, and Wallace DG: A mitochondrial DNA mutation as a cause of Leber's hereditary optic neuropathy, N Engl J Med 320:1300-5, 1989.

Sklar GS and King BD: Endotracheal intubation and Treacher-Collins syndrome, Anesthesiology 44:247-49, 1976.

Steenson A and Torkelson RD: King's syndrome with malignant hyperthermia, Am J Dis Child 141:271-73, 1987.

Steward DJ: Manual of pediatric anesthesia, ed 2, New York, 1985, Churchill Livingstone.

Trapp LD and others: Anesthetic management of the pediatric patient with multiple congenital anomalies including severe hemifacial hypertrophy, Anesthesia Progress (Nov-Dec):162-66, 1981.

Yee LL, Gunter JB, and Manley CB: Caudal epidural anesthesia in an infant with epidermolysis bullosa, Anesthesiology 70:149-51, 1989.

18

ANESTHETIC MANAGEMENT OF PEDIATRIC AND NEONATAL EMERGENCIES

Mary M. Stenger

Rock-a-bye, baby, on the tree top,
When the wind blows the cradle will rock;
When the bough breaks the cradle will fall,
Down will come baby, cradle, and all.
ANON

GENERAL PROBLEMS ASSOCIATED WITH THE EMERGENT PATIENT

Securing the Airway

Anesthetic management of the neonate, infant, or child for emergency surgery often necessitates a rapid-sequence induction or awake intubation of the trachea. Like adults, pain, trauma, anxiety or a variety of drugs can slow gastric emptying in children despite their NPO status. Therefore, they should be treated as having a "full stomach."

The Neonate

In a vigorous neonate with an uncomplicated airway and secure IV access a rapid-sequence induction may be considered. Most neonates undergoing emergency procedures are critically ill (lethargic, septic, premature) and lack the physiologic respiratory reserve to tolerate the 30 to 40 seconds of apnea present in a rapid sequence. For this majority an awake intubation of the trachea is appropriate. (See the box on p. 200, in Chapter 10, for technique of awake intubation.)

The Infant and Child

1. Unless contraindicated in the awake state (e.g., open globe, epiglottitis) an IV should be secured. Preoxygenation may be difficult in the uncooperative child but should be attempted. Induction may then proceed with ketamine or thiopental and succinylcholine, with cricoid pressure maintained until correct endotracheal tube placement is verified. After the airway is secured the stomach is emptied.
2. When a delay of 1 to 2 hours is anticipated before the surgical procedure, the child can be given cimetidine (7.5 mg/kg) and metaclopromide (0.2 to 0.4 mg/kg) IV to decrease gastric volume and acidity.
3. In certain situations the concern for securing the airway takes precedence over the concern regarding the full stomach (e.g., epiglottitis or aspirated foreign body). Other occasions may arise when positive pressure ventilation should be avoided (e.g., congenital lobar emphysema, bronchogenic cyst). In these cases a gentle inhalation induction using halothane and oxygen is preferable, with maintenance of spontaneous ventilation. Induction in the Trendelenburg and lateral decubitus positions will prevent passive entry of regurgitated stomach contents into the lungs.

Vascular Access

1. A secure, large-bore IV catheter is necessary for fluid resuscitation and transfusions.
2. If potential veins cannot be seen or palpated, access may be secured "blindly" in common anatomic locations, particularly the dorsal hand between middle and ring metacarpals and the saphenous vein. The saphenous vein nearly always can be found 0.5 to 1.0 cm superior and anterior to the medial melleolus running parallel to the tibia (Fig. 18-1).
3. Lower-extremity IV catheters should be avoided when the inferior vena cava may be compromised.

Monitors

Noninvasive

1. Temperature—rectal, esophageal, or skin temperature
2. ECG
3. Blood pressure (oscillometric)
4. Precordial or esophageal stethescope
5. Pulse oximeter
6. Capnography

Invasive

1. Foley catheter for urine output
2. Arterial catheter—in the neonate a preductal site is preferred (i.e., right radial or right superficial temporal arteries); if an umbilical artery catheter is placed at birth it may be replaced by a right radial artery catheter
3. Central venous catheter—usually through the external or internal jugular or subclavian veins

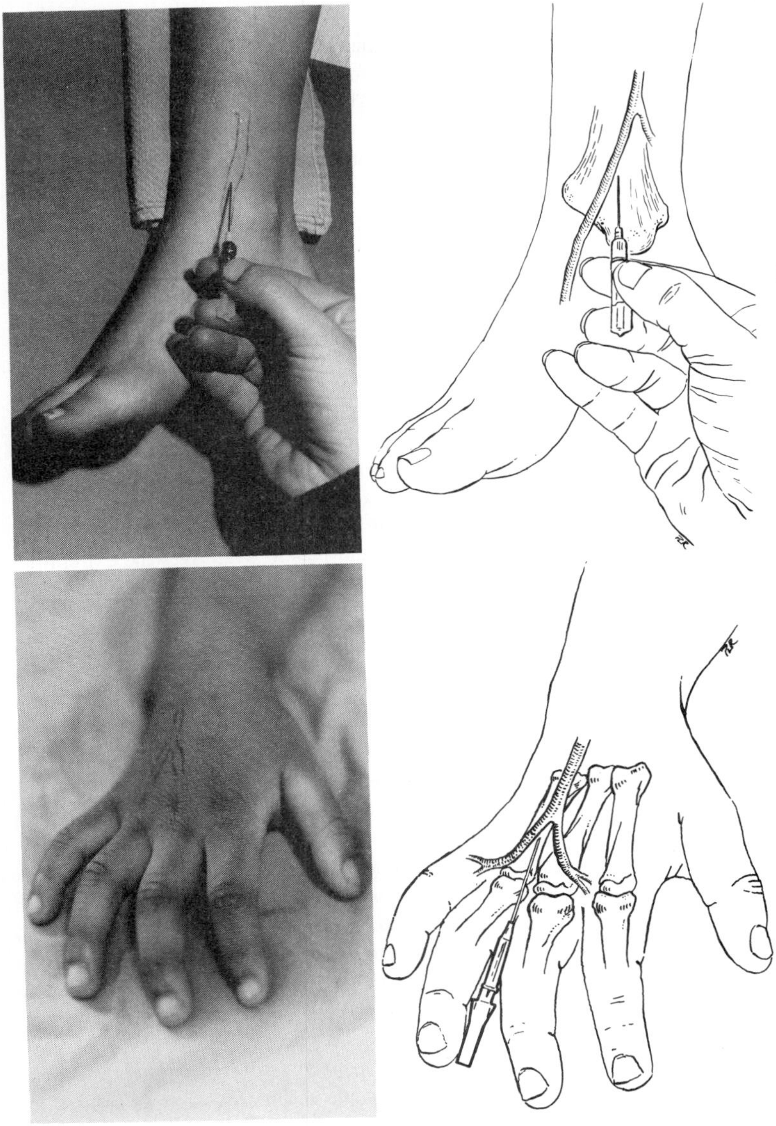

Fig. 18-1. Intravenous access. Intravenous access may be secured even when the vein is not visualized by knowing venous anatomy. The saphenous vein can almost always be cannulated 0.5-1.0 cm superior and anterior to the medial malleolus running parallel to the tibia (**A** and **B**). A vein is also usually found on the mid-dorsum of the hand between the middle and ring metacarpals (**C** and **D**).

Temperature Regulation

Temperature regulation is critical in the emergent pediatric patient. Heat loss can be extremely rapid, increasing morbidity, particularly in the smaller infant with a large surgical incision. The high body surface area-body mass ratio and the presence of a thin layer of subcutaneous fat increase susceptibility to hypothermia. Infants do not shiver, and thermogenesis is maintained by brown fat metabolism, substantially increasing oxygen consumption.

Steps to Maintain Normothermia

1. Continually monitoring temperature
2. Transporting the infant in a temperature controlled incubator to maintain neutral temperature
3. Increasing the ambient temperature of the operating room
4. Warming and humidifying inspired gases
5. Using heating mattresses for infants less than 10 kg or for long procedures
6. Using radiant warmers before draping
7. Warming preparatory solutions and irrigation
8. Warming IV solutions and infused blood
9. Using a stocking cap on the head and plastic wrap over the extremities

RESPIRATORY EMERGENCIES

Congenital Upper Airway Obstruction

Choanal Atresia

1. Choanal atresia usually is not associated with other anomalies. It occurs in approximately 1:8000 births when the bony or membranous portions of the nasopharynx fail to perforate during development.
2. Unilateral obstruction may be unrecognized, but bilateral obstruction can cause acute respiratory distress, because the neonate is an obligate nose breather.
3. The diagnosis usually is made shortly after birth, when a catheter fails to pass into the nasopharynx, or when the infant chokes and becomes cyanotic from aspiration during feeding.
4. Early surgical repair is necessary to prevent respiratory distress and aspiration. If respiratory distress develops the airway should be secured by an oral airway or endotracheal intubation.

Laryngeal or Tracheal Webs

Laryngeal or tracheal webs can cause acute respiratory distress and stridor at birth. It may be possible to break through this incomplete fibrous web with an endotracheal tube stented by a stylette. If ventilation through an ETT is unsuccessful, cricothyroid puncture with an IV catheter may serve temporarily, until the web can be resected.

Congenital Subglottic Stenosis

Congenital subglottic stenosis may cause neonatal respiratory distress that usually is less acute than with a web. The severity of stenosis usually is determined by bronchoscopy, which may require general anesthesia. Mask inhalation induction with gentle assisted ventilation helps keep the airway from further soft-tissue obstruction. Lidocaine aerosol or spray can be applied directly to the trachea during laryngoscopy to minimize airway reactivity. A 3-ml syringe with an IV catheter attached can be used for lidocaine spray. (Maximum dosage: 0.5 ml/kg of 1% solution or 5 mg/kg.)

Congenital Pulmonary Defects

Bronchogenic Cysts

Congenital bronchogenic cysts are formed by primordial respiratory tissue isolated from the rest of the developing lung. The location and size of the cyst are critical. Carinal cysts can cause dramatic respiratory decompensation, as the cyst enlarges to obstruct the mainstem bronchi and cause air trapping. This situation may occur in the neonate and require emergency decompression of the cyst to allow adequate ventilation. Bronchogenic cysts of the hilum or parenchyma often cause chronic infections with abscess formation. The cyst should be resected in late infancy or early childhood to prevent recurrent pulmonary infections.

Lobar Emphysema

Congenital lobar emphysema occurs in the neonatal period as progressive respiratory distress. Chest radiographs reveal unilateral thoracic hyperexpansion with mediastinal shift and contralateral atelectasis. High intrathoracic pressures generated by the emphysematous lobe may decrease cardiac output. Because usually only one lobe is affected (most commonly the left upper lobe) the condition can be treated successfully by lobectomy.

Anesthetic Management

1. Anesthesia should be induced by mask inhalation with spontaneous ventilation. If assisted ventilation is necessary, low peak inspiratory pressures should be used with adequate time allowed for exhalation. Positive pressure ventilation may increase intrathoracic pressure and worsen air trapping.
2. N_2O should be avoided because it can cause expansion of the emphysematous lobe or cyst. Oxygen and air mixtures should be used to attain an adequate F_IO_2 and saturation.
3. One-lung ventilation may be useful to isolate an infected cyst or to improve visualization of the surgical field. In the neonate it may be necessary to advance the endotracheal tube into the selected bronchus under direct vision of the surgeon. Alternatively, a Fogarty catheter may be placed in the bronchus through the surgical field. Usually, flow to the ipsilateral pulmonary artery also must be restricted during the procedure to decrease shunting.

Tracheoesophageal Fistula

General Considerations

1. There are five major presentations of esophageal atresia and tracheoesophageal fistula (TEF; Fig. 18-2 on the next page). The most common type is IIIB, which consists of an esophageal blind pouch connected to

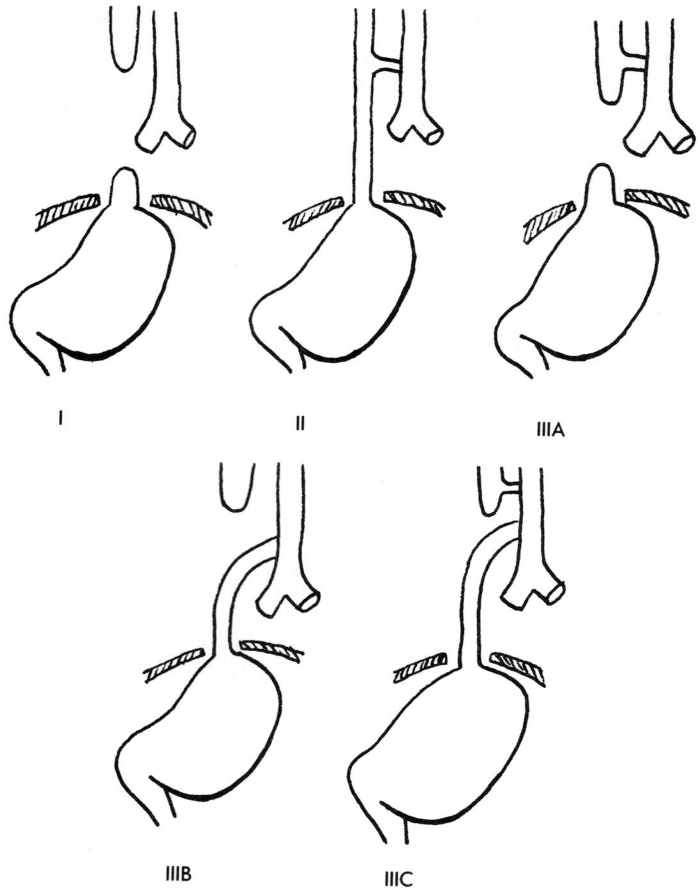

Fig. 18-2. Classification of tracheoesophageal fistula. (Adapted from Dierdorf SF and Krishna G: Anesthetic management of neonatal surgical emergencies. Anes Analg 60:208, 1981.)

the lower esophagus by a fistula. As a result, gastric secretions reflux into the trachea and lungs, producing severe chemical pneumonitis.

2. The diagnosis of TEF usually is made at birth upon failure to pass a catheter into the stomach, or when the infant chokes or becomes cyanotic with the first feeding. Chest radiographs show a catheter coiled in the blind esophageal pouch. When TEF is suspected, the infant's head should be elevated to prevent aspiration, oral feeding should be stopped, and an IV catheter placed. Gastric distention that impairs respiratory excursions should be avoided by early placement of a gastrostomy tube.
3. Approximately 20% of patients with TEF have an associated cardiac anomaly such as the tetralogy of Fallot, coarctation, VSD, or ASD. TEF

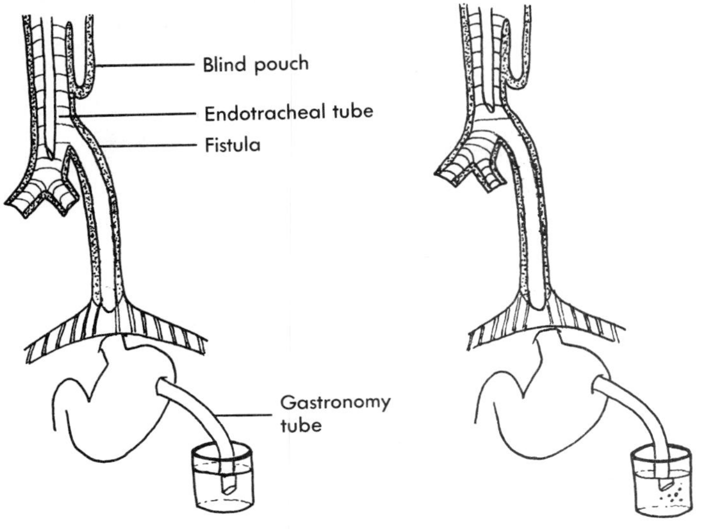

Fig. 18-3. Correct positioning of the endotracheal tube (ETT) for patients with tracheoesophageal fistula is facilitated by prior placement of the gastrostomy tube. With the end of the gastrostomy tube under water, bubbles will appear when the ETT is above the fistula (right), and will disappear as the ETT is advanced beyond the fistula (left). (Adapted from Dierdorf SF and Krishna G: Anesthetic management of neonatal surgical emergencies, Anes Analg 60:208, 1981.)

is part of VATER syndrome (vertebral defects, anal atresia, TEF, radial anomalies, and renal dysplasia). Thirty to forty percent of infants with TEF are born prematurely.

Preoperative Considerations

Many surgeons prefer to perform a gastrostomy under local anesthesia when the diagnosis of TEF is made, and delay thoracotomy and definitive repair for 48 to 72 hours. This allows adequate time to diagnose and treat associated congenital anomalies and pulmonary complications.

Anesthetic Management

Securing the airway. The gastrostomy should be performed under local anesthesia or with ketamine, with the infant maintaining spontaneous ventilation. After the gastrostomy tube is placed, secretions and excess gas that may enter the stomach can be vented. The trachea is then intubated with the infant awake. The tip of the endotracheal tube must be above the carina but below the fistula, which usually enters the trachea 1 to 2 cm above the carina. Tube position may be checked by placing the end of the gastrostomy tube in a beaker of water (Fig. 18-3). Bubbles will appear when the endotracheal tube is above the fistula, but will disappear as the endotracheal tube (ETT) is advanced beyond the fistula. Alternatively, the ETT may be advanced intentionally into the right mainstem bronchus, and then withdrawn until bilateral breath sounds are audible. Inadvertently leaving the endotracheal tube in the right mainstem bronchus intraoperatively may result in severe hypoxia, because the right lung is compressed during thoractomy. Another technique involves intentionally intubating the left mainstem bronchus and maintaining one-lung ventilation throughout the repair.

Monitoring. Monitoring should consist of the standard monitors and an arterial catheter for serial blood gases. The precordial stethoscope should be placed over the left chest as the repair is performed through the right thoractomy. A pulse oximeter is critical in maintaining proper positioning of the endotracheal tube.

Maintenance of anesthesia. Maintenance of anesthesia can be provided with a narcotic and muscle relaxant or inhalation agent as tolerated. No N_2O should be used before gastrostomy.

Postoperative Considerations

1. Early extubation is desirable postoperatively to minimize stress on suture lines. If early weaning and extubation is not feasible, the infant should be sedated, relaxed, and ventilated. Tracheomalacia is a common finding, and the infant must be observed carefully after extubation of the trachea for signs of tracheal collapse.
2. Aspiration pneumonitis from chronic gastroesophageal reflux may occur following repair of TEF.
3. Esophageal strictures commonly occur in infancy and childhood following repair and often require multiple procedures for esophageal dilation.

Diaphragmatic Hernia (DH)

1. Diaphragmatic hernia, the herniation of abdominal contents into the chest in utero, occurs with hypoplasia of the lungs in 1 in 5000 live births. Males are affected more often than females (2:1), and more frequently on the left than the right. The hernia itself is usually relatively easy to repair, but the pulmonary hypoplasia and subsequent respiratory dysfunction remain and are responsible for the high perioperative mortality rate (30% to 60%). Associated anomalies include malrotation of the gut and cataracts.
2. Embryologically, DH occurs when the gut returns to the abdominal cavity from the body stalk before the diaphragm has separated the pleural and peritoneal cavities. Because the pulmonary system develops concurrently, the degree of hypoplasia is related to the timing of herniation. Prognosis primarily depends on the severity of pulmonary hypoplasia and the involvement of one or both lungs.
3. Signs of DH include scaphoid abdomen, barrel chest, bowel sounds in the chest, respiratory distress, and cyanosis, though a small hernia may be asymptomatic. A chest radiograph reveals mediastinal shift and bowel in the chest.

Preoperative Treatment

1. The stomach should be decompressed with an orogastric or nasogastric tube.

2. Mask ventilation should be avoided, because it may increase the stomach volume and further compromise pulmonary function.
3. Early intubation may be necessary for ventilatory support.
4. Positive pressure ventilation should be used judiciously; it may cause a contralateral pneumothorax, with immediate decompensation.

Anesthetic Management

1. After the stomach is decompressed the infant should be preoxygenated and intubated awake.
2. Maintenance of anesthesia with narcotic and muscle relaxant usually is tolerated well. Inhalation agents may be used. However, the ability of the infant heart to tolerate the depressant effects of volatile agents may be compromised secondary to mediastinal distortion and underlying acidosis. N_2O should be avoided both because of the imminent danger of pneumothorax and because the infant usually requires a high F_IO_2.
3. Standard monitors and a right radial or right temporal (preductal) arterial catheter are indicated. Airway pressures also should be monitored with peak inspiratory pressure maintained at less than 20 cm H_2O.
4. After hernia reduction the temptation to "expand" the hypoplastic lung, which may lead to a contralateral pneumothorax, must be avoided. Because the opposite lung is responsible for nearly all respiration, pneumothorax can cause immediate and profound decompensation.
5. The abdominal wall is often hypoplastic and attempts at primary closure may impair diaphragmatic excursion or venous return. It may be necessary to create a ventral hernia using a silastic silo similar to the repair for omphalocele or gastroschesis.
6. The infant will require mechanical ventilation postoperatively, using muscle relaxants to decrease movement and the work of breathing, and narcotics or sedatives. Frequent, low tidal volume breaths should be used to decrease peak pressures. Classically, the postoperative course is heralded by a "honeymoon" period of 1 to 24 hours where improvement is seen, followed by rapid deterioration with hypoxemia, acidosis, and even death. Because of the presence of the hypoplastic lung, pulmonary vascular resistance (PVR) is high. Acidosis, hypercarbia, and hypoxemia contribute to the increase in PVR, and persistent pulmonary hypertension (PPH) develops with right-to-left shunting. The major determinant of outcome is the degree and reversibility of pulmonary hypertension.

Treatment for High PVR

1. The PVR may be lowered pharmacologically with tolazoline, isoproterenol, prostaglandin E, and NTG. Mixed success has been achieved with these agents, and dopamine often is required to support systemic circulation.
2. Hyperventilation to a pH value of 7.50 to 7.60 may decrease PVR.
3. Ligation of the PDA has been unsuccessful and associated with sudden RV failure.
4. Initial reports on the use of extracorporeal membrane oxygenation (ECMO) in DH were dismal, as it was only used on moribund infants

who died despite treatment. As indications have broadened, and more infants are treated, reports have been more optimistic and ECMO may prove to be the best treatment available for infants with severe DH.

GASTROINTESTINAL EMERGENCIES
Omphalocele and Gastroschesis

Omphalocele and gastroschesis (see Table 18-1 for characteristics) are defects of the anterior abdominal wall with herniation or evisceration of bowel contents through the defect.

Preoperative Considerations

The prevention of infection and minimization of heat and fluid loss are major concerns. The following measures should be instituted at birth, and continued until the defect is closed.

1. The herniated viscus should be covered with sterile saline soaked gauze and plastic wrap.
2. A neutral thermal environment should be maintained.
3. A nasogastric tube should be placed to prevent regurgitation and aspiration.
4. Systemic antibiotics should be started early.
5. Intravenous hydration should be maintained aggressively.
6. In patients with gastroschesis and ruptured omphalocele, considerable protein loss and fluid translocation can occur because of the absence

TABLE 18-1. Characteristics of bowel wall defects

	Omphalocele	Gastroschesis
Defect	Herniation of the viscera into the base of the umbilical cord through a central defect; membranous sac covers and protects gut, however, the sac may rupture	Evisceration of gut through 2-5 cm–long defect in abdominal wall lateral to the umbilicus; no sac covers viscera; viscera directly exposed to amniotic fluid and environment
Embryologic process	Failure of the gut to migrate back into abdominal cavity and thus failure of abdominal wall to develop	Intrauterine occlusion of the omphalomesenteric artery, resulting in a defect of the abdominal wall lateral to the umbilicus
Incidence	1/5000-1/10,000	1/15,000-1/30,000
Incidence of prematurity	33%	58%
Associated congenital anomalies	Frequent (76% incidence): cardiac defects (20%); Beckwith Wiedemann syndrome; extrophy of the bladder	Rare

of a protective membranous sac. Colloid should be given to maintain normal oncotic pressure. Hemoconcentration and metabolic acidosis may be evident and therapy should be guided by urine output and measurement of serial hematocrit and arterial blood gases.

Anesthetic Management

1. After decompression of the stomach and preoxygenation the awake infant's trachea is intubated.
2. Because prolonged postoperative ventilation usually is required, a narcotic technique is reasonable for maintenance of anesthesia. Inhalation agents may be used judiciously in the well-hydrated infant. Muscle relaxants are used to facilitate closure of the defect. N_2O should be avoided because of bowel distention.
3. Closure of the defect depends on the size of the defect and the development of the anterior abdominal wall. Small defects can be closed primarily. Larger defects require a staged reduction over several days or weeks.
4. Changes in pulmonary compliance will help guide the surgical repair. When the abdomen is closed tightly, peak inspiratory pressures rise, impairing diaphragmatic excursion. A tight repair can impede venous return and therefore reduce cardiac output by caval compression. Bowel ischemia and eventual wound dehiscence may result. Airway pressures, oxygen saturation, and arterial blood gases should be observed carefully upon closure of the defect.
5. In a staged procedure a dacron-reinforced silastic silo is placed over the defect and reduced gradually. These procedures can be performed on the intubated infant quite expeditiously with small doses of ketamine. Inhalation agents or narcotics and muscle relaxation may be required.
6. In addition to standard monitoring, all infants should have airway pressures followed carefully. The use of invasive monitoring depends upon the size of the defect. A large defect requires arterial cannulation for blood gas analysis to guide fluid resuscitation and respiratory support.

Postoperative Management

1. Most infants require postoperative mechanical ventilation. Airway pressures, oxygenation, and respiratory efforts should be observed carefully, and sedation and muscle relaxation provided as needed.
2. Prolonged postoperative ileus is not unusual and may necessitate parenteral alimentation.

TRAUMA

Major Trauma

Trauma continues to be the major cause of death in the pediatric population. Victims of major trauma usually sustain injuries to more than one organ system, making rapid assessment and evaluation of the entire patient essential. Life-threatening injuries must be identified and treated rapidly; young trauma patients often can stabilize vital signs with initial resuscitation and then rapidly decompensate if the injury is not repaired.

Potentially salvageable but life-threatening injuries fall primarily into two categories: head trauma and massive hemorrhage.

Head Trauma

1. The most common cause of morbidity and mortality in salvageable head injuries is caused by obstruction of the airway by the tongue and subsequent hypoxia in the unconscious patient.
2. Immediate intubation assures a patent airway, limits the risks of aspiration, and allows for hyperventilation to decrease intracranial pressure.
3. Cervical spine injuries often accompany head trauma. Although cervical spine radiographs are very helpful for determining possible fractures, airway management should never be neglected while films are being obtained. A trained assistant can hold the head in a neutral position with traction during intubation if necessary. Blind nasal intubations may cause bleeding or further intracranial trauma through undiagnosed facial fractures. Fiberoptic or awake intubations are difficult in an uncooperative child.
   a. If cervical spine injury is clinically apparent, it is important to document the level of spinal cord injury and the extent of deficit before performing intubation or operative procedures.
   b. Intraoperatively, neuromuscular blockade may interfere with the surgeon's assessment of cord injury. Somatosensory-evoked potentials may be useful to monitor nerve and spinal cord integrity in the presence of neuromuscular blockade.
4. The presence of elevated intracranial pressure (ICP) should be determined quickly (hypertension, bradycardia, pupil dilatation, posturing).
   a. The most common initial finding on computerized tomography (CT) is diffuse cerebral swelling, which mandates early and aggressive treatment. As with adults these measures include hyperventilation and diuresis.
   b. Systemic hypertension must be avoided, and the head should be carefully positioned, elevated, and without any obstruction to venous outflow.
   c. Patients with high ICP should be intubated with atropine 0.02 mg/kg, thiopental 5 to 10 mg/kg, and succinylcholine 2 mg/kg with cricoid pressure. Thiopental should not be used in the presence of hypovolemia, hypotension, or shock. Succinylcholine should be avoided in crush injuries because of the potential for hyperkalemia.
5. It is rare to have hypotension with head injury except as a terminal event. Other sources of bleeding should be suspected.
6. Neurologic function after injury can be described and documented by the *Glasgow Coma Scale* (see the box on the next page). In the younger nonverbal child the *Neonatal Arousal Scale* (see the box on p. 446) should be used. These scales allow uniformity in evaluating level of consciousness, but they do not necessarily correlate with the CT scan findings or predict outcome. They are best used for following the progression of neurological symptoms.

GLASGOW COMA SCALE

Eye opening	
Spontaneous	4
To speech	3
To pain	2
None	1
Verbal response	
Oriented	5
Confused conversation	4
Inappropriate words	3
Incomprehensible sounds	2
Nil	1
Best motor response	
Obeys	6
Localizes	5
Withdraws	4
Abnormal flexion—decorticate	3
Extensor response—decerebrate	2
Nil	1
Total	**3-15**

From Teasdale G and Jennett B: Aspects of coma after severe head injury, Lancet 1:878, 1972. Used with permission.

Massive Hemorrhage

Patients with massive hemorrhage usually will stabilize briefly with crystalloid infusion. If necessary, type-specific blood is given. Time is of the essence. It usually is not possible to replace volume losses from an unrepaired major vascular injury continuously. The anesthesiologist must be prepared for rapid volume replacement and transport to the operating room.

Anesthetic Management of Trauma

Fluid resuscitation

- In general, trauma patients should be resuscitated with Ringer's lactate (which converts to bicarbonate in the hepatic circulation).
- Glucose should be avoided because it may worsen CNS injury if ischemia occurs.
- Also, trauma causes physiologic stress that increases catecholamine levels. Consequent hyperglycemia and hyperosmolarity lead to diuresis and worsen hypovolemia.

Monitoring

- The anesthesiologist is an important member of the trauma team throughout the resuscitation process and during surgery and must continuously monitor the patient while performing resuscitation.

NEONATAL AROUSAL SCALE

Best response to bell	
Facial and extremity movements	5
Grimaces/blinks	4
Increase in RR/HR	3
Seizures/extensor posturing	2
No response	1
Best response to light	
Blink and facial/extremity movements	4
Blink	3
Seizures/extensor posturing	2
No response	1
Best motor response	
Spontaneous	
Periods of activity alternating with sleep	6
Occasional spontaneous movements	5
Sternal rub	
Extremity movements	4
Grimace/facial movements	3
Seizures/extensor posturing	2
No response	1
Total	**3-15**

From Duncan CC and others: A scale for the assessment of neonatal neurologic status, Child's Brain 8:300, 1981. Used with permission.

- In addition to transport monitors (particularly ECG, oximetry, and blood pressure), invasive monitors (arterial and central venous catheter) are usually needed to rapidly assess blood pressure and intravascular volume.
- When speed is essential, some monitors can perform more than one function. An oximeter with plethysmograph can give heart rate, oxygen saturation, and a rough estimate of peripheral perfusion. Capnography supplies both end-tidal CO_2 measurements and an estimate of cardiac output. Rapidly applying these two monitors may allow the surgical team to proceed in a life-threatening situation while the anesthetists continue to resuscitate and apply remaining monitors.
- Temperature monitoring often is overlooked in a crisis situation. However, hypothermia from exposure and massive infusion of cold fluids is a common problem in trauma victims. Besides increasing acidosis, overlooked hypothermia may result in cardiac fibrillation or arrest.

Anesthetic agents. If hemodynamically unstable, trauma patients may tolerate very little anesthesia. Volatile agents may worsen hypotension. Ketamine or fentanyl may be used judiciously. At the very least, amnestic agents (scopolamine, benzodiazepines) should be administered.

Burns

Burn injuries in the United States claim the lives of 3000 children and disable 9000 others under the age of 15 each year. Because of the prolonged treatment process, intense pain and suffering, and potential for disfigurement, both children and their parents require special support and attention. The anesthesiologist has the expertise in fluid resuscitation, transfusion therapy, and pain management to assist in the ongoing management of these patients, as well as caring for them in their frequent trips to the operating room.

History

1. The history must include details of the burn injury, especially the amount of time elapsed since the burn and the type of burn.
2. In an electrical burn the extent of injury often is greater than seen externally.
3. A fire in an enclosed space raises the suspicion of smoke inhalation and suggests the need to check carboxyhemoglobin levels and perform bronchoscopy.
4. Evidence of associated injuries (cervical spine injury, fractures, internal organ injury) should be sought, as well as any pertinent data from the child's medical history.

Physical Examination

1. The physical examination should focus immediately on the airway. With head and neck burns, hoarseness and wheezing may indicate upper airway involvement. The presence of carbonaceous sputum suggests smoke inhalation injury.
2. The extent and depth of the burn should be documented to calculate fluid resuscitation (see Fig. 18-4 on the next page to calculate burn percentage).
3. Sites for potential vascular access should be identified.

Securing the Airway

1. If any airway compromise is anticipated the trachea should be intubated immediately. Airway edema following a major burn can be extremely rapid, distorting the anatomy.
2. If prolonged endotracheal intubation is anticipated, a nasal tube often is tolerated better.
3. The endotracheal tube must be secured without further compromise to the burned skin.
    a. Tape should be avoided.
    b. Circumferential ties should be observed and readjusted frequently to allow for swelling of the face and neck.
    c. The endotracheal tube may be sutured to the nasal septum or wired to a secure tooth.
    d. A bite block, soft but secure restraints, and adequate sedation are useful in preventing accidental extubation.

Fluid/Electrolyte/Blood Requirements

Fluid requirements are proportional to the extent and depth of the burn.

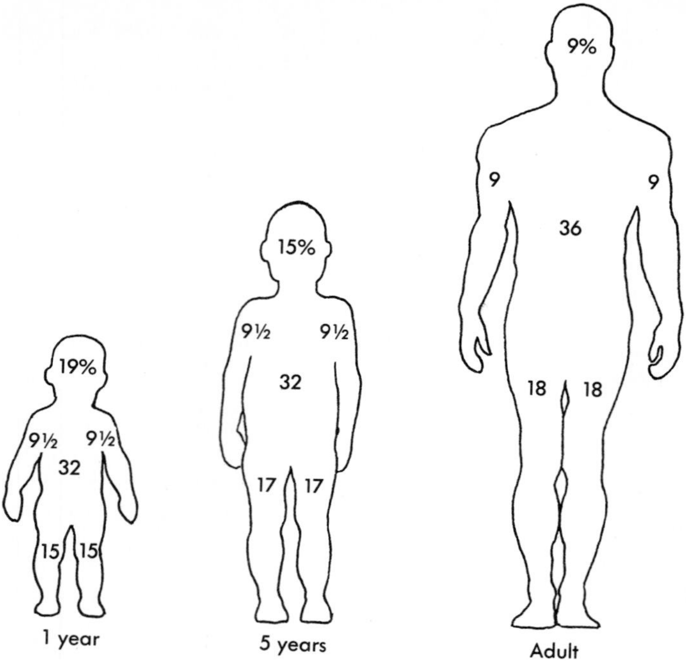

Fig. 18-4. The age of the patient must be considered when calculating the percent of body surface involved in a burn injury. (Adapted from Smith EI: Acute management of thermal burns in children, Surg Clin North Am 50:807-14, 1970.)

1. The Parkland formula for initial resuscitation:
   a. 4 ml/kg/% burn of Ringer's lactate in the first 24 hours.
   b. Half of the above in the first 8 hours (from time of injury).
2. Electrolytes, glucose, BUN and creatinine, hematocrit, platelet count, PT, and PTT must be checked frequently.
3. The best estimate of adequate volume replacement is urine output of at least 1.0 ml/kg/hr.
4. Appropriate amounts of blood and blood factors must be available before major debridement or grafting procedures.

Intravenous Access

Adequate IV access must be established for debridement and grafting procedures. In severely burned children, areas that escaped injury such as the axilla or web spaces of the digits may be used. A cutdown may be necessary, or even percutaneous placement of an IV through eschar, though this should be replaced as soon as possible to avoid infection. A central venous catheter is desirable to monitor CVP and replace large volumes. The surgeon may insert a large-bore cannula into the femoral vein and transfusions given with a bypass pump.

Monitoring

1. ECG leads can be wired onto the chest wall if the skin is burned, or an esophageal lead can be used.
2. Information from a pulse oximeter usually is extremely valuable; the probe is attached to the ear, the bridge of the nose, nasal alae, cheek, or even tongue. It is best to use an oximeter probe that is sterilizable (immersible) and can be applied without tape (Fig. 18-5 on pp. 450 and 451). Pulse oximeters generally measure the percentage of oxygenated hemoglobin present in the total of oxygenated and deoxygenated hemoglobin. If a large percentage of the total hemoglobin is carboxyhemoglobin, falsely elevated readings will be obtained. Cooximetry should be used to measure both oxyhemoglobin and carboxyhemoglobin in burn patients with inhalation injuries.
3. In major burn injuries an arterial catheter should be placed to facilitate blood pressure monitoring and to obtain laboratory data frequently.
4. Temperature must be monitored carefully, because burned children are extremely vulnerable to heat loss. A warm operating room, a heating blanket, warmed fluids, and warm humidified gases are essential for maintaining the child's temperature.

Anesthetic Agents

Choice of anesthetic agents depends upon the underlying condition of the patient, the extent of injury, and the surgery planned.

1. Succinylcholine administration should be avoided with the burn patient. From 5 days to 6 months following thermal injury, extrajunctional receptors develop on the skeletal muscle, causing a massive release of potassium when depolarized with succinylcholine.
2. Volatile agents may be used with caution in the postburn period. Cardiac output may be decreased by hypovolemia, and myocardial depression from anemia, sepsis, and increased metabolic demands. Further depression from a volatile agent may not be tolerated.
3. Ketamine may be used for acutely painful dressing changes. Narcotics and benzodiazepines are indicated for analgesia and sedation during the long, painful recovery process.

Poisoning and Overdose

1. Poisoning in childhood usually involves the accidental ingestion of toxic substances. Overdoses usually occur in adolescence from abuse of alcohol or drugs or from suicide attempts.
2. Problems encountered in these patients involve systemic toxicity, need for airway protection, and local skin and mucosal damage from a toxic substance.
3. The trachea should be intubated and ventilation assisted as necessary. The level of responsiveness must be ascertained before laryngoscopy to prevent aspiration. All equipment necessary for a rapid-sequence induction must be assembled before intubation. The patient should be preoxygenated, and cricoid pressure should be applied until the airway is secured.

A

B

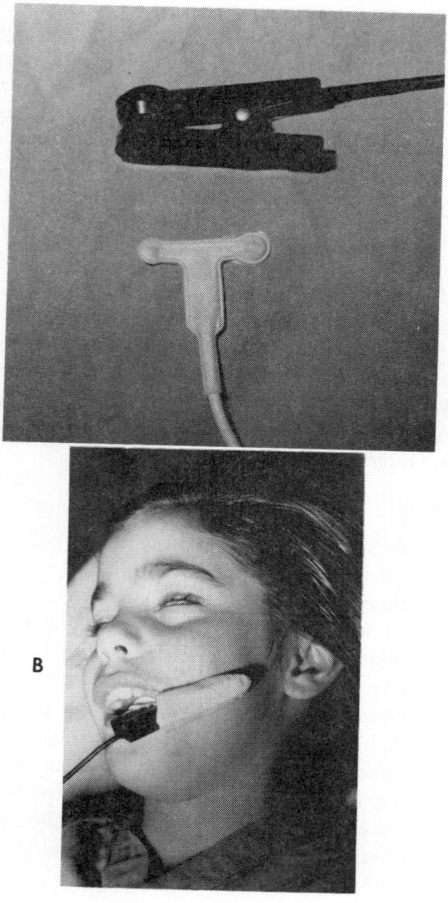

Fig. 18-5. The use of oximeter probes, which are immersible and/or can be sterilized, is particularly important for the pediatric burn patient or any patient with a loss of skin integrity. The ability to secure the probe without the use of adhesives is also advantageous. Probe 1 (Ohmeda) (**A,** *top*) is not immersible but can be rendered sterile by covering it with the finger cut from a sterile surgical glove (**B**). No adhesives are required for this spring-loaded clip model. The highly vascular cheek is an ideal location for oximetry in the patient with multiple trauma or burns. Probe 2 (Ohmeda) (**A,** *bottom*) may be completely sterilized by soaking in antibacterial solution. A flat piece of aluminum, removed from the nose of a surgical mask, can be placed between two pieces of adhesive dressing upon which the probe is mounted with double-stick tape (**C**). The probe can now be molded to the desired location, including the digits (**D**), ear helix (**E**), tongue, or nasal septum, without using adhesives.

C

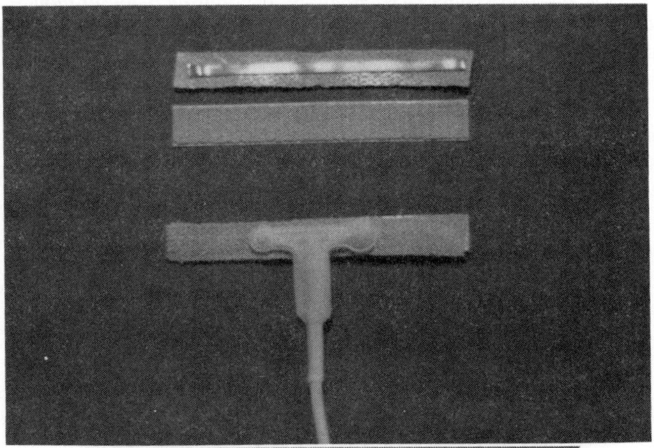

D

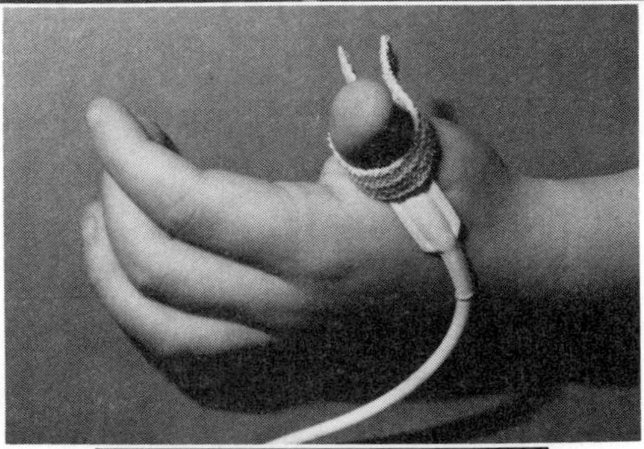

E

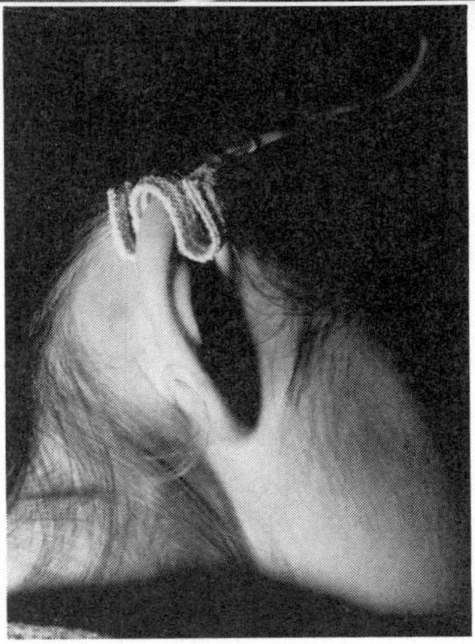

4. Ingestion of a corrosive substance can cause severe burns of the mouth, oropharynx, and esophagus. No attempt should be made to induce vomiting. The airway should be secured if there is any danger of decreased airway reflexes or edema from the mouth or oropharynx. The child may require intubation for endoscopy to evaluate the extent of the burn.
5. A thorough history should be elicited and a urine and serum drug screen performed if appropriate. The poison index or regional poison control center should be consulted to provide specific treatment of the child.
6. Systemic toxicity of poisons and drugs may manifest as cardiac, respiratory, neurologic, hepatic, or renal failure. Because of the anesthesiologist's knowledge of physiology and pharmacology, he or she may provide valuable assistance to the pediatrician in the treatment of poisoned and overdosed children.

BIBLIOGRAPHY

Dierdorf SF and Krishna G: Anesthetic management of neonatal surgical emergencies, Anesth Analg 60:209, 1981.

Duggan CP: Burns. In Greene MG, editor: The Harriet Lane Handbook: a manual for pediatric house officers, ed 12, St Louis, 1991, Mosby–Year Book.

Heiss K and others: Reversal of mortality for congenital diaphragmatic hernia with ECMO, Ann Surg 209(2):225-230, 1989.

Holl JW: Anesthesia for gastrointestional and abdominal wall disorders. In Gregory GA, editor: Pediatric anesthesia, ed 2, New York, 1989, Churchill Livingstone.

Steward DJ: Diseases of the gastrointestinal system. In Katz J and Steward DJ, editors: Anesthesia and uncommon pediatric diseases, Philadelphia, 1987, WB Saunders Co.

Striker TW: Anesthesia for trauma in the pediatric patient. In Gregory GA, editor: Pediatric anesthesia, ed 2, New York, 1989, Churchill Livingstone.

Szyfelbein SK and others, editors: Burns. In Ryan JF and others, editors: A practice of anesthesia for infants and children, Orlando, Fla, 1986, Grune & Stratton.

Todres ID and Berde CB: Pediatric emergencies. In Ryan JF and others, editors: A practice of anesthesia for infants and children, Orlando, Fla, 1986, Grune & Stratton.

Todres ID and Firestone S: Neonatal emergencies. In Ryan JF and others, editors: A practice of anesthesia for infants and children, Orlando, Fla, 1986, Grune & Stratton.

19

ANESTHESIA FOR PEDIATRIC TRANSPLANT SURGERY

A. Pamela Reichheld
Roberta H. Hines
Christine S. Rinder

Star light, star bright,
First star I've seen tonight,
Wish I may, wish I might
Have the wish I wish tonight.
ANON

RENAL TRANSPLANTATION

Infants with end stage renal disease (ESRD) exhibit severe growth retardation and neurologic deficits that cannot be mitigated by dialysis. Successful renal transplantation is usually followed by sustained catch-up growth, particularly in recipients less than 7 years of age.

Improved immunosuppression protocols and blood transfusion preceding transplantation have improved graft survival. If the recipient shares at least one HLA-DR antigen with the blood donor, the graft fares much better than it would if the HLA-DR antigens were mismatched or if no transfusion were given. (See Chapter 6.)

Causes of ESRD

- Children with ESRD and cessation of growth are candidates for renal transplantation. Common causes of ESRD that require transplantation and the potential for disease recurrence are listed in the box on p. 454.
- The pathophysiology shared by patients with ESRD is described in the box on p. 455.

CAUSES OF END STAGE RENAL DISEASE WITH THEIR POTENTIAL FOR RECURRENCE AFTER TRANSPLANTATION

High potential

Dense deposit disease
IgA nephropathy
Metabolic disorders: oxalosis

Moderate potential

Focal segmental glomerulosclerosis
Membranoproliferative glomerulonephritis (GN)
Crescent GN (idiopathic)
Membranous nephropathy
Interstitial nephritis

Low potential (rare)

Hereditary nephritis
Medullary cystic disease
Alport's syndrome
Primary reflux pyelonephritis
Posterior urethral valves (often require undiversion of previously diverted urinary tract to allow the urethra and bladder the capability of effective storage and voiding; otherwise prognosis is made worse by reduced bladder compliance)
Wilm's tumor (requires 1-year period after resection and chemotherapy without recurrence before transplantation can be considered)
Metabolic disorders:
Cystinosis
Diabetes mellitus

No potential

Renal hypoplasia/dysplasia

Pharmacology in Patients With ESRD

See Table 19-1 on pp. 456 and 457.

1. The loading dose of a drug is similar for patients with or without ESRD. Digitalis is an exception by virtue of its decreased capacity to bind to myocardial receptors in the presence of uremia. The patient with ESRD should receive two thirds of the normal digitalis loading dose.
2. Drugs that rely on renal clearance display a prolonged $T_{1/2}$, including diazepam, pancuronium, gallamine, metocurine, and normeperidine (the metabolic product of meperidine that causes CNS stimulation).
3. Drugs that normally bind to albumin have less affinity for albumin. In the nephrotic syndrome, less albumin is available with which to bind, resulting in more circulating free drug (e.g., diazepam, morphine sulfate, thiopental).
4. Chronic anemia alters the blood-brain barrier for inhalation anesthetics.
5. Inhalation anesthetics are useful in both controlling blood pressure and potentiating muscle relaxation. In addition, their elimination is rapid and predictable.

PATHOPHYSIOLOGY OF END STAGE RENAL DISEASE (ESRD)

Organ System	Effects of ESRD
Endocrine	Diminished growth Hyperparathyroidism Diabetes
Neurologic	Depression Psychosis Peripheral neuropathy Delayed development
Cardiac	Hypertension Left ventricular hypertrophy Heart failure Volume overload Pericarditis High output failure caused by dialysis fistulas
Pulmonary	Pulmonary edema due to volume overload
Gastrointestinal	Anorexia Nausea Vomiting Delayed gastric emptying
Hematopoietic	Anemia Hemolysis Decrease in platelet number and function
Renal	Unpredictable intravascular volume Nephrotic syndrome with decreased serum albumin Uremia Metabolic acidosis Increased serum potassium and magnesium Decreased serum calcium levels
Musculoskeletal	Osteomalacia Osteosclerosis Osteoporosis Osteitis fibrosa cystica Aluminum and magnesium toxicity Hypophosphatemia
Infectious	Chronic hepatitis B surface antigen from dialysis

TABLE 19-1. Implications of ESRD for anesthesia pharmacology

Drugs	Effects of ESRD
Neuromuscular blockers	• Blockade may be potentiated by: 1. Acidosis 2. Increased serum magnesium 3. Hypocalcemia 4. Hyponatremia 5. Mycin antibiotics • Usual doses of atropine and neostigmine, edrophonium, or pyridostigmine can be used for reversal.
Succinylcholine	• If serum potassium is greater than 5.5 mmol/L, use of succinylcholine is prohibited because potential exists for hyperkalemia.
Pancuronium, d-tubocurare	• $T_{1/2}$ increased up to 500%. • The same initial loading dose (Pancuronium 0.1 mg/kg, d-tubocurare 0.5 mg/kg) is needed to produce intubating conditions. • Interval dosing requires adjustment to avoid prolonged relaxation.
Vecuronium	• Normally 10% to 25% excreted in urine, the remainder in bile. • Accumulation can occur as $T_{1/2}$ is increased about 30% in patients with ESRD. • Interval dosing should be titrated to twitch response.
Atracurium	• Essentially unaffected by hepatorenal function. • No cumulative effect with dosing.
Intravascular agents	
Thiopental	• Induction dose is unchanged. • Twice as much thiopental exists in the unbound state in patients with ESRD. • An increased volume of distribution and increased clearance cause no change in $T_{1/2}$.
Midazolam	• Primarily metabolized by the liver. • No change in clearance or $T_{1/2}$ of a single dose.
Etomidate, fentanyl, alfentanil	• Short acting, with minimal change in duration caused by ESRD.
Inhalation anesthetics	
Enflurane	• Metabolized to fluoride, which is nephrotoxic and relies on glomerular filtration for elimination.

TABLE 19-1. Implications of ESRD for anesthesia pharmacology—cont'd

Drugs	Effects of ESRD
Halothane	• Metabolized to fluoride but to a much lesser extent than enflurane. • May cause myocardial depression and subsequent hypotension, which decreases glomerular filtration rate.
Isoflurane	• No known renal side effects and therefore useful for anesthetic maintenance.

Graft Selection

1. Renal transplantations have been performed in children as young as 7 months.
2. Living related-donor grafts have been more successful than cadaveric grafts in infants and young children. It is generally held that cadaveric transplants should not be performed in children under 1 year of age because of the enhanced immune responsiveness seen in the uremic child.
3. The living related donor should be ABO and HLA-A, B, and C compatible.
4. The cadaveric donor should be ABO and HLA-DR compatible.
5. A high rate of primary nonfunction accompanies grafts from anencephalic donors.
6. Grafts from donors under 6 years old often yield suboptimal results.

Pretransplant Nephrectomy

1. Preservation of the native kidney is preferred, because it facilitates erythropoietin and vitamin D production.
2. Nephrectomy preceding transplantation is indicated for the following conditions:
   - Renal malignancy
   - Ureterovesical reflux
   - Goodpasture's syndrome
   - Severe hypertension
   - Massive proteinuria
   - Hydronephrosis

Harvesting and Preservation

1. The left kidney is preferred to the right because of its longer renal vein.
2. The operations on the living related donor and the recipient are performed simultaneously. The donor is generously hydrated and diuresis is forced, after which the kidney is removed, immersed in ice, and flushed with cold electrolyte solution.
3. The cadaver is heparinized before kidney removal en bloc, with attachments to the aorta and vena cava. It is kept cold with iced saline and perfused with a preservation solution; commonly used solutions are listed in Table 19-3 on p. 465.

Surgical Procedures

1. Pediatric donors are preferable for recipients under 10 kg, although an infant weighing 5 to 6 kg can accommodate an adult kidney placed transabdominally.
2. With patients weighing less than 15 kg, the renal artery and vein are anastomosed to the aorta and vena cava respectively. This technique, referred to as the transperitoneal approach, carries an increased risk of small bowel obstruction.
3. With the larger patient, the renal artery and vein are anastomosed to the common iliac vessels extraperitoneally, in the pelvis.
4. The donor ureter is anastomosed to the native ureter whenever possible, or to the bladder using an antireflux technique.
5. Institutions vary in their immunosuppressive protocol. The most frequently used drugs are prednisone, methylprednisolone, cyclosporin-A, azathioprine, and antilymphoblast globulin.

Anesthetic Management

Preoperative Evaluation

In addition to the usual pediatric anesthesia evaluation (see Chapter 3), special attention should be paid to the following:

- Primary renal disease.
- Review of systems, noting pathology associated with ESRD.
- Whether patient is dialyzed, and if so, how often, any complications, pre- and postdialysis weights, highest BUN and creatinine levels, and date of last dialysis.
- Recent BUN, creatinine, electrolytes, glucose, and hematocrit.
- Dialysis sight location and function (presence of shunts or fistulas).
- Current medications (e.g., antihypertensives and steroids). Perioperative stress steroid coverage may be needed.
- Previous transfusions and hepatitis profile.
- Availability of blood for intraoperative transfusion.
- ECG and chest X-ray results.
- Physical assessment of hydration.

Monitoring and Equipment

Routine monitors

- ECG
- Temperature probe
- Blood pressure (BP) cuff
- Oximetry
- Capnography
- Gas humidifier and warmer

Monitors and equipment of particular importance in renal transplantation.

- Foley catheter—Even if the patient is anuric preoperatively, measurement of urine output will be necessary soon after unclamping.
- Large-bore intravenous access and blood warmers. Permanent vascular shunts should be protected and IV access avoided in that extremity.
- Intraarterial catheter is useful for taking blood samples from the very ill patient and for hemodynamic monitoring in either the very small patient or the poorly controlled hypertensive.

- Central venous pressure (CVP) monitoring may be critical. After unclamping, a large percentage of cardiac output will be directed to the transplanted kidney. This percentage will increase if a child receives an adult kidney. Raising the CVP just before unclamping will prevent hypotension and hypoperfusion to the new organ. Some institutions avoid inserting CVP catheters because of the added risk of sepsis.
- Special care should be taken in the use of forearm veins and arteries because they may be needed for future shunts or fistulas.
- Pulmonary inflation pressures (peak inspiratory pressure) require close monitoring. Use of large ring abdominal retractors and bowel packs under the diaphragm will raise intrathoracic pressure and falsely elevate CVP. This may convince the anesthesiologist that intravascular volume is actually sufficient for unclamping, and marked hypotension may result.

Induction and Maintenance of Anesthesia

1. Strict asepsis is necessary to protect the immunosuppressed patient. Also, operating room personnel should take appropriate precautions against becoming infected, because many dialysis patients carry hepatitis virus.
2. Sodium thiopental or etomidate may be used in their usual doses for induction of anesthesia in patients with ESRD. Preoxygenation is beneficial in those with anemia. A rapid-sequence induction with preoxygenation is often indicated because of decreased gastric emptying time and/or urgent surgery.
3. Succinylcholine is acceptable if potassium is less than 5.5 mEq/L with ECG monitoring. Because of minimal requirements for renal excretion, atracurium or vecuronium are recommended for muscle relaxation. However, pancuronium can be used in a single dose to last the duration of the procedure. Use of a neuromuscular blockade monitor is required for repeat dosing or for assessing the efficacy of reversal.
4. If there is no vascular access and the risk of aspiration is deemed minimal, an inhalation induction with halothane or isoflurane is acceptable. Because the inhalation anesthetics and nitrous oxide (N_2O) are rapidly eliminated, they are preferred to an intravenous technique for maintenance of anesthesia. If bowel distension is present, N_2O should be avoided.
5. The patient is ventilated to maintain normocapnia with 30% to 50% oxygen.
   - Hyperventilation results in a shift of the oxyhemoglobin curve to the left with decreased oxygen availability, and hypocapnia decreases renal perfusion.
   - Hypoventilation increases $PaCO_2$ and further increases intravascular potassium.
6. Once anesthetized, the patient is positioned so that fistula sites are protected. Function of fistula sites should be rechecked frequently during the procedure.

Intraoperative Considerations

1. ''Bucking'' and coughing should be suppressed because they may compromise vascular anastomoses.
2. Room temperature should be maintained at 32° C and irrigation fluids and blood products warmed to 32° to 35°.

3. Intraoperative doses of immunosuppressive agents and antibiotics are administered according to protocol. These can be prepared preoperatively.
4. Electrolytes, glucose, pH, and oxygen tension are monitored frequently. Note that the perfusion solution is rinsed out of the donor kidney and replaced with cold lactated Ringer's before transplantation in order to prevent high serum potassium concentrations.
5. Blood pressure, CVP, venous PO_2, and urine output are monitored to assess volume status and replaced with warmed crystalloid or blood as needed.
6. Before releasing the vascular clamps, the CVP should be raised with crystalloid to 12 to 16 cm H_2O to prevent hypotension with ischemic injury to the kidney and/or vascular thrombosis. A higher CVP may be needed if false elevations exist because of abdominal retractors or packs.
7. Furosemide (1 mg/kg) may be given before clamp release to improve urine output. Ischemic injury may be attenuated by furosemide's inhibition of cell transport activity.
8. Mannitol (125 to 200 mg/kg) given before clamp release increases plasma volume, filling pressures, and cardiac output and decreases systemic vascular resistance. It is a renal vasodilator, has osmotic action in the tubules, and slightly increases plasma potassium.
9. Acidosis may be prevented with bicarbonate (1 mEq/kg) before unclamping.
10. Vascular clamps are released slowly. After unclamping, a fall in CVP with resultant hypotension is due to the following factors:
    - Up to 300 ml of blood can be sequestered in an adult kidney when perfused. If the infant's blood volume is 80 ml/kg, the 10-kg infant will have a fall in CVP of 3 to 7 cm H_2O.
    - When the kidney begins to function, CVP falls as urine output increases. Urine should be replaced ml for ml with crystalloid.
    - Third space fluid loss will need replacement.
    - Blood loss should be replaced with red cells because these patients are anemic, maintaining a hematocrit of 24% to 25%.
    - Hypertension is rarely seen after unclamping but should be treated with inhalation anesthetics or antihypertensives if it should occur.
    - Fluid overload in young children can cause congestive heart failure and pulmonary edema.
11. After surgery, neuromuscular blockade is reversed with standard doses of reversal agents. Prolonged ventilation is not usually needed except in situations of residual muscle relaxation or inadequate oxygenation/ventilation. Rarely, a large kidney placed in a small child compromises pulmonary function in the immediate postoperative period and necessitates gradual weaning from mechanical ventilation.

Postoperative Management

1. The hourly urine output in the postoperative period may exceed the estimated blood volume. This is replaced at 15-minute intervals with 2.5% dextrose 0.45% NaCl.

2. Insensible loss is managed with 5% or 10% dextrose in water at 500 ml/M^2/day.
3. Levels of serum sodium, potassium, chloride, bicarbonate, and glucose are measured every 2 to 4 hours.
4. Serum calcium, magnesium, and phosphorous should be checked every 8 to 12 hours.
5. Urine glucose is checked hourly.
6. CVP should be monitored as an additional indication of volume status.

Complications of Transplantation

Complications may occur acutely in the postoperative period or after initial recovery has taken place (see box below). *Rejection* can occur at any time.

1. The diagnosis of rejection is made by the following:
   - Increase in serum creatinine, which may be subtle in small children who have received large kidneys

COMPLICATIONS OF RENAL TRANSPLANT

Acute complications of renal transplant in the immediate postoperative period

Hypertension
Hypotension
Pulmonary edema
Congestive heart failure
Hyperkalemia
Hypocalcemia
Arrhythmias, cardiac arrest
Coagulation defects
Bleeding
Urine or lymph leakage
Infection, sepsis
Acute graft loss

Late complications of renal transplant

Graft loss
- Acute tubular necrosis
- Rejection
- Vascular thrombosis (more common in small children who receive cadaveric transplants)

Small bowel obstruction
Pancreatitis
Cyclosporine toxicity
Side effects of steroid therapy
- Decrease in growth rate
- Aseptic necrosis
- Gastric ulcers
- Cataracts
- Infection
- Malignancies

- Fever
- Graft tenderness
- Irritability
- Renal ultrasound, with or without biopsy

2. An increase in immunosuppression may successfully treat the rejection episode. If treatment is not successful, the nonfunctioning organ must be removed.

PEDIATRIC LIVER TRANSPLANTATION

Liver transplantation has been performed in children as young as 3 months of age. Selection of candidates for liver transplantation is based primarily on the anticipated clinical course of the underlying disease process. Patients who undergo liver transplantation before hepatic failure possess greater physiologic reserve and a greater chance for survival.

Indications for Liver Transplantation

Congenital biliary atresia is the condition that most frequently necessitates liver transplantation in children. Most patients have undergone Kasai procedure (hepatic portoenterostomy) and may have multiple intraabdominal adhesions. Surgical dissection is more difficult as a result, requiring a lengthier procedure and necessitating greater red cell transfusion. The box "Indications for Liver Transplantation" lists other disease processes that may require liver transplantation. Regardless of the underlying disease process, patients with endstage liver disease share a characteristic pathophysiology (Table 19-2).

INDICATIONS FOR LIVER TRANSPLANTATION

Congenital biliary atresia
Inborn errors of metabolism
- Tyrosinemia
- α_1 antitrypsin deficiency
- Neonatal hemochromatosis
- Wilson's disease
- Glycogen storage disease
- Familial hypercholesterolemia
- Crigler-Najjar syndrome type I (absence of bilirubin UDP-glucuronyl transferase)

Intrahepatic cholestasis
- Byler's disease
- Alagille's syndrome

Hepatitis
- Infectious, neonatal, toxin or drug induced

Congenital hepatic fibrosis
Postnecrotic cirrhosis
Primary biliary cirrhosis
Budd-Chiari syndrome
Sclerosing cholangitis
Malignancy
Failed liver transplant

TABLE 19-2. Pathophysiology of end stage hepatic disease

Clinical conditions	Pathologic manifestations
Coagulopathy	• Increased protime (PT) and partial thromboplastin time (PTT), thrombocytopenia • Disseminated intravascular coagulation (DIC) • Diminished hepatic synthesis of factors I, II, V, VII, IX, X • Dysfibrinogenemia • Fibrinolysis • Increased levels of fibrinogen and factor VIII
Anemia	• Decreased red cell production as a result of chronic disease, renal failure, malnutrition • Variceal bleeding
Cardiovascular changes	• Hyperdynamic circulation • Decreased peripheral vascular resistance and increased cardiac output from vasoactive polypeptides and large portosystemic shunt • Increased intraabdominal pressure from ascites impeding venous return • Increased SVO_2 and decreased A-V O_2 difference from A-V shunting • Cardiomyopathy • Decreased sensitivity to catecholamines
Hypoxemia	• Clubbing and cyanosis • Restrictive defect from ascites • Increased alveolar-arterial O_2 difference from pulmonary A-V shunting • Right-to-left shunts with increased risk of air emboli • Decreased pulmonary diffusing capacity
Renal failure	• Increased renin, ADH, angiotensin, aldosterone • Decreased effective plasma volume • Hepatorenal syndrome with sodium retention • Acute tubular necrosis (ATN)
Encephalopathy	• Increased blood ammonia • Cerebral edema
Glucose	• Decreased stores of glucose and glycogen • Insulin resistance • Hypoglycemia
Electrolyte disorders	• Hyponatremia • Hypokalemia • Hyperphosphatemia • Hypocalcemia • Hypomagnesemia • Alkalosis or acidosis
Prior abdominal surgery	• Increase in red cell transfusion because of more difficult dissection

Continued.

TABLE 19-2. Pathophysiology of end stage hepatic disease—cont'd

Clinical conditions	Pathologic manifestations
• Increased infection rate • Adhesions are not a problem in retransplants occurring within 2 to 4 weeks	
Changes in pharmacokinetics	• Decreased protein binding • Increased volume of distribution • Decreased hepatic blood flow and hepatic enzyme activity resulting in decreased clearance and increased half-life of drugs dependent on liver metabolism

General Preoperative Preparation

Three aspects of liver transplant surgery warrant special consideration:

1. Timing of the procedure—With new methods of preservation, the donor liver can be safely preserved for up to 24 hours. A favorable prognosis necessitates coordination of the harvesting team and surgical transplant team with anesthetic, nursing, perfusion, blood bank, and laboratory personnel.
2. Aseptic technique must be scrupulously followed because these patients are immunosuppressed.
3. The anesthesia staff on hand should consist of at least one staff anesthesiologist and two experienced nurse anesthetists or residents, because the procedure can be lengthy and complicated.

Surgical Management

1. The donor liver must be matched with the recipient for ABO compatibility and for size in order to fit in the hepatic cavity.
2. Hypothermia is the most important technique for successful organ preservation. Hypothermic cell swelling is inhibited with organ preservation solutions which contain impermeant substances. University of Wisconsin (UW) solution contains raffinose and lactobionate anion to suppress cell swelling. The UW solution allows for preservation times of up to 24 hours with good transplant results. Note that the potassium concentration in the UW solution is 125 mM/L (see Table 19-3). Therefore, on reperfusion of the new liver, acute symptomatic hyperkalemia may occur.
3. The actual surgical procedure is divided into three phases: preanhepatic, anhepatic and reperfusion, and postreperfusion (see Table 19-4 on p. 466).

Anesthetic Management

Preoperative Evaluation and Preparation

1. A preoperative assessment should be made with an emphasis on recent history; present medications; cardiac, pulmonary, renal, and coagulation status; previous operations; allergies; and last oral intake.
2. Recent laboratory data, ECG, chest X-ray, height, and weight should be noted.

TABLE 19-3. Characteristics and constituents of preservation solutions for donor organs

	EC*	UW*	UM3*
Anions			
Bicarbonate (mM/L)	10	—	—
Chloride (mM/L)	15	—	5
Lactate (mM/L)	—	—	—
Phosphate (mM/L)	57.5	25	0.72
Lactobionate (mM/L)	—	100	90
Cations			
Calcium (mM/L)	—	—	0.6-1.4
Sodium (mM/L)	10	30	1
Potassium (mM/L)	115	120	124
Magnesium (mM/L)	—	5	7.8
Colloids and osmotically active agents			
Hydroxyethyl starch (gm/L)	—	50	—
Proteins (gm/L)	—	—	65
Mannitol (gm/L)	—	—	—
Raffinose (gm/L)	—	17.8	48
Glucose (gm/L)	194	—	99
Others			
Adenosine (gm/L)	—	1.34	—
Glutathione (gm/L)	—	0.922	—
Insulin (units)	—	100	—
Allopurinol (gm/L)	—	0.136	—
Antibiotics and steroids			
Ampicillin (mg)	—	—	50
Sulfamethoxazole (mg)	—	40	—
Trimethoprim (mg)	—	8	—
Dexamethasone (mg)	—	8	—
Methyl prednisolone (mg)	—	—	500
Osmolality (mOsm/L)	375	320	301
pH	7.4	7.4	7.4

Adapted from Todo S and others: Clin Transplant 3:253-59, 1989.
*EC, Euro-Collins; UW, University of Wisconsin; UM3, University of Minnesota III.

3. The patient should be examined and venous access evaluated.
4. The patient and/or family should already have been well prepared during the selection process and made aware of the procedural risks involved. The visit should enable the anesthesiologist to meet the patient and family, review anesthetic implications, and answer remaining questions.
5. As soon as the operation is scheduled, oral intake ceases except for necessary preoperative medications.
6. Premedication is dependent on the mental and physical status of the patient. Agents to relieve anxiety and pain should be employed. If the patient does not have a coagulopathy, intramuscular injections may be given. Alternatively, intravenous medication can be titrated to effect under supervision in the operative area.

TABLE 19-4. Stages of liver transplantation

Stages	Surgical procedures	Anticipated sequelae
I Preanhepatic	1. Bilateral subcostal T-incision 2. Liver freed to its vascular pedicle 3. Veno-venous bypass (patients > 20 kg) by cannulating and draining portal/femoral veins into axillary vein 4. Preparation of donor homograft	• Hypotension due to surgical bleeding or drainage of ascites • Arrhythmias from diaphragmatic irritation • Hypothermia from massive fluid exchanges, use of veno-venous bypass, evaporative loss
II Anhepatic and reperfusion	1. Diseased organ's vessels are clamped and bile duct transsected 2. Vascular anastomoses: a. suprahepatic IVC b. infrahepatic IVC and portal vein after completely flushing perfusate 3. Liver perfused by unclamping supra- and infrahepatic IVC and portal vein 4. Hepatic artery anastomosed (may require aortic cross-clamp in small children)	• Reduced renal perfusion from cross-clamping • Cardiovascular changes after reperfusion: - Hypotension - Arrhythmias (bradycardia or tachycardia, heart block, arrest) - Decreased SVR - Cardiac decompensation - Pulmonary edema • Hypoxemia from diaphragmatic retraction, emboli, pulmonary edema • Hyperkalemia after reperfusion • Hypothermia • Hypoglycemia
III Postreperfusion	1. Hemostasis 2. Biliary anastomosis—duct to duct or roux en y—choledochojejunostomy 3. Intraoperative cholangiogram to check patency 4. Incision closure	• Worsened coagulopathy from massive transfusion • Hypotension due to histamine release by OKT3, PGE_1, bleeding, hyperacute rejection, DIC, shock, anaphylaxis • Refractory hypertension (nitroprusside toxicity may occur because of inadequate rhodanase in the new liver to clear cyanide) • Respiratory insufficiency caused by large donor liver after incision closure • Persistent myocardial depression from lowered calcium levels, hypotension, acidosis, etc.

7. The blood bank and laboratory personnel should be notified as soon as the procedure is scheduled. A minimum of 10 to 20 units of packed red blood cells (PRBC), 10 to 20 units of fresh frozen plasma (FFP), and 10 units of platelets should be made ready for the operating room before the patient is incised. Frequent requests to the hematology and chemistry laboratories will be made, with the results needed by the anesthesia team as rapidly as possible.
8. There should be continuous communication with the harvesting team to allow prediction of a starting time. Approximately 1 to 2 hours will be needed for induction and catheter insertions before the incision.

Monitoring and Equipment

Routine

- Air and oxygen supply
- Suction
- Anesthesia machine with appropriate pediatric circuit and ventilator
- Appropriate endotracheal tube (ETT) and airway equipment, including PEEP valves
- ECG
- Blood pressure cuff
- Precordial and esophageal stethoscope
- Oxygen saturation monitor
- Neuromuscular blockade monitor
- Padding for pressure points and plastic wrap for extremities

Special

- Heated humidifier
- End-tidal CO_2 monitor
- Mass spectrometer for nitrogen detection
- Transducers for two or three pressure lines, and monitors
- Cardiac output machine if indicated
- Four large-bore intravenous catheters, arterial catheter, and central venous or pulmonary artery catheters
- Four volume lines primed with Normosol or Plasmalyte solution, all connected to blood warmers
- Two to four drug infusion pumps
- Nasogastric tube
- Warming blanket
- Pediatric tubes for blood sampling and heparinized syringes for blood gases (labeled with patient's name and hospital number)
- Flow sheets to record laboratory values and amount and type of volume replacement
- Rapid transfusion device. This device is used for rapid volume replacement in larger patients. It consists of a 3-L reservoir, large blood filters, heat exchanger, roller pump, and bubble detector (which will shut off the pump if air is detected). The unit is connected to the patient via one or two large-bore (i.e., 8.5 French) catheters to provide flows of 800 ml/min. The standard solution in the reservoir is 2 units of PRBC, 2 units of FFP, and up to 500 ml of crystalloid with a resultant hematocrit of 28% to 30%.

No bicarbonate or heparin is needed. Separate access must be used for cryoprecipitate and platelet infusion.

- Cell saver. The cell saver is not often used because of the potential for bowel contamination. Also, the small size of the patient may lead to inadequate volume production. If the cell saver is used, 1 unit of processed red blood cells can be substituted for 1 unit of packed red blood cells either in the rapid transfusion device or through a peripheral line.

Drugs

The drugs listed in the box below should be readily available to the anesthesia team.

DRUGS FOR LIVER TRANSPLANTATION

Induction agents

Thiopental, ketamine

Muscle relaxants

Succinylcholine, pancuronium, atracurium

Narcotics

Fentanyl, morphine

Benzodiazepines

Diazepam, midazolam

Resuscitative drugs

Bolus—atropine, calcium chloride, epinephrine, sodium bicarbonate, lidocaine, phenylephrine
Infusions—dopamine, epinephrine

Vasodilators

Nitroprusside, nitroglycerine

Special

Potassium
Furosemide
Mannitol
Insulin
D_{50}
Epsilon aminocaproic acid
Vasopressin
Antibiotics according to protocol
Immunosuppressants according to protocol

Anesthetic Induction and Vascular Access

Intravenous inductions are common in children because IV access is usually in place for the purpose of preoperative medication.

1. Before induction, the room temperature should be increased, and

the usual ECG, BP cuff, precordial stethoscope, and pulse oximeter applied.

2. A rapid-sequence induction with either thiopental or ketamine is used when food or cyclosporine has been recently ingested, or in the presence of a distended abdomen.
3. Awake intubation may be required in small infants or in the presence of a difficult airway.
4. If a rapid-sequence induction is not required, either intravenous or inhalation agents may be used.
   a. Halothane may be used for inhalation induction because it precipitates less airway reactivity. Its potential for hepatoxicity should preclude its use for maintenance of anesthesia.
   b. Enflurane results in increased fluoride concentrations during long procedures and should be avoided.
   c. Isoflurane is preferred to both halothane and enflurane because it requires minimal hepatic metabolism.
5. After induction and initiation of mechanical ventilation with heated humidification, the following are placed:
   a. Esophageal stethoscope, rectal or esophageal temperature probe, urinary catheter, nasogastric tube (nasal trauma may precipitate epistaxis in the presence of coagulopathy)
   b. Two to four large-bore intravenous catheters in the upper extremities or the jugular veins (one jugular vein is needed for central venous access)
   c. Central venous pressure catheter through an internal or external jugular vein or a pulmonary artery catheter in larger patients
   d. Intraarterial catheter, preferably placed in a radial artery because the aorta may be cross-clamped during the hepatic artery anastomosis
6. If the rapid-transfusion device is to be used, two 8.5 French catheters should be inserted into central and/or antecubital veins, connected to three-way stopcocks and then directly to the transfusion tubing.
7. In this case, all other venous and arterial catheters are placed in the right upper extremity. The left axillary vein is usually cannulated for veno-venous bypass.
8. In the presence of veno-venous bypass or clamping of the IVC, intravenous catheters should not be placed in the lower extremities.
9. Preparations for the prevention of hypothermia should be made early in the procedure; that is, warming all fluids and inspired gases, maintaining room temperature, and using the warming blanket.
10. Extremities should be padded and wrapped in cellophane to prevent heat loss and pressure necrosis. The head should also be wrapped and the eyes protected.

Maintenance of Anesthesia

1. Anesthesia is maintained either by inhalation agents (isoflurane) or by using a narcotic/amnesic technique (fentanyl or morphine and a benzodiazepine).

2. Decreased clearance and increased half-life of morphine sulfate may or may not be manifested in these patients because of the continual replacement of intravascular volume.
3. No significant change occurs in the pharmacokinetics of fentanyl in patients with cirrhosis.
4. Nitrous oxide should be avoided because it causes bowel dilatation, which adds to the technical difficulties of the surgical procedure. Additionally, the risk of air embolism is always present.
5. Muscle relaxation is achieved with pancuronium or atracurium.
   a. Use of a neuromuscular blockade monitor is crucial for the continual assessment of muscle relaxation.
   b. In patients with liver failure, pancuronium has a greater volume of distribution and half-life, and decreased clearance.
   c. Atracurium may show a decreased response because of increased binding to globulin.
6. Laboratory data are procured hourly.
   a. Equipment to perform the following determinations should be available in the operating room for rapid analysis:
      - Arterial blood gases
      - Hemoglobin
      - Sodium
      - Potassium
      - Ionized calcium
   b. Access to the following laboratory values should be available in 30 to 45 minutes:
      - Glucose
      - Platelet count
      - Prothrombin time
      - Partial thromboplastin time
      - Fibrinogen
   c. A thromboelastograph of whole blood may be used to diagnose coagulopathies.

Intraoperative Anesthetic Management

The anesthetic management of these patients often becomes a form of organized resuscitation. Many of the complications are ongoing: others are associated with a specific stage of the surgical procedure.

Blood loss

1. Preoperative coagulopathy, portal hypertension, and previous abdominal surgery will increase the volume of blood loss. Replacement of as much as ½ to 25 blood volumes may be required.
2. Replacement of blood products and fluids requires constant assessment of numerous patient variables. These include coagulation status, hematocrit, blood pressure, filling pressures, cardiac output, and urine output.
3. Filtered and warmed packed red blood cells and fresh frozen plasma are administered in a 1:1 ratio by either rapid transfusion device or large-bore IV catheters to maintain a hematocrit of 30% to 35%.
4. Separate lines are used to administer platelets and cryoprecipitate.

Coagulopathy

1. Etiologies:
   - Initial depletion of coagulation factors and thrombocytopenia
   - Dilutional coagulopathy
   - Primary fibrinolysis
   - Disseminated intravascular coagulation (DIC) along with secondary fibrinolysis
   - Activity from heparin given during donor organ harvesting
2. Treatment:
   - Replacement therapy should be initiated at the start of the surgical procedure. The goal is to keep the platelet count greater than 100,000 mm^3 and to normalize the PT and PTT: ⅔ units of platelets and 1 unit of FFP to 1 unit of packed red cells is the replacement ratio usually required. Cryoprecipitate is used for low fibrinogen levels.
   - Although rare, if severe fibrinolysis should occur as demonstrated by thromboelastogram, epsilon aminocaproic acid (20 mg/kg IV) should be given. Inappropriate use, however, can result in lethal thrombosis.
   - If present, heparin activity may be reversed by the titration of protamine.
   - The use of vasopressin (0.1 U/min IV infusion) may decrease portal hypertension and hence bleeding.
3. Normalization:
   The coagulation status should begin to normalize after perfusion of the new liver with a combination of replacement therapy, restoration of physiologic variables, and pharmacologic treatment.

Citrate intoxication

1. Citrate intoxication, a result of massive blood transfusion in patients with liver disease, is potentiated by hypothermia. A low ionized calcium is the result, and is manifested by a prolonged QT interval, A-V dissociation, myocardial depression, hypotension, and asystole.
2. Treatment is based on measured ionized calcium levels and consists of calcium chloride IV bolus (10 to 20 mg/kg) or infusion (approximately 10 mg/kg/hr). Calcium chloride should be given through a central catheter. (Calcium gluconate is not used because it is metabolized by the liver.) Increased citrate levels resolve with reperfusion of the new liver.

Potassium

1. Unless symptomatic, hypokalemia should not be treated before reperfusion of the donor liver. Although the liver is flushed before reperfusion to remove the potassium-rich preservation solution, acute hyperkalemia is always anticipated (7 to 11 mEq/L), and the occurrence of a cardiac arrest is possible.
2. Treatment should consist of glucose, insulin, and bicarbonate (see Table 6-4 on p. 103), and if necessary, CPR. After reperfusion of the new liver, it will begin to take up potassium. Low levels of potassium at this time may necessitate replacement.

Glucose

1. Glucose levels remain normal or high during retransplantation as a result of decreased use and the continuous infusion of blood products (1 unit packed red cells contains 0.5 g of glucose).

2. Levels should be checked often, although glucose infusions are rarely required.
3. Hyperglycemia is insulin resistant during the anhepatic phase and should not be treated until the new liver is functioning. The high glucose levels decrease spontaneously after revascularization as the new liver begins effective metabolism. Osmotic diuresis from hyperglycemia should not be mistaken for adequate intravascular volume or cardiac output.

Acid-base balance

1. Before revascularization, mild metabolic acidosis increases progressively. The conservative use of bicarbonate is recommended.
2. With reperfusion, metabolic alkalosis results from the metabolism of citrate to bicarbonate and furosemide-induced chloride loss. The alkalosis usually persists postoperatively and occasionally requires treatment.

Hypothermia. Methods to prevent hypothermia should be instituted early. Esophageal temperatures below 35.5° C are common. If necessary, radiant warmers can be used even if the surgical team must wait while rewarming is being effected.

Cardiovascular changes

Often an ongoing hemodynamic resuscitation is performed by the anesthesiologists during liver transplantation because of the occurrence of numerous physiologic and metabolic changes. Besides continuous blood loss, changes in ionized calcium, serum potassium, and pH, hypothermia, drainage of ascites, manipulation of major vessels, and/or compression of the diaphragm and heart can result in decreased venous return and hypotension during any stage of the procedure.

1. If veno-venous bypass is used (the patient must be large enough to maintain flows of 800 ml/min for thromboembolism to be avoided), it is easier to maintain preload to the heart and adequate cardiac output.
2. In smaller children, the inferior vena cava (IVC) is clamped, resulting in decreased preload, increased pressure of systemic venous and portal beds, and increased blood loss. Treatment should include increasing the preload, vasopressors, calcium chloride, and/or removal of the IVC clamps.
3. When partial hepatic circulation is reinstituted with the unclamping of the inferior vena cava and the portal vein, an increase in the volume of the intravascular beds should be anticipated. Transient hypotension may be attenuated by increasing preload. If hypotension persists, treatment with calcium chloride and dopamine are instituted. It is important to remember that the simultaneous occurrence of a large potassium flux during reperfusion can also depress cardiac output.

Air embolism

1. The likelihood of an air embolism occurring is increased by the use of veno-venous bypass and the presence of a large venous anastomosis. The preexisting right-to-left shunts increase the risk that these emboli will become systemic.
2. Embolization occurs most commonly during the anhepatic phase and reperfusion.
3. An index of suspicion, end tidal CO_2 and nitrogen, and pulmonary artery pressures are used to make the diagnosis.

4. A positive end-expiratory pressure of 5 cm H_2O and the avoidance of N_2O during the anhepatic phase are recommended.

Pulmonary changes

1. Hypoxemia from parenchymal disease, pulmonary arteriovenous shunting, and pleural effusions may exist preoperatively.
2. If possible, the oxygen concentration should be maintained below 50% to prevent further pulmonary damage from oxygen toxicity and atelectasis.
3. PEEP is useful if tolerated by the cardiovascular system.
4. PaO_2 and $PaCO_2$ are maintained within the normal range.
5. Pulmonary edema may occur with reperfusion of the donor liver and should be treated with PEEP, diuretics, and decreasing volume replacement.
6. The proximity of the surgical field makes pneumothorax a potential problem.
7. Abdominal closure may be impossible because of gut distention and a large donor liver, resulting in increased airway pressure and inadequate ventilation. In this situation, a temporary closure can be used.

Renal function

1. Low urine output at the start of the procedure is usually caused by hepatorenal syndrome or acute tubular necrosis. Most patients are anuric or oliguric during the anhepatic phase because of increased venous pressure in the renal beds. Urine output usually improves after revascularization.
2. In attempting to maintain urine output, dopamine (0.3 μg/kg/min) and furosemide (0.5-1 mg/kg) are used, and adequate intravascular volume is maintained.

Conclusion of surgery

1. Toward the end of surgery, with the restoration of physiologic variables and decreased surgical manipulation, the patient begins to stabilize. The new liver will begin to make bile 2 to 4 hours after reperfusion.
2. At the conclusion of the operation the patient is disconnected from the rapid-transfusion device, and the lines are flushed with heparinized saline.
3. Muscle relaxants are not reversed, and prolonged mechanical ventilation is anticipated.
4. The patient is transported to the intensive care unit with 100% O_2 and continuous monitoring.

Postoperative Considerations

1. Ideally, the ETT is removed as soon as possible, typically on the first, second, or third postoperative day. Patients who are either very young or severely malnourished require longer durations of assisted ventilation. The occurrence of large pleural effusions, pulmonary edema, lobar atelectasis, and occasionally ARDS necessitates appropriate treatment. Temporary paralysis of the right hemidiaphragm is a rare complication.
2. Hypertension is common in the pediatric group, often beginning intraoperatively and persisting for months. This problem does not appear to be related to pain or intravascular volume levels, but steroid treatment, cyclosporine, catecholamine levels, underlying renal dysfunction, and

hypomagnesemia have been implicated. If untreated, seizures, subarachnoid hemorrhage, and coma may result. Treatment should therefore be aggressive, employing sodium nitroprusside, hydralazine, diazoxide, β-blockers, clonidine, nifedipine, and/or captopril.

3. Hypotension is rare but may occur as a result of abdominal distention, hypovolemia, intraabdominal sepsis or acute hepatic necrosis.
4. The patient usually awakens on the first or second postoperative day as hypothermia resolves and the anesthetic agents dissipate.
   a. If recovery of neurological function appears to be slower than anticipated, patients with reversible metabolic encephalopathy or preoperative hepatic encephalopathy must be distinguished from those with irreversible cerebral edema.
   b. Postoperative seizures are not uncommon and may be due to hypoglycemia, hyponatremia, hypomagnesemia, hypocalcemia, hypertension, cerebral infection, intracranial hemorrhage or air embolism.
5. Adequate urine output should be maintained, although there is a wide range in acceptable postoperative renal function. It should be noted that cyclosporine is nephrotoxic and may require dosage adjustment.
6. Citrate metabolism, diuretic therapy, and nasogastric tube drainage contribute to metabolic alkalosis. A base excess of 10 mEq/L is common and generally tolerated. The patient should be weaned from mechanical ventilation according to pH, not $PaCO_2$.
7. Hypocalcemia, hypomagnesemia, hypokalemia, and hyperglycemia are common postoperatively and should be corrected.
8. The hematocrit should be maintained at a level of approximately 30%.
9. An elevated PT and PTT (up to 1.5 times normal) and platelet counts of 50,000/uL are common on arrival in the intensive care unit and should not be treated unless significant bleeding occurs. The PTT will normalize over a period of 24 to 72 hours, the PT in about 1 week, and the platelet count in a few days. Replacement therapy can be considered if the PT and PTT are greater than 1.5 times normal or the platelet count is less than 30,000/uL.
10. Parenteral or enteral alimentation is instituted early in the postoperative period.
11. Complications
    a. Serious problems include sepsis, rejection, and vascular compromise of the donor liver, and biliary tract dehiscence, leak, or obstruction. Intraabdominal sepsis or acute hepatic necrosis is characterized by fever, acidosis, abdominal tenderness, and hepatic dysfunction. Thrombocytopenia, hyperkalemia, and hypoglycemia are also seen with hepatic necrosis.
    b. More common in the pediatric population because of the small size of the vessels is thrombosis of the hepatic artery and the portal vein, resulting in rapid graft destruction. Rapid correction of coagulopathies is consequently avoided. Prophylactic therapy consists of hemodilution to a hematocrit level of about 30% and possible administration of dextran, low-dose heparin, aspirin, and persantine.
    c. If the donor liver fails, retransplantation should be considered.

d. Early infectious complications are usually bacterial in origin, with viral infections occurring later. Most deaths occur within the first 6 months and are due to sepsis. Common infectious agents are *Pneumocystis carinii*, cytomegalovirus, Epstein-Barr virus, respiratory syncytial virus, adenovirus, herpes simplex, herpes zoster, HIV, candidiasis, and aspergillus. Most of these occur more commonly in the immunosuppressed patient.

PEDIATRIC CARDIAC TRANSPLANTATION

The principal indication for pediatric cardiac transplantation is the hypoplastic left heart syndrome (HLHS). Because this syndrome is rapidly fatal at birth, anesthetic management must encompass problems of the neonate with transitional circulation, the infant with heart failure and cyanosis, and anesthesia for open heart surgery.

Preoperative Management

Recipient

1. Children with HLHS require patency of the ductus arteriosus for the continued ejection of blood from the right ventricle into the aorta and the systemic and pulmonic circulations. They are maintained on prostaglandin infusions preoperatively, and vital to their survival is management of the ratio of systemic to pulmonary resistance. Agents that increase pulmonary vascular resistance (PVR) must be avoided because of the resulting further decrease in pulmonary flow (see Chapter 11).
2. Although increasing F_IO_2 does not improve oxygenation with a fixed shunt, high concentrations of inspired oxygen will dilate the pulmonary vasculature, decreasing PVR and improving pulmonary blood flow. An F_IO_2 sufficient to maintain an oxygen saturation of 80% (PaO_2 approximately equal to 40 mm Hg in a 3-week-old infant) should be used for adequate tissue oxygenation.
3. Spontaneous ventilation or positive pressure ventilation at low pulmonary pressures improves pulmonary blood flow.
4. Hypocarbia decreases PVR. The $PaCO_2$ should be maintained at around 30 mm Hg.
5. When cardiovascular stability is maintained with inotropic support, drugs should be used that do not increase systemic vascular resistance to improve aortic outflow. Use of isoproterenol, epinephrine, and dopamine is recommended. The use of agents such as phenylephrine and norepinephrine should be avoided.
6. Immunosuppressive therapy—cyclosporine (0.25 to 1 mg/kg) with serum levels confirmed by radioimmunoassay—is administered preoperatively.

Donor

1. The donor must be diagnosed as brain dead according to the Uniform Brain Death Code.
2. Normal levels of pH, $PaCO_2$, PaO_2, and normothermia must be maintained.
3. Blood pressure should be maintained primarily with fluid administration.

4. If pressor support is required, dopamine is infused at rates less than 5 μg/kg/min.
5. Transfusions may be necessary to keep the hematocrit over 30%.
6. Methylprednisolone (125 mg IV) should be given to maintain graft cell membrane integrity before harvesting along with heparin (500 μg/kg/IV) and cefazolin (20 to 25 mg/kg IV).

Intraoperative Management—Recipient

Vascular access

1. A central venous catheter placed in the internal jugular vein is used for fluid and vasopressor administration. The left side of the neck should be cannulated, if possible, to allow for the frequent postoperative myocardial biopsies through the right internal jugular vein.
2. A radial arterial catheter inserted either percutaneously or by surgical cutdown is necessary for blood pressure monitoring and for obtaining blood gases and laboratory samples.
3. A second peripheral intravenous cannula is required for volume administration.

Monitoring

Along with standard monitoring, the following monitors are requisite to this procedure: urinary catheter, esophageal and rectal (or tympanic membrane temperature), esophageal stethoscope, pulse oximeter, and a capnograph or mass spectrometer. Heat lamps and a heating blanket/cooling blanket are required.

Anesthetic agents

1. Fentanyl is commonly used as an induction and maintenance agent because it provides cardiovascular stability, particularly in infants with HLHS.
2. Ketamine may be used as an induction agent in doses of 1 to 2 mg/kg IV.
3. Inhalation anesthetics should be avoided because of their direct myocardial depressant effects.
4. Muscle relaxation
   - Either pancuronium (0.1 mg/kg) or vecuronium (0.1 mg/kg) may be used as the primary muscle relaxant.
   - In higher doses, atracurium may cause histamine release, which increases pulmonary vascular resistance.

Surface cooling

Surface cooling to achieve hypothermia should be instituted after placement of all monitors and intraarterial and intravenous catheters. To achieve cooling, the temperature of the heating blanket is lowered, room temperature is decreased, and an ice pack is placed around the patient's head. Core temperature should be 33° to 35° C before bypass.

Cardiopulmonary bypass (CPB)

- Before bypass, heparin is administered at 3 to 4 mg/kg. Adequacy of heparinization must be assured by an activated clotting time (ACT) greater than or equal to 450 sec before initiating bypass.
- Before circulatory arrest, which is usually performed in infants less than

10 kg, core temperature should be approximately 16° C. Transplantation in larger infants is accomplished using CPB at traditional flows.

Postbypass pharmacologic support

Since the transplanted heart is denervated, transvenous pacing or isoproterenol must be used to increase heart rate after bypass. Atropine is ineffective because vagal continuity no longer exists. Isoproterenol, epinephrine, or dopamine, used alone or in combination, can provide inotropic support.

PEDIATRIC HEART LUNG TRANSPLANTATION

Indications

The major indication for heart lung transplantation in the pediatric population is cystic fibrosis. An additional indication is Eisenmenger's syndrome (pulmonary hypertension) from long-standing congenital heart disease.

Preoperative Management

- See discussion on heart transplantation.
- Immunosuppressive therapy is administered according to institution protocol.

Intraoperative Management

For general considerations, see also section on heart transplantation.

Pulmonary Vascular Resistance

The key to successful intraoperative anesthetic management is maximum reduction in pulmonary vascular resistance (PVR). Many children who are to receive heart-lung transplants come to the operating room receiving infusions of pulmonary vasodilators. (See box below.)

VARIABLES AFFECTING PULMONARY VASCULAR RESISTANCE

Increase PVR

Decreased PaO_2
Increased $PaCO_2$
N_2O
Dopamine
Norepinephrine
Phenylephrine

Decrease PVR

Increased PaO_2
Decreased $PaCO_2$
Inhalation anesthetics
Nitroprusside
Tolazoline
Isoproterenol

Intubation

- Intubation must be performed with meticulously sterile technique. Use of a sterile disposable laryngoscope is ideal; a sterilized reusable laryngoscope is also acceptable. To minimize bacterial contamination, the patient's head should be prepared and sterilely draped before intubation.
- Use of the largest ETT that can be accommodated by the trachea is advisable to allow for postoperative bronchoscopy.
- A fiberoptic bronchoscope must be available for the dual purpose of verifying placement of the ETT and manipulating the tube following the tracheal anastomosis. The ETT is repositioned just proximal to the suture line after completion of the tracheal anastomosis.

Fluid Management

- Fluid volume administration is strictly minimized in both the donor and recipient. Hemodynamic control is achieved with vasopressors.
- Blood products are preferred to crystalloid if fluid resuscitation is absolutely necessary.

Oxygenation

- Parenchymal damage to the new lungs may be caused by oxygen toxicity (free radical formation).
- Toxicity is limited by maintaining as low an F_IO_2 as possible, preferably less than 40%.

Cardiopulmonary Bypass

See section on isolated heart transplantation, p. 476.

Pharmacologic Support

1. The transplanted heart is denervated. Control of the heart rate must therefore be accomplished with the use of a β agonist such as isoproterenol or epinephrine or mechanically by intravenous pacing. Atropine is ineffective without vagal continuity.
2. Isoproterenol, epinephrine, or dopamine may be used for inotropic support, separately or in combination.
3. Prostaglandins (PGE_1) are frequently used after lung transplantation to maintain normal levels of PVR.

Anesthetic Management of Heart Transplant Patients for Noncardiac Surgery

1. Preoperative assessment of current cardiopulmonary function, exercise tolerance, and current medications is obtained.
2. Meticulous aseptic technique is observed in the immunosuppressed patient. Endocarditis prophylaxis is required.
3. Isoproterenol or epinephrine should be available for chronotropic support in the denervated heart. Atropine is not effective in the absence of vagal continuity.
4. Transvenous pacing may also be used to control heart rate. External thoracic pacing is useful in children over 10 kg.

5. Anesthetic agents that maintain heart rate are ideal (e.g., ketamine). Inhalation agents that may cause myocardial depression or slow conduction should be used with caution.
6. Because of the small population of pediatric patients who have received heart transplants, not all of the reactions or sequelae to anesthetic agents are known. Cardiology and intensive care support should be readily available in the postoperative period.

BONE MARROW TRANSPLANTATION

Indications

Bone marrow transplantation (BMT) is the treatment of choice for severe combined immunodeficiency syndrome (SCIDS), aplastic anemia, Wiskott-Aldrich syndrome, and other lethal hematopoietic disorders when a histocompatible donor is available.

For hematologic malignancies, BMT is used after failure of traditional chemotherapy or for "poor risk" leukemias in first remission.

Anesthesia for Donors

1. Major complications occur rarely in the donor (0.3% incidence).
2. Donors are generally healthy, HLA-matched siblings from 5 to 6 months of age and older.
3. The volume of marrow required for transplantation is 10 ml/kg body weight of the recipient. To minimize dilution of the marrow aspirate by peripheral blood, individual aspirates are limited to 2 to 3 ml per puncture, necessitating 100 to 400 separate aspirates per harvest depending on the size of the recipient.
4. Use of either general or regional anesthesia is appropriate. The possibility that use of nitrous oxide will depress hematopoiesis in the transplanted marrow is of theoretical concern, particularly if the operation is expected to last longer than 2 hours.
5. It is often necessary to harvest bone marrow from both anterior and posterior iliac crests, making it necessary to adjust the patient's position during the operation from supine to prone or vice versa.
6. Volume of marrow taken should be replaced as if it were blood lost directly from the intravascular space.

Anesthesia for Recipients

Marrow is given to the recipient intravenously after suitable marrow ablation with high-dose chemotherapy and/or total body irradiation. Should the recipient require surgery following transplantation, certain BMT complications are of concern.

1. Effective hematopoiesis does not begin until 3 to 5 weeks after BMT, which gives rise to a prolonged period of profound immunosuppression.
2. Acute graft-versus-host disease (GVHD) can appear 10 days to 6 weeks post-BMT causing skin, liver, and GI complications.
   - Chronic GVHD also involves the skin, liver, and GI tract and is associated with more profound immunosuppression post-BMT.

- GVHD has a very low incidence among young children, but the incidence increases with age.

3. There is a 50% incidence of interstitial pneumonitis after a bone marrow transplant, which may result in severe hypoxemia. Opportunistic infections are most serious in the first weeks immediately following transplant, before effective granulopoiesis.
4. Chemotherapeutic toxicity (see Table 12-1, pp. 260-262) may be particularly severe, in part because of the marrow-ablative doses required. The most commonly used agent is cyclophosphamide, associated with pulmonary, GI, hepatic, and renal toxicity. Total body irradiation may lead to hypothyroidism in approximately 50% of transplant recipients.

ANESTHESIA AND THE IMMUNOSUPPRESSED PATIENT

As experience increases, patients are surviving longer after the immediate posttransplant period. Consequently, more patients will be candidates for nontransplant surgery after successfully receiving a heterologous organ. Of primary concern for the anesthesiologist is the function of the graft and related organ systems and the effects of immunosuppression (see following section, "Immunosuppressant Drugs").

Formal immunosuppression protocols not only vary from institution to institution but must be flexible enough to treat the individual patient's needs. The ultimate goal of therapy is to prevent rejection and minimize side effects. Ideally, the host will develop some adaptation to the graft, which will allow levels of suppression to be decreased with fewer complications. If severe rejection occurs, survival has been increased by the early use of retransplantation before total host compromise occurs.

Immunosuppressant Drugs

Cyclosporine A

Pharmacology

1. Interferes with release of interleukin-2, which normally stimulates antigen-activated helper and cytotoxic T cells to begin DNA synthesis; inhibits activation of B and T lymphocytes and certain macrophage functions.
2. Cyclosporine A is extensively metabolized in the liver to inactive metabolites by the cytochrome P450 microsomal enzyme system, with 99% undergoing biliary elimination and 1% renal elimination.
3. 90% is normally bound to serum proteins.
4. When given simultaneously, the following drugs increase the nephrotoxic potential of cyclosporine: trimethoprim, amphotericin B, aminoglycosides, melphalan, cotrimoxazole, indomethacin.
5. The following drugs increase cyclosporine levels by enzyme inhibition: ketoconazole, allopurinol, phenylbutazone, chloramphenicol, ethanol, cimetidine, erythromycin.
6. The following drugs decrease cyclosporine levels by enzyme induction: phenytoin, barbiturates, carbamazepine, rifampin, griseofulvin, primidone, glutethimide.

7. Cyclosporine may increase resistance to nondepolarizing muscle relaxants.
8. Cyclosporine is insoluble in water. Oral preparations are mixed with olive oil and ethanol and intravenous preparations with ethanol. Because of the ethanol vehicle, nausea and vomiting may result when administered with metronidazole, cefamandole, moxalactam, and chlorpropamide. Intravenous preparation should be given slowly over 2 to 4 hours because hypotension can occur. Desired whole blood levels are 200 to 600 ng/ml.

Side effects

- Nephrotoxicity
- Hepatotoxicity
- Increased susceptibility to infection
- Bone marrow toxicity
- Tremors, hyperesthesia
- Encephalopathy and seizures have been reported in patients with low serum cholesterol after liver transplantation
- Gingival hyperplasia
- Hirsutism
- Gastrointestinal upset: nausea, vomiting, diarrhea (usually mild)
- Hyperuricemia
- Lymphadenopathy and adenotonsillar hypertrophy
- Hypertension and myocardial fibrosis may be associated with cyclosporine
- Increased incidence of lymphoid tumors.

Glucocorticoids

Pharmacology

1. May act synergistically with other immunosuppressants, possibly by inhibiting interleukin production; alone, will not prevent rejection.
2. Decreases number of antigen-activated lymphocytes.
3. Preferentially removes helper-inducer lymphocytes (OKT-4) from circulation.
4. A daily high dose is given during the first posttransplant week.
5. Doses are rapidly tapered. Transition eventually to an alternate-day regimen to promote growth is ideal.
6. Intravenous high-dose boluses are used during episodes of rejection.

Side effects

- Suppression of pituitary adrenal function requiring perioperative steroid coverage
- Fluid and electrolyte disturbances
- Hyperglycemia and glycosuria
- Infection
- Peptic ulcer disease
- Osteoporosis
- Myopathy
- Behavioral changes
- Cataracts
- Cushing's habitus
- Inhibition of growth in children

Azathioprine

Pharmacology

1. Derivative of 6-mercaptopurine.
2. Interferes with DNA synthesis of rapidly dividing cells.
3. Used primarily to decrease the dose of cyclosporine.
4. Dose: 1.5-5 mg/kg/day IV or PO.
5. Clearance is reduced in the presence of renal insufficiency.

Side effects

- Myelosuppression (dose related and reversible)
- Cholestatic jaundice (dose related and reversible)
- Hepatitis
- Infrequent side effects: stomatitis, dermatitis, fever, alopecia, gastrointestinal disturbances

Antilymphocyte Globulin (ALG)

Pharmacology

1. ALG is primarily used for treatment of acute rejection unresponsive to steroids and cyclosporine.
2. Derived from animals inoculated with human lymphocytes.
3. Varies widely in potency and effectiveness.
4. Polyclonal composition allows for repeated use without development of resistance.
5. Pretreatment with steroids, antihistamines, and acetaminophen will attenuate side effects.

Side effects

- Shares side effects of heterologous serum transfusion
- Fever, chills, rash, dyspnea, anaphylaxis
- Thrombocytopenia

Monoclonal Antibodies (OKT-3)

Pharmacology

1. Murine-derived antibody that recognizes the gamma portion of the T cell.
2. Complete disappearance of circulating T cells occurs within 15 minutes of administration.
3. Development of antimurine antibodies limits its repeated use.
4. The antibody does not fix complement.

Side effects

- Flu syndrome often present at initial dosage, decreases with time
- Pulmonary edema
- Histamine release (blocked by pretreatment with H_1 and H_2 antagonists)

BIBLIOGRAPHY

Bailey LL and others: Baboon to human cardiac xenotransplantation in a neonate, JAMA 254:3321-29, 1985.

Bailey LL and others: Cardiac allotransplantation in newborns as therapy for hypoplastic left heart syndrome, N Engl J Med 315:949-51, 1986.

Bailey LL and others: Host maturation after orthotopic cardiac transplantation during neonatal life, Heart Transplantation 3:265-67, 1984.

Borland LM, Roule M, and Cook DR: Anesthesia for pediatric orthotopic liver transplantation, Anesth Analg 64:117-24, 1985.
Churchill BM and others: Factors influencing patient and graft survival in 300 cadaveric pediatric renal transplants, J Urol 40:1129-33, 1988.
Cuervas-Mons V and others: Does previous abdominal surgery alter the outcome of pediatric patients subjected to orthotopic liver transplantation? Gastroenterology 90:853-57, 1986.
deGroen PC and others: Central nervous system toxicity after liver transplantation: the role of cyclosporine and cholesterol, N Engl J Med 317:861-66, 1987.
Ettenger RB and others: Successful cadaveric renal transplantation in infants and young children, Transplant Proc 21:1707-8, 1989.
Fine RN: Renal transplantation of the infant and young child and the use of pediatric cadaver kidneys for transplantation in pediatric and adult recipients, Am J Kidney Dis 12:1-10, 1988.
Fine RN and Tejani A: Renal transplantation in children, Nephron 47:81-86, 1987.
Graybar GB and Jarpay M: Kidney transplantation. In Gelman S, editor: Anesthesia and organ transplantation, Philadelphia, 1987, WB Saunders, 61-110.
Guidelines for the determination of death: report of the medical consultants on the diagnosis of death to the President's Commission for the Study of Ethical Problems in Medicine and Biomedical and Behavioral Research, JAMA 246:2184-86, 1981.
Hansen DD and Hickey PR: Anesthesia for hypoplastic left heart syndrome: use of high-dose fentanyl in 30 neonates, Anesth Analg 65:127-32, 1986.
Jamieson NV: A new solution for liver preservation, Br J Surg 76:107-8, 1989.
Kalia A and others: Renal transplantation in the infant and young child, Am J Dis Child 142:47-50, 1988.
Kang Y and others: Intraoperative coagulation changes in children undergoing liver transplantation, Anesthesiology 71:44-47, 1989.
Lagaaij EL and others: Effect of one-HLA-DR-antigen matched and completely HLA-DR-mismatched blood transfusions on survival of heart and kidney allografts, N Engl J Med 321:701-5, 1989.
Lin HY and others: Cyclosporin-induced hyperuricemia and gout, N Engl J Med 321:287-92, 1989.
Martin RD and others: Anesthesia for neonatal orthotopic cardiac xenograft, J Cardiothorac Anesth 1:132-135, 1987.
Martin RD and others: Anesthetic management of neonatal cardiac transplantation, J Cardiothorac Anesth 3d:465-69, 1989.
Myer III CM and Reilly JS: Airway obstruction in an immunosuppressed child, Arch Otolaryngol Head Neck Surg 111:409-11, 1985.
Myers BD and others: Cyclosporin-associated chronic nephropathy, N Engl J Med 311:699-705, 1984.
Paradis KJG, Freese DK, and Sharp HL: A pediatric perspective on liver transplantation, Pediatr Clin North Am 35:409-433, 1988.
Perlmutter D and others: Liver transplantation in pediatric patients, Adv Pediatr 32:177-196, 1985.
Rappaport JM: Bone marrow transplantation. In Oski FH and Nathan DG, editors: Hematology of infancy and childhood, Philadelphia, 1987, WB Saunders.
Report of special task force: guidelines for the determination of brain death in children, Pediatrics 80:298-300, 1987.
Rettke SR and others: Anesthesia approach to hepatic transplantation, Mayo Clin Proc 64:244-31, 1989.
Sheldon CA, McLorie GA, and Churchill BM: Renal transplantation in children, Pediatr Clin North Am 34:1209-32, 1987.

Sommerauer J and others: Intensive care course following liver transplantation in children, J Pediatr Surg 23:705-8, 1988.
Starnes VA and others: Cardiac transplantation in children and adolescents, Circulation 76(suppl V):43-47, 1987.
Thompson AE: Aspects of pediatric intensive care after liver transplantation, Transplant Proc 19:34-39, 1987.
Todo S and others: Extended preservation of human liver grafts with UW solution, JAMA 261:711-714, 1989.
Van Thiel DH: Liver transplantation, Pediatr Ann 14:474-480, 1985.
Zitelli BJ and others: Evaluation of the pediatric patient for liver transplantation, Pediatrics 78:559-565, 1986.

20

ANESTHESIA FOR REMOTE LOCATIONS

Cindy W. Hughes

TRAVELING TO REMOTE LOCATIONS

Socioeconomic changes that limit the cost of patient hospitalizations and advances in modern technology have produced a rapid explosion in the number of procedures performed outside of the operating room (Table 20-1). Many procedures that formerly required a surgical incision can now be accomplished transdermally or percutaneously (e.g., angiographic embolization, lithotripsy, and umbrella occlusion). Furthermore, equipment necessary for these procedures and for new diagnostic studies sometimes cannot be moved to an operating room (e.g., magnetic resonance imaging [MRI] and computerized tomography [CT]). Many of these procedures or studies could be done with little or no analgesia, but require patient cooperation and absence of movement, which make their success nearly impossible in the awake child.

Therefore, it is not unusual for many pediatric anesthesiologists to administer anesthesia in remote locations of the hospital where equipment is unfamiliar or unavailable and there are no colleagues to assist in an emergency. Additionally, radiology suites, MRI centers, CT scanners, and fluoroscopy rooms are all built to optimize imaging. They are not constructed for the needs of an anesthetized patient, so that flexibility and creativity are required of the anesthesia teams. Many of these patients are outpatients; the anesthesiologist will be primarily responsible for their care during their hospitalization.

PLANNING THE ANESTHETIC

The Four Ps

Knowledge of the four Ps is essential when planning an anesthetic for a remote location: the procedure, the problems, the patient, and the plans.

TABLE 20-1. Some common non–operating room sites and procedures

Sites	Procedures
Cardiac catheterization laboratory	Cardiac catheterization ASD umbrella closure PDA umbrella closure Valvuloplasty Angioplasty
CT scan	Diagnostic imaging
MRI	Diagnostic imaging
Radiation center	Radiation therapy of neoplastic disease Bone marrow ablation for transplant
Clinic areas	Endoscopy Bone marrow biopsy Percutaneous biopsy Lumbar puncture with or without intrathecal chemotherapy
Radiology	Angiography Myelography Arthrography Lithotripsy (biliary, renal) Angioplasty Percutaneous nephrostomy Percutaneous biliary drainage

The Procedure

Rapid technological advances in each medical specialty make it progressively more difficult for physicians to stay "current" and knowledgeable about new procedures outside of their area of expertise. Chances are that the physician who usually does not work in an operating room is as unfamiliar with anesthetic procedures as the anesthesiologist is with the planned study. The following points should be clarified well in advance of the procedure:

1. What is the specific *technique*? For example, is heparinization required for catheter placement? Is the procedure painful or stimulating?
2. Will radiopaque dye (intravenous contrast) be used? If so, will ionic or nonionic compounds be chosen?
3. What is the anticipated *duration* of the procedure? What is the anticipated recovery time after the procedure? Will the patient be hospitalized or discharged?
4. What *position(s)* will the patient be in? Will he or she need to be moved during the procedure? Is the patient accessible to the anesthesiologist? Must the patient be absolutely motionless (e.g., cerebral angiographic embolization) or can some movement be tolerated (e.g., bone marrow aspiration)?
5. What are the anticipated *complications* and sequelae? Pain? Bleeding? Nausea or vomiting?

TABLE 20-2. Equipment for anesthesia in remote locations

Equipment	Comments
Suction	If no wall suction is available a portable suction machine should be placed at the site.
Oxygen	Even if central oxygen is available a full oxygen tank and Ambu bag or Jackson-Rees circuit is necessary as a back-up system and for transport.
Monitors	Check for the availability of monitors at the site; some radiology suites will already have ECG, oximetry, or noninvasive blood pressure monitors; all monitoring needed to fulfill ASA standards should be available; electrical adapters and multiple outlet extension cords may be needed.
Machines	An anesthesia machine is useful if there is sufficient space available; wall suction for scavenging gases, and wall oxygen are required.
Cart	A fully stocked cart on casters can be taken to the site with appropriate drugs, IV equipment, circuits, probes, etc.

The Problems

Physical set-up (Table 20-2). Oxygen, suction, the appropriate number and type of electrical outlets, and space for an anesthesia machine and monitors often are not available. The anesthesiologist should inspect the site before beginning the planned procedure.

1. Wall oxygen should be accessible.
2. Wall suction is necessary both for patient care and to scavenge gases if inhalation agents will be used. Portable suction is sufficient for patient care but cannot be used to scavenge gases.
3. Isolated electrical outlets usually are not available. Electrical converters or adapters may be needed to plug in monitoring equipment. Extension cords should be available.

Staffing. Technicians and nurses trained to assist with the procedure are unfamiliar with the needs of the anesthesiologist or the care of the anesthetized patient. A two-person anesthesia team will ensure a smooth induction, emergence, and transport to recovery. It also will guarantee that help is nearby if an untoward event occurs away from the operating room.

Radiation exposure. The problems of excessive exposure are well recognized. All precautionary measures should be taken including wearing a radiation badge that measures cumulative exposure, leaded glasses, a lead apron, and a thyroid shield. If possible the anesthesiologist should leave the area during periods of high radiation (i.e., plain films, cinematography, dye injection). The patient and monitors can still be observed continuously from behind leaded glass shields during these periods. Radio stethoscopes are available for listening to heart and breath sounds outside of the room.

Similarly the patient should be protected by covering the most sensitive areas (i.e., the eyes, thyroid, and genital areas).

Limited access to the patient

1. A crowded work space, lead shields, and fluoroscopy tubes often make it impossible to get to the patient. Intravenous tubing, breathing circuits,

and monitors should have adequate extensions to allow for movement of the table without disconnecting equipment.

2. During CT scans and radiation therapy it is impossible to be present in the room with the patient. All monitors should be observed easily through a leaded glass window or from a video camera. An emergency plan should be made with the radiologist in the event that the procedure must be stopped to treat the patient.

Dim lighting. The lights are dimmed in order to intensify the images being observed. A spot light or flashlight is useful to check the patient and monitors and to complete charting.

Cold rooms. Many of the sites are kept cold to accommodate the computers that are used to reconstruct the images. Warming blankets cannot be used because they interfere with the imaging. Alternative methods for warming the patient include the use of warming fluids, warming and humidifying gases, wrapping the head and limbs in plastic wrap, keeping the patient dry, and using radiant heat lamps.

Terrible tables. Fluoroscopy tables are hard and flat to accommodate film plates and cannot be placed in the Trendelenburg position if hypotension or vomiting occur. Hypotension should be treated with intravenous volume expansion or a vasopressor. A large-bore suction in case emesis occurs must be readily available. Pressure points will require extra padding.

Monitoring. The same ASA standards of monitoring should be employed for all anesthetics, regardless of where they are administered. Monitoring in the MRI scanner has been the most challenging problem to date, but many companies are now making MRI-compatible equipment so that monitoring in a magnetic field is becoming less problematic (Table 20-3). The high magnetic fields generated by the MRI do not tolerate ferrous material to be present without drawing it into the magnet, causing extensive damage to the magnet or injury to persons in the room. Most hospitals are now using 1.5-tesla magnets, which are much stronger than the original 0.6-tesla scanners. It is important to know the type of scanner and the field strength in order to purchase compatible monitoring equipment. Suction and central wall oxygen attachments are available for most MRI units. Pass-through shielded port holes can be built for monitoring cables. ECG telemetry units have been designed specifically for MRI as well. It is best to have monitoring equipment and the scanners installed simultaneously after consultation with the radiologists and engineers.

Radiofrequency (RF) waves are another troubling aspect of monitoring in the MRI. A high magnetic field is induced and then RF waves are directed at the patient. Images are constructed from the RF waves reflecting back out of the patient. Electric cables and cords from monitoring equipment function as antennae for the RF, causing monitor dysfunction. Furthermore the images are degraded by the interference caused by monitoring equipment with the RF signals. Any electrical cables or cords should be shielded. Nonferrous aluminum foil is wrapped easily around cables or stuffed into port holes to shield them from RF.

TABLE 20-3. Monitoring during magnetic resonance imaging*,[1-4]

ASA standard	Monitor	Comments
Oxygenation	1. Skin color	1. Very unreliable because of poor lighting and the patient's position in tunnel, obscured from view
	2. Pulse oximeter	2. Cables need shielding with aluminum foil; the limb with the oximeter must be outside the bore of the magnet; a probe with a light source can burn a patient in MRI; plastic drapes can shield the patient from direct contact with the probe
Ventilation	1. Auscultation of breath sounds	1. Breath sounds are obscured during RF pulse sequencing; a system of amplifiers and filters can augment breath sounds/heart tones and delete outside noises
	2. Observation	2. A rising chest is not a reliable monitor of adequate ventilation
	3. End tidal CO_2	3. Monitors are available; some only denote the presence of CO_2 and do not quantitate the amount
Circulation	1. Auscultation of heart sounds	1. As with breath sounds the RF pulse sequencing can obscure sounds; a system of filters and amplifiers can be made to augment physiologic sounds and filter outside noise; these must be installed by biomedical engineers on site
	2. ECG	2. Telemetry units are available for specific MRI manufacturers, which grossly detect the presence of a QRS complex, but not specific changes in complex configuration; the ECG always will be distorted because of magnetized blood flowing through the heart, creating an electrical current that distorts the ECG vector
	3. Perfusion	3. Monitors of perfusion include: (a) plethysmography; (b) Doppler flow systems; (c) noninvasive blood pressure monitoring; (d) fiberoptic pressure transducer (in development); (e) capillary perfusion by laser-Doppler velocimetry
Temperature	1. Thermometer	1. Heat-sensitive adhesive thermometers are ideal for MRI; RF can cause hyperthermia during an MRI scan

*Some companies presently involved in the manufacture of MRI compatible equipment include: In-Vivo Research Labs, Ohmeda, Biochem, Monaghan, CMS Medical, GEc.

The Patient

1. Often the physician doing the procedure is a consultant not acquainted with the patient. It is important to identify the patient's primary physician and request a preanesthetic history and physical examination.
2. Routine preanesthetic laboratory data as well as any special tests pertinent to the patient should be obtained.
3. Any contraindications to the administration of sedatives should be noted, including altered mental status, increased ICP, the presence of a difficult airway, compromised respiratory function, and hemodynamic instability.
4. For outpatients it is best to speak with the parent or guardian before the procedure about anesthetic procedures, risks, and plans. NPO times should be reinforced and critical medications continued. Plans for recovery, discharge, and at-home care should be detailed. This can be accomplished by telephone or a preoperative visit.

The Plan

1. The anesthetic plan must be safe for the child given the physical plant and environment, the child's underlying pathology, and the expertise of the medical team. Common choices include monitored sedation, dissociative anesthesia (i.e., ketamine), or general anesthesia. Regional anesthesia is used rarely.
2. The anesthetic plan should be agreeable to the parents and the older child.
3. Children's procedures should be scheduled as the first case in the morning to help guarantee NPO status and allow time for recovery.
4. If the child is to be sedated by either PO or IM routes, sufficient time should be allowed for drug administration before the onset of the procedure (1 to 2 hours).
5. Details of the anesthetic plan should be understood by those performing the procedure. They should realize the importance of communicating with the anesthesia team before moving the patient and before conducting different phases of the procedure that may require an increase in anesthetic depth.
6. Arrangements to recover the child must be made in advance. If the child will recover on site the area must have appropriate staff, suction, oxygen, monitoring, and supervision by anesthesia personnel. If on-site recovery is not possible, it is necessary to transport the child to the postanesthesia recovery unit.

   The anesthesiologist must be available for postanesthesia teaching and discharge planning with the family. A responsible adult should be home with the child for 24 hours after receiving sedation. The primary-care physician should be aware of discharge plans, the possible need for admission, and any anticipated sequelae.

ANESTHETIC TECHNIQUES

Monitored Sedation

1. Preprocedure interview and laboratory data should be obtained as discussed previously.
2. The appropriate NPO schedule should be applied (see Chapter 4).

3. Monitored sedation is most appropriate for nonpainful, simple diagnostic examinations (e.g., CT or MRI scans) that require the child's cooperation. However, this method may not be useful for daily radiation therapy because the child must be motionless during these treatments.
4. Monitoring standards apply (ECG, blood pressure, pulse oximetry, temperature).
5. Common drug choices for sedation include: (see Table 20-4)
   a. Chloral hydrate
   b. Barbiturates
   c. Benzodiazepines
   d. Narcotic/sedative combinations (Table 20-5)

Dissociative Anesthesia (Ketamine)

Standards

All standards used for general anesthesia in the operating room apply, including the following:

1. Preoperative interview and laboratory data
2. Appropriate NPO schedules
3. Routine monitoring
4. Indwelling intravenous catheter

Indications

This technique is only considered for a child who can maintain his or her own airway or when the airway is not compromised during the course of the procedure. Ketamine is used in children who must lie still or who are having painful procedures including MRI scans, cardiac catheterization, angiography, valvuloplasty, and radiation therapy.

Technique

1. Induction with ketamine, 4 to 5 mg/kg IM or 6 mg/kg PO
2. Placement of indwelling intravenous catheter after induction
3. An antisialagogue (glycopyrrolate or atropine 0.01 mg/kg) is used to decrease secretions
4. Anesthesia is maintained with small IV boluses of ketamine, 0.5 to 1.0 mg/kg
5. Concurrent use of a benzodiazepine usually prevents emergence delirium, but may depress ventilation; Diazepam 0.1 mg/kg IV, or Midazolam 0.03 to 0.05 mg/kg IV may be used.

Advantages

1. Spontaneous respiration usually is preserved.
2. Anesthesia may be induced by IM injection without prior placement of an intravenous catheter.
3. Heart rate and blood pressure usually are increased.

Disadvantages

1. Increased airway irritability
2. Prolonged, unpredictable, or delirious emergence
3. Increased intracranial pressure

TABLE 20-4. Drugs for monitored sedation

Classification drug	Primary effect	Dose/route	Onset	Duration	Advantages	Disadvantages
NONBARBITURATE SEDATIVES Chloral hydrate Triclofos	Sedation	30-75 mg/kg PO	1-1.5 hr	30-60 min	• Reliably sedates most children • Minimal cardiac or respiratory depression	• Paradoxic excitation • Long half-life (8-12 hr) • Unpleasant taste • Irritating to skin and GI tract
BARBITURATES Pentobarbital (Nembutal) Secobarbital (Seconal)	Sedation	2-4 mg/kg PO, IM, PR	1-1.5 hr	30-60 min	• Reliably sedates most children • Minimal cardiac or respiratory depression • Little nausea or vomiting	• Paradoxic excitation • Painful if IM injection • Contraindicated in patients with porphyria or history of hypersensitivity
BENZODIAZEPINES	Sedation/anxiolysis		1 hr	2-4 hr	• Amnestic • Minimal cardiac depression • Lorazepam has antiemetic properties	• Diazepam and lorazepam have very long half-lives • Hallucinations with lorazepam have been reported in children <6 years of age
Diazepam (Valium)		0.1-0.5 mg/kg PO				
Midazolam (Versed)		0.06-0.08 mg/kg IM				
Lorazepam (Ativan)		0.05 mg/kg PO not to exceed 2 mg in children 4 mg in teens				

BUTYROPHENONE Droperidol (Inapsine)	Ataractic/neuroleptic	30-75 μg/kg IM	0.5-1 hr	Prolonged	• Antiemetic • Minimal cardiac or respiration depression	• Hypotension • Dysphoria (occurs less if used with fentanyl) • Extrapyramidal symptoms
PHENOTHIAZINES Chlorpromazine (Thorazine) Promethazine (Phenergan)	Sedation	0.3-0.5 mg/kg IM, PO	0.5-1 hr	2-3 hr	• Antiemetic • Minimal cardiac or respiratory depression	• Hypotension • Extrapyramidal symptoms
NARCOTICS Morphine Meperidine Fentanyl	Analgesia	 0.1-0.15 mg/kg IM 1-2 mg/kg IM/PO 1-2 μg/kg IM	0.5 hr	1.5-2 hr	• Reliably sedates most children • Ideal for painful procedures • Reversible with naloxone • May be combined with sedatives or anxiolytics	• May cause respiratory depression • May cause nausea and vomiting • May increase ICP, by causing hypoventilation • Should not be used with a history of hypersensitivity • Fentanyl is minimally effective when used alone, but useful as neurolept analgesic when combined with droperidol (Innovar)

TABLE 20-5. Drug combinations for monitored sedation*

Combination	Drugs and doses
Narcotic and barbiturate	Meperidine (Demerol) 1 mg/kg and pentobarbital 4 mg/kg IM Morphine 0.1 mg/kg and pentobarbital 4 mg/kg IM
Narcotic and butyrophenone (neuroleptanalgesia)	Fentanyl 1 μg/kg and droperidol 50 μg/kg
Narcotic and phenothiazine	Meperidine 1 mg/kg and promethazine (Phenergan) 0.25 mg/kg IM, PO
Narcotic and antihistamine	Meperidine 1 mg/kg and hydroxyzine (Vistaril) 0.5 mg/kg IM or PO

*Advantages: (1) More reliable sedation because of the additive effect of the drugs; and (2) provides analgesia and sedation or anxiolysis. Disadvantages: (1) Respiratory depression; and (2) long and unpredictable duration of action.

General Anesthesia

Indications

General anesthesia with tracheal intubation is the only choice for many procedures.

1. When a patent airway cannot be assured because of positioning (e.g., myelography)
2. When the procedure is lengthy and painful
3. When the airway must be protected (e.g., upper endoscopy)
4. When the airway may be inaccessible to the anesthesiologist for a lengthy procedure (e.g., cerebral angiography)
5. When the patient must remain motionless for a lengthy procedure or when neuromuscular blockade is needed (e.g., percutaneous ASD closure)
6. When the use of sedation or ketamine is contraindicated (e.g., airway compromise)

Techniques

1. If the location is suitable for an anesthesia machine, any appropriate technique may be used.
2. If an anesthesia machine is not available, alternative choices include the following:
   a. Narcotic and amnestic (benzodiazepine)
   b. Continuous narcotic infusion and amnestic
   c. Propofol infusion
   d. Ketamine and benzodiazepine

USE OF RADIOPAQUE DYE

1. Ionic contrast media (sodium meglumine, salts of iodinated acids, or their combinations) commonly are used for IV imaging.

TABLE 20-6. Treatment for allergic reactions to intravenous contrast

Drug	Dose	Administration
Prophylaxis		
Methylprednisolone	0.5 mg/kg PO	Two doses: 12 hr preprocedure, 2 hr preprocedure
Diphenhydramine	0.5-1.0 mg/kg PO/IV	1-2 hr preprocedure
Treatment of anaphylaxis		
Epinephrine	Bolus 10 μg/kg IV Infusion 0.1-1.0 μg/kg/min IV	Can be given by peripheral vessel until central venous access is established

TABLE 20-7. Properties of intravenous contrast

Compound	Iodine (mg/ml)	Osmolarity (mOsm/L)	Sodium content	Recommended dose in children*
Ionic				
Hypaque Conray Renograffin	~300	1000-2000	May be significant	2 ml/kg of 30% or 60% (maximum dose 5 ml/kg)
Nonionic				
Hexabrix Iopamidol Iohexol	~300	700-900	Insignificant	2 ml/kg (maximum dose <4 ml/kg)

*The dye is excreted over time, and doses may be repeated during lengthy procedures with careful attention to hydration.

2. The hyperosmolarity of these compounds causes a typical reaction probably caused by endothelial disruption and the subsequent nonimmunologic release of vasoactive substances from mast cells. These non–allergy related reactions are characterized by flushing, tachycardia, and nausea.
3. A small percentage of patients will exhibit true allergy to the iodine modality. Although a history of iodine or shellfish allergy, asthma, or drug allergies may help elucidate which patients are susceptible, anaphylaxis can occur without significant history.
4. Pretreatment with corticosteroids is most effective in ameliorating allergic reactions. The use of H_2 blockers (cimetidine) has not been found to be helpful. The use of diphenhydramine alone is not recommended, although it is useful as an adjuvant (Table 20-6).
5. If ionic dyes are used for procedures in children, concentrations of 30% to 60% are preferred to reduce osmolality (Table 20-7).
6. Volume contraction and high urine osmolality can be anticipated after using ionic contrast because of the hyperosmolarity and high iodine and sodium concentration.

7. Nonionic compounds are significantly less osmolar than their ionic counterparts and are associated with a decreased incidence of dye reactions. Their use is preferred in children, although they are substantially more expensive.

REFERENCES

1. Shellock FG: Monitoring during MRI: an evaluation of the effect of high field MRI on various patient monitors, Med Electr 17:93-97, 1986.
2. Roos CF and Canole FE: Fiber optic pressure transducer for use near MR magnetic fields, Radiology 156:547, 1985.
3. Watkinson WP, Gordon CJ: An improved technique for monitoring electrocardiograms during exposure to radiofrequency radiation, Am J Physiol 250:H320-24, 1986.
4. Shellock FG, Schaifer DJ, and Crues JV: Effect of a 1.5 Tesla static magnetic field on body temperature of humans, Clin Res 34:383A, 1986.
5. Van Hoff J and Olszewski D: Lorazepam for the control of chemotherapy-related nausea and vomiting in children, J Pediatr 113:146-49, 1988.

SUGGESTED READINGS

Barnett G, Ropper A, and Johnson K: Physiologic support and monitoring during magnetic resonance imaging, Anesthesiology 62:80-83, 1985.

Boutrous A and Pavlicek W: Anesthesia in an NMR scanner, Anesth Analg 66:367-74, 1987.

McCardle CB and others: Monitoring of the neonate undergoing MR imaging: technical considerations, Radiology 159:223-26, 1986.

Rao CC, McNeice WL, and Emhardt J: Modification of an anesthesia machine for use during magnetic resonance imaging, Anesthesiology 68:640-41, 1988.

Roth JL and others: Patient monitoring during magnetic resonance imaging, Anesthesiology 62:80-83, 1985.

Shellock FG: Biological effects of MRI, Diagn Imag Feb 96-101, 1987.

21

PEDIATRIC OUTPATIENT ANESTHESIA

Tae Hee Oh

There I was, inside the house,
   So fuddled up I could shout,
When I got a hunch,
   A Happy Hunch,
That I shouldn't be *in* . . . but *OUT!*

DR. SEUSS
HUNCHES IN BUNCHES

In 1970 the first free-standing outpatient surgical center, the Phoenix Surgicenter, opened in the United States. Since then health care cost containment concerns have resulted in an explosive increase in outpatient surgery. In response to the rapid growth in outpatient surgery, many pediatric surgical procedures also have been performed on an ambulatory basis.

ADVANTAGES OF OUTPATIENT SURGERY

1. Rarely do life-threatening complications occur after surgery.
2. It minimizes the length of hospitalization time and promotes active parental involvement in the postoperative recovery.
3. It may attenuate the stress and behavioral responses associated with hospitalization.
4. It may lessen the risk of nosocomial infection and iatrogenic illness.

DISADVANTAGES OF OUTPATIENT SURGERY

1. The child and family have insufficient time to adjust to the hospital environment.

Modified from Oh TH and Davis PJ: Pediatric outpatient anesthesia. In Motoyama EK and Davis PJ, editors: Smith's anesthesia for infants and children, ed 5, St Louis, 1990, CV Mosby.

2. Anesthesiologists, surgeons, and other trained medical personnel have limited time for assessment and interviewing of patients.
3. Parents and patients frequently are unable to see their surgeon or meet their anesthesiologist.
4. Often patients and parents are forced to make extra visits to the hospital or laboratory facilities for preoperative screening and consultations.
5. The need for parents to stay with children throughout the surgical procedures may mean potential loss of income and arranging of care for siblings at home.

SELECTION OF PATIENTS

Selection of patients for outpatient surgery varies from institution to institution. In general the criteria include the following points:

1. Minimal bleeding anticipated
2. No infection present
3. No major body cavity entered
4. No special postoperative nursing care required
5. Parents or guardians committed to participation in care

Selected patients usually are rated as ASA Class 1 or 2. ASA Class 3 patients with well-controlled systemic illness are reasonable candidates. Prematurely born infants require special consideration because of the risk for postoperative cardiopulmonary complications.

1. Preterm infants are at a higher risk for developing postoperative respiratory dysfunction and apnea because of immature central nervous system control and respiratory physiology.
2. There is an increasing number of surviving preterm infants, and increasing medical and economic pressure to use day surgery facilities for infants having uncomplicated procedures.
3. Although it is impossible to predict accurately which infants will develop postoperative apnea, the following factors correlate highly:
   a. A postconceptual age (PCA) of less than 42 weeks, and possibly as high as 60 weeks.
   b. A preoperative history of apnea.
   c. A preoperative history of patent ductus arteriosus (closed at time of operation).
   d. Previous respiratory distress syndrome.
   e. Preoperative pneumogram positive for abnormal breathing.
4. Recommendations for infants
   a. Delay nonessential surgery until preterm infants are beyond 60 weeks PCA.
   b. Defer elective procedures in term infants until the PCA is greater than 44 weeks.
   c. Infants who require operation at ages less than those above should be admitted to the hospital for 24 hours of cardiorespiratory monitoring.
   d. If postoperative apnea occurs, monitoring should continue for at least 12 hours free of apnea.

TYPE OF SURGERY

The type of surgery also has a strong influence in outpatient selection. Anticipated perioperative complications, postoperative nursing involvement, and duration of surgery are all factors that help in determining which child is appropriate for outpatient surgery.

The commitment of the family also must be considered for outpatient selection. The parents must feel comfortable providing postoperative care for the performance of successful ambulatory surgery.

PREPARATION FOR OUTPATIENT SURGERY

1. It is essential that proper evaluation of patients, including physical examination and appropriate laboratory tests, be done before the induction of anesthesia.
2. Appropriate counseling of the patients and parents must also be provided before surgery.
3. Records regarding the patient's medical conditions, anesthetic plan, important findings, and so forth, should be documented accurately, just as for inpatients. For patients with repeated admissions a review of previous hospital records provides important information regarding emotional as well as medical problems of which the patient or parents might be unaware or reluctant to discuss.
4. Explanation of events in the preoperative period should be reasonable and truthful. Anticipated fear and the anxiety of surgery are often so intense that they remain until the real experience of surgery is completed.
5. Rapport developed during the preoperative visit and evaluation may prevent physiologic, intellectual, social, or emotional damage.

ANESTHETIC MANAGEMENT

1. Anesthetic considerations as well as operating personnel, anesthesia monitoring, equipment, and facilities must be equivalent to the standard of care provided for inpatient surgery.
2. The margin of error in terms of sedation and tolerance for postoperative nausea and vomiting should be less than that of inpatients.
3. The anesthetic used should produce a rapid and smooth induction, intraoperative analgesia and amnesia, good operating conditions, a rapid emergence, and a short postoperative recovery period with minimal adverse effects.

NPO

1. The minimum acceptable duration of NPO is a frequently debated issue among anesthesiologists.
2. Children do not understand why they cannot eat or drink before surgery so that fasting cannot be enforced strictly without the parent's cooperation.
3. The importance of fasting must be conveyed to the parents with clear, specific instructions on when and what the patient can or cannot eat or drink.

4. The following NPO schedule is recommended:
   a. No solid food, milk, or milk products after midnight.
   b. Clear liquids as much as tolerated up to:

4 hours	0-12 months
6 hours	1-3 years
8 hours	older than 3 years

   c. A longer period of fasting may be better for prevention of aspiration, but oral intake should not be interrupted unnecessarily. Most children are less tolerant of thirst than hunger.

Premedication

1. Premedication should be ordered only when clear beneficial effects are possible.
2. Role of premedication (see Chapter 4)
   a. With adequate time for premedication, a combination of oral agents has proven very effective.
   b. Intranasal and rectal administration of premedication may be more useful in the outpatient setting because of faster onset.
   c. Premedication by intramuscular injection may be counterproductive because IM injection usually is the most painful, unpleasant event the child experiences and remembers during the entire period of hospitalization.

General Anesthesia

1. Anesthetic induction techniques vary with the child's age and his individual response or cooperation.
2. Anesthesia generally is induced with inhalation of halothane.
3. Intravenous attempts and intramuscular injections are unpleasant experiences according to hospitalized children.
4. Anesthesia usually is maintained with halothane or isoflurane in a nitrous oxide and oxygen mixture, but isoflurane has shown a higher incidence of coughing and breath holding.
5. Intravenous narcotics can be used either to decrease the required inhalational anesthetic or to act as an anesthetic with nitrous oxide and oxygen.

Regional Anesthesia

The commonly used regional blocks include ilioinguinal and iliohypogastric nerve block, or penile block by the surgeon. The anesthesiologist usually places the caudal block using bupivacaine 0.25%, 2 mg/kg, or lidocaine 0.5%, 5 mg/kg. This technique has been reported to be particularly effective after orchidopexy without delaying ambulation before discharge from the hospital. Details of the techniques and indications are discussed in Chapter 22.

Endotracheal Intubation

1. Indications for endotracheal intubation during ambulatory anesthesia do not differ from those for inpatient anesthesia.

2. In the neonate, endotracheal intubation and controlled ventilation are used.
3. For older children the relative risks of intubation such as sore throat, croup, and hoarseness must be weighed against the potential benefits of protecting the airway against aspiration.
4. No data are available on the incidence of complications directly related to endotracheal tube sizes and duration of anesthesia in the ambulatory setting.

Postoperative Care

Recovery

1. Postoperative care is the same as for inpatients.
2. Patients must awaken from anesthesia.
3. They should demonstrate stable vital signs, resume normal activity, and be able to swallow and retain oral fluids.
4. The expedient use of narcotics for pain may shorten the recovery period.
5. The routine use of a pulse oximeter for early detection of oxygen desaturation and supplying supplemental oxygen by mask is recommended.
6. Oral fluids should be offered gradually. Because thirst is not necessarily a sign of gastrointestinal activity, oral fluid should not be given until a child feels hungry.

Criteria for Discharge

1. Patient's condition assessed by an anesthesiologist
2. Age-appropriate level of alertness
3. Age-appropriate level of ambulation
4. Stable vital signs
5. Absence of vomiting
6. Tolerance of oral fluids
7. Absence of bleeding
8. Written instructions for postoperative care
9. Names and phone numbers of person to contact with questions

COMPLICATIONS AND ADMISSION

The overall incidence of complications may be as high as 35%, including vomiting, sleepiness, fever, sore throat, coughing, mild croup, and hoarseness. Nausea and vomiting are the most frequent complications.

1. The incidence of vomiting ranged from 41% after circumcision to 76% after strabismus repair in premedicated patients.
2. In unpremedicated patients, as many as 85% experience nausea and vomiting following nitrous oxide, oxygen, and halothane anesthesia for strabismus surgery.
3. Protracted vomiting accounts for one-third of the unscheduled overnight admissions.
4. Vomiting can be prevented by giving droperidol, 0.075 mg/kg, either at induction or 30 minutes before the end of surgery.

The rate of hospital admissions following ambulatory surgery was reported to be less than 1.0% in the United States. Besides severe vomiting, the reasons for unscheduled hospital admission include postoperative croup, fever, bleeding, sleepiness, family request, and surgical complications. When there is any doubt it is safest to admit the patient to the hospital for overnight observation.

SUMMARY

In pediatric ambulatory surgery and anesthesia the surgical procedure itself is considered relatively minor, but the anesthetic administration is not. Actually it demands more skillful hands.

BIBLIOGRAPHY

Abramowitz MD and others: The antiemetic effect of droperidol following outpatient strabismus surgery in children, Anesthesiology 59:579-583, 1983.

Berry FA: Pediatric outpatient anesthesia. In Hershey SG, editor: ASA Refresher Courses in Anesthesiology, 10:17, Philadelphia, 1982, JB Lippincott.

Brzustowicz RM and others: Efficacy of oral premedication for pediatric outpatient surgery, Anesthesiology 60:475, 1984.

Hannallah RS and others: Comparison of caudal and ilioinguinal/iliohypogastric nerve block for control of postorchiopexy pain in pediatric ambulatory surgery, Anesthesiology 66:832, 1987.

Kingston HGG: Halothane and isoflurane anesthesia in pediatric outpatients, Anesth Analg 65:181, 1986.

Kurth CD and others: Postoperative apnea in preterm infants, Anesthesiology 66:483, 1987.

Liu LMP and others: Life-threatening apnea in infants recovering from anesthesia, Anesthesiology 59:506, 1983.

Motoyama EK and Glazener CH: Hypoxemia after general anesthesia in children, Anesth Analg 65:267, 1986.

Patel RI and Hannallah RS: Anesthetic complications following pediatric ambulatory surgery: a 3 year study, Anesthesiology 69:1009, 1988.

Shandling B and Steward DJ: Regional analgesia for postoperative pain in pediatric outpatient surgery, J Pediatr Surg 15:477, 1980.

Steward DJ: Outpatient pediatric anesthesia, Anesthesiology 43:268, 1975.

22

PEDIATRIC PAIN MANAGEMENT

Stephen A. Eige
Charlotte Bell

They scooped up lots of snow
and rolled it round and round.
They built two forts and in between
was their battleground.

Suddenly a snowball
landed right on Ethan's head.
"I don't want to play.
I think I'm sick," he said.

MARGUERITE RUSH LERNER, M.D.
DEAR LITTLE MUMPS CHILD

EVALUATION OF PAIN IN CHILDREN

The perception of pain is primarily a subjective phenomenon, influenced by sensory and emotional input. What is perceived as pain by one individual is not necessarily perceived to the same degree, or even at all, by another, although the nociceptive reception may be the same for both. Both infants and children are like adults in that they appear to be subject to this basic tenet of pain perception.

Children's perception of their pain closely parallels their intellectual and social development. The ability to understand, quantitate, and communicate are key factors underlying the expression of pain. A preverbal child cannot articulate analgesic requirements.

Traditionally, the treatment of children has relied upon physiologic signs to determine analgesic requirements. More sophisticated methods by which the degree of pain in children can be quantitated are essential for determining when to initiate treatment and for evaluating its effectiveness. Three types of assessment techniques are available: self-reporting scales, behavioral observation scores, and physiologic monitoring.

Self-Reporting Scales

Self-reporting scales require that a child have sufficient cognitive ability to indicate degree of pain on a relative scale. These scales have been modified and put into a format children can understand. Comparison of scores before and after initiating treatment helps to determine any necessary adjustments in the treatment protocol. Three types of self-reporting scales are used.

1. Visual analog scale (VAS)

   No Pain |————————————————| Worst Pain

   The child is asked to mark the line at a point that corresponds to his or her pain. The VAS is easy to understand and may be useful with preschool children.

2. Numerical rating score (NRS)

   0 1 2 3 4 5 6 7 8 9 10

   The child is asked to choose the number that corresponds to the intensity of his or her pain. Because of the use of numbers, the NRS is best used in young school-age children or children who can count.

3. Graphic rating scales (GRS)
   - One scale employs a series of cartoon faces or photographs of children depicting a range of facial expressions from a sad or crying face to one that is happy or smiling. The child is asked to select the face that best describes his or her pain.
   - The Oucher scale is a type of GRS. It consists of a photographic progression of facial expressions on a number scale, with 0 representing no pain and 100 representing the worst pain (screaming child).
   - Another type of GRS presents children with an opportunity to choose from a range of colors the one that best represents their pain and to color a picture of a child that further describes their pain.

Behavioral Observation Scores

For preverbal children, behavioral observation scores can be used. These make the assumption, however, that certain behavior correlates with certain types and degrees of pain, a theory that has not been completely validated. See Table 22-1 for an example of a behaviorally based scoring system.

Physiologic Monitoring

Physiologic monitoring as a technique of pain assessment is based on the principle that the perception of pain initiates a stress response, which in turn triggers changes in the sympathoadrenal system.

Changes in heart rate, blood pressure, and respiration may represent increased sympathetic activity and are presumed to correlate with stress or discomfort.

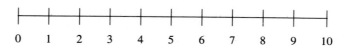

TABLE 22-1. Pain-discomfort scale based on behavioral observation

Observation	Criteria	Points
Blood pressure	Within 10% of preoperative value	0
	>20% of preoperative value	1
	>30% of preoperative value	2
Crying	No	0
	Crying but can be calmed	1
	Crying and cannot be calmed	2
Movement	None	0
	Restless	1
	Thrashing	2
Agitation	Asleep or calm	0
	Mild	1
	Localizing pain	2
Posture	Relaxed	0
	Flexing legs and thighs	1
	Localizing pain	2
Verbalization	Asleep or describes no pain	0
	Cannot localize	1
	Can localize	2

When total pain score exceeds 7 twice during a 5-minute period, increased analgesia is needed.

Adapted from Hannallah RS and others: Comparison of caudal and ilioinguinal/iliohypogastric nerve blocks for control of postorchiopexy pain in pediatric ambulatory surgery, Anesthesiology 66:832-34, 1987.

TREATMENT MODALITIES

Several therapeutic measures are employed for the management of pain in children. These include systemic drug therapy, regional techniques, and nonpharmacologic approaches.

SYSTEMIC DRUG THERAPY

Nonnarcotic Analgesics

- Nonnarcotic analgesics (Table 22-2) act peripherally to block afferent pain impulses, probably by inhibiting prostaglandin types of mediators.
- These drugs all have a ceiling of efficacy (i.e., dosing beyond the ceiling, or threshold, does not improve analgesia and may increase side effects).
- Nonnarcotic analgesics are useful for the treatment of mild to moderate pain or as adjuvant therapy to diminish narcotic side effects (nausea, pruritus, dysphoria). With the exception of acetaminophen, these agents are particularly useful for pain caused by inflammation.

Opioids (Table 22-3)

- Opioids are potent analgesics and provide an increased tolerance to pain.
- Side effects can be predicted on the basis of pain type, dose of drug

TABLE 22-2. Nonnarcotic analgesics in children

Oral agents	Dosages	Comments
Acetaminophen	10-15 mg/kg/dose q4h PO 10-20 mg/kg/dose q4h PR*	• Maximum 2,600 mg/24 hr or 120 mg/kg/day • Inconsistent rectal absorption • Nephropathy and hepatotoxicity not seen with short-term use
Aspirin	10-20 mg/kg/dose q4h PO	• Associated with Reye's syndrome • Side effects include gastritis and platelet dysfunction
Choline-magnesium salicylate (Trilisate)	10-15 mg/kg/dose q6-8h PO	• Questionable association with Reye's syndrome • Minimal effect on platelet dysfunction or gastric lining • Limited experience in young children
Ibuprofen (Motrin)	4-10 mg/kg/dose q6-8h PO	• May cause gastritis and platelet dysfunction • Nephrotoxicity and hepatotoxicity can occur with chronic use
Naprosyn (Naproxen)	5-7 mg/kg/dose q8-12h PO	• As with ibuprofen
Tolectin (Tolmetin)	5-7 mg/kg/dose q6-8h PO	• As with ibuprofen

*PR, per rectum; PO, per oral.
Data from Shannon and Berde (1989); Greene (1991).

TABLE 22-3. Narcotics for analgesia in children

Name	Relative potency	Dosage	Comments
Morphine	1	0.02-0.05 mg/kg IV 0.1-0.2 mg/kg/dose q2-4h IM	• Duration: Child 2-3 hr Neonate 14 hr
	1	0.3-0.5 mg/kg/dose q4h PO	• Enterohepatic circulation is important for elimination
Sustained-release morphine (MS-Cotin)	1	0.3-0.6 mg/kg/dose q12h PO	• Bid dosing useful in out-patient care
Hydromorphone (Dilaudid)	6	0.05-0.1 mg/kg/dose q6h PO (Max: 5 mg/dose)	• Possibly less dysphoria, nausea, vomiting
Meperidine (Demerol)	0.1	1-1.5 mg/kg/dose q4h PO, IM 0.1-0.25 mg/kg/dose IV	• Duration: Child 3-4 hr Neonate 24 hr • Risk of CNS toxicity from normeperidine metabolite accumulation • Increased euphoria, dysphoria
Fentanyl	80	1-1.5 μg/kg/dose q1-2h IV	• Duration: 3-4 hr
Methadone (Dolobid)	1 0.5	0.1 mg/kg/dose q6-12h IV 0.2 mg/kg/dose q6-12h PO	• Duration: 12-24 hr • Less sedation, nausea, and dysphoria than morphine
Propoxyphene (Oxycodone)	1	0.05-0.15 mg/kg/dose q4-5h PO	• Duration: 4-5 hr • Lower dependence liability
Codeine	0.8	0.5-1 mg/kg/dose q4-6h PO (Max: 5 mg/dose)	• Duration: 3-4 hr • High incidence of constipation

Data from Greene (1991); Koren and Maurice (1989).

administered, patient characteristics (including tolerance), and specific narcotics selected.

Administration

- Route of administration is determined by the needs of the patient.
- It is important to maintain continuous pain relief by avoiding decreases in plasma narcotic levels below the analgesic threshold through the following techniques (see Table 22-5 for techniques of maintaining continuous pain relief):
  1. Continuous infusions
  2. Avoidance of prn dosing (Although its occurrence is rare in children, addiction is much more likely when pain relief is not consistent.)
  3. Use of standard dosage guidelines for initial dosing only, and then dosing to effect
  4. Patient controlled analgesia (PCA)
  5. Increasing dosages gradually to compensate for physiologic tolerance and gradually tapering (10% to 20% daily), as pain subsides
  6. Use of long-acting agents such as methadone

Side Effects

- Anticipated side effects include pruritus, nausea and vomiting, constipation, and respiratory depression, all of which can be treated without discontinuing pain relief.
- Respiratory depression from opioid use can be detected by appropriate apnea monitoring and oximetry and should be anticipated in the following populations:
  1. Patients with acute or chronic respiratory dysfunction (e.g., cystic fibrosis, asthma)
  2. Patients receiving other sedatives such as benzodiazepines or barbiturates
  3. Neonates and premature infants
     a. Morphine has a prolonged elimination half-life in infants, particularly after abdominal surgery.
     b. The increased permeability of the blood:brain barrier in neonates permits more morphine to enter the brain.
     c. Narcotic administration may exacerbate the already depressed ventilatory response of neonates to hypoxia and hypercarbia.
     d. See box on p. 509 for neonatal narcotic dosages.
     e. Narcotics may be used in high doses in the anesthetic management of infants remaining intubated and mechanically ventilated. Hemodynamic stability and a lack of physiologic response to surgical stimulation have been shown with doses of fentanyl from 10 to 50 μg/kg.

Adjuvant Drugs

Also effective in the overall management of pain are some agents not commonly considered analgesics (Table 22-6). These include the tricyclic antidepressants, neuroleptics, anticonvulsants, corticosteroids, benzodiazepines, and some stimulants.

Text continued on p. 514.

RECOMMENDED NARCOTIC DOSAGES FOR NEONATES

Not intubated (requires apnea monitoring)

Morphine initial dose: 50 μg/kg IV
Morphine infusion: 10-15 μg/kg/hr IV

Intubated

Morphine infusion: 10-30 μg/kg/hr
Fentanyl infusion: 1-3 μg/kg/hr
Sufentanil infusion: 0.1-0.4 μg/kg/hr

TABLE 22-4. Drugs useful for managing narcotic side effects

Drug	Dose	Route	Side effect to be treated
Naloxone	0.5-1.0 μg/kg/hr 0.5-1.0 μg/kg/dose IV bolus, then 5-10 μg/kg/hr IV infusion	IV infusion	• Itching, urinary retention • Respiratory depression
Benadryl	1.25 mg/kg/dose	IV/IM	• Itching
Droperidol	10-20 μg/kg/dose 30-50 μg/kg/dose	IV IM	• Nausea and vomiting
Bethanecol	0.05 mg/kg/dose	SC	• Urinary retention

TABLE 22-5. Methods for maintenance of continuous analgesia in children with parenteral narcotics

Drug/technique	Initial loading dose	Maintenance	Weaning	Advantages	Disadvantages
Methadone	IV: 0.1 mg/kg in saline over 20 min: may repeat loading dose in 3 hr SC: 0.2 mg/kg	For IV, sliding scale, doses given q4-6h (*not* prn) unless patient is somnolent or shows signs of toxicity as follows: • Mild pain: 0.03 mg/kg in saline over 20 min • Moderate pain: 0.05 mg/kg in saline over 20 min • Severe pain: 0.07 mg/kg in saline over 20 min For SQ: 0.1 mg/kg q4-8h unless somnolent	• As methadone accumulates, dosing frequency is decreased to q6h, then q8h and q12h as tolerated. • In short courses of therapy, drug may be discontinued abruptly and will "self-wean" because of the long half-life.	• Long half-life (infrequent dosing, self-weaning) • Less euphoria and dysphoria than with other narcotics	• Potent respiratory depressant • Difficult to titrate because of prolonged time to onset
Morphine/PCA	Postoperative pain: 0.05-0.1 mg/kg IV (optional, based on narcotics received intraoperatively) Sickle cell crisis: 0.10-0.15 mg/kg IV	Postoperative pain: • Total hourly dose: 0.05-0.1 mg/kg/hr • Optional background infusion: ¼-⅓ of total hourly dose • PCA bolus: remaining hourly dose divided into equal doses at 6-15-min intervals			

		Sickle cell crisis: • Total hourly dose: As for postoperative pain • Background infusion: ⅔-¾ of total hourly dose • PCA bolus: As for postoperative pain [Promethazine (2-5 mg) may be added to 30 ml of morphine if needed for nausea and vomiting.]	• Decrease dose by 20%-30% on first 2 days and then 10%-20% daily.	• Less respiratory depression seen • High patient satisfaction • Many patients "self-wean" by decreasing dosage frequency	• Requires specialized equipment and training • Requires patient participation and cooperation
Continuous infusion					
Morphine	0.05-0.1 mg/kg IV	0.05-0.06 mg/kg/hr	As for morphine PCA	• Patient cooperation and participation not required • Easy to titrate to effect	• Potential for respiratory depression • Increased incidence of side effects (nausea, vomiting, constipation) • Frequent nursing and medical observation required
Fentanyl	1-1.5 μg/kg IV	2-4 μg/kg/hr	As for morphine PCA	As for continuous infusion morphine	As for continuous infusion morphine

Data from Berde (1989); Koren (1985).

TABLE 22-6. Adjuvant drugs useful in pediatric pain management

Drug class	Uses	Drug and dosages	Comments
Tricyclic antidepressants	• Decrease pain by central action on pain inhibitory systems • Improve sleep cycles • Improve mood	Amitriptyline (Elavil): 0.1 mg/kg qhs PO advanced as tolerated to 0.5-2 mg/kg Doxepin: As for amitriptyline Imipramine (Tofranil): 1.5 mg/kg/day tid PO	• Anticholinergic effects (morning somnolence and dry mouth) diminished by starting with small doses. • Contraindicated in patients with cardiac conduction defects • Imipramine causes photosensitization, lowers seizure threshold, and has lower metabolism in the presence of methylphenidate (Ritalin)
Stimulants	• Increase analgesia and decrease sedation caused by chronic use of opioids (e.g., cancer therapy) • Provide some euphoria	Methylphenidate: 0.1-0.3 mg/kg/dose bid PO Dextroamphetamine: 0.1-0.2 mg/kg/dose bid PO	• Given in early morning and midday to avoid nighttime insomnia
Neuroleptics	• Used with continuous opioid infusions to diminish nausea and increase sedation • May increase patient cooperation for single painful procedures when used with narcotics	Droperidol: 30-50 μg/kg/dose IM 10-30 μg/kg/dose IV	• May cause dysphoria, dystonic reactions, and hypotension (by α blockade)

Anticonvulsants	• Used for neuropathic pain (trigeminal neuralgia) and migraine • Appear to alter neuronal excitability	Phenytoin (Dilantin): modified adult doses used in older children Carbamazepine (Tegretol): as for phenytoin Clonazepam (Klonopin): as for phenytoin	• Side effects include sedation, ataxia, dysphoria, GI symptoms, and hepatotoxicity • Drug level must be monitored
Corticosteroids	• Relieve pain associated with swelling and inflammation	Dexamethasone: variable, as per patient requirements Hydrocortisone: as for dexamethasone Prednisone: as for dexamethrasone	• Dosage and route determined by patient's medical condition
Benzodiazepines	• Decrease anxiety when given as premedication • Provide amnesia • Most useful for very short-term use or for single procedures	Diazepam (Valium): as per patient requirements (see Chapter 4 for dosage guidelines) Midazolam (Versed): as for diazepam Lorazepam (Ativan): as for diazepam	• Increased respiratory depression when given with opioids • Do not provide analgesia • Lorazepam has antiemetic qualities and causes hallucinations in children under 6 years of age

REGIONAL TECHNIQUES

Indications

- Regional anesthesia may be used in the following populations without concurrent general anesthesia or heavy sedation:
  1. Premature infants at risk for postoperative apnea undergoing lower abdominal or lower extremity operations (most commonly, inguinal herniorrhaphy)
  2. Older children with significant neuromuscular or pulmonary disease in whom general anesthesia may substantially worsen respiratory dysfunction (e.g., cystic fibrosis or muscular dystrophy)
  3. Children with a history of malignant hyperthermia (MH) or at risk for MH
  4. Older children who fear loss of consciousness and have the ability to cooperate during a regional technique
- Regional blockade may be placed during general anesthesia to decrease intraoperative anesthetic requirements and postoperative pain (e.g., caudal with local anesthetic and/or narcotics).

Contraindications

- The use of regional techniques should be limited by the technical expertise of the anesthesiologist.
- If the duration of blockade is intended to last beyond the operative period, skilled personnel must be available on a 24-hour basis to manage any complications that may arise.
- Consent of the parent(s) (and patient, if age appropriate) must be obtained before the procedure.
- Regional techniques should usually be avoided in patients with coagulopathy, infection, or anatomic abnormalities at the site of injection, severe hypovolemia or poorly controlled seizures (seizure threshold may be lowered with local anesthetics).

Preparation for Placement of Regional Blockade

Whether for intraoperative anesthesia, chronic pain, or procedures out of the operating room, the following are required for placement of regional blockade:

- NPO status and the absence of airway abnormalities that could prevent the airway from being rapidly secured if necessary
- Standard monitoring of cardiorespiratory function during the procedure and recovery
- Intravenous access
- Resuscitative capability, including suction, oxygen, circuits (mask and intubation equipment), and emergency drugs

Pharmacologic Principles of Local Anesthetics in Children

- Because of decreased albumin in the infant less than 2 months of age, less bupivacaine will be bound to protein, which results in higher concentrations of free drug.
- Although infants less than 6 months of age have lower levels of plasma cholinesterase, there seems to be little effect on the duration of ester anesthetics.
- The effects of incomplete myelination on local anesthetic activity in infants less than 1 year of age are unknown.
- Maximum doses of lidocaine (Table 22-7) are identical for infants and adults despite the infant's increased volume of distribution and lowered hepatic metabolism.

TABLE 22-7. Maximum recommended doses of local anesthetics commonly used in children

	Injection dose	
Drug	**Plain**	**With epinephrine**
Tetracaine	1.5 mg/kg	1.5 mg/kg
Chloroprocaine	8.5 mg/kg	9 mg/kg
Procaine	7 mg/kg	8.5 mg/kg
Lidocaine	4 mg/kg	7 mg/kg
Bupivacaine	2.5 mg/kg	3.6 mg/kg

From Scott DB and Cousins MJ: Clinical pharmacology of local anesthetic agents. In Cousins MJ and Bridenbaugh CO, editors: Neural blockade in clinical anesthesia and management of pain, Philadelphia, 1980, JB Lippincott Co. With permission.

Spinal Anesthesia

Isobaric Bupivacaine 0.5%

Patient selection

- Procedures at or below T_{10}
- Infants less than 6 months of age with weight between 1.5 and 7 kg

Technique

- The infant is placed in lateral decubitus position, with the chin extended for optimal ventilation.

- A 22-gauge, 3.5- or 4-cm spinal needle is placed in the L_4 to L_5 interspace using a 1-ml tuberculin syringe for injection.
- To allow for dead space in the needle, 0.04 ml of additional anesthetic is added to the syringe.
- Anesthetic loss through the needle track may be minimized by leaving needle and syringe in place for 5 seconds after injection.

Dosages

- No clinically significant change in level, duration of block, or hemodynamics with or without epinephrine has been reported.

Weight	Dosage
<2 kg	1.25 mg or 0.25 ml
2-5 kg	3.75 mg or 0.75 ml
>5 kg	5.0 mg or 1 ml

Parameters

- T_1 to T_6 level within 10 minutes of injection
- Complete motor blockade of a 70- to 80-minute duration
- 15% to 20% decrease in heart rate and 20% to 25% decrease in blood pressure

Hyperbaric Tetracaine 0.5 %

Patient selection

- As for isobaric bupivacaine

Technique

- As for isobaric bupivacaine

Dosages

- Solution: 1% tetracaine plus equal volume of D_{10} to yield 0.5% solution
- Preterm infants: 0.8 to 1 mg/kg (T_2 level)
- Less than 1 year of age: 0.2 to 0.5 mg/kg (T_4 level)
- Over 1 year of age: 0.2 mg/kg (T_4 level)

Parameters

- Sensory level achieved of T2 to T4
- Onset of motor blockade within 2 minutes
- Duration of motor blockade:
  - With epinephrine: average of 110 min (range: 80-145 min)
  - Without epinephrine: average of 80 min (range: 50-135 min)
- No reports of hypotension or bradycardia in children less than 3 years of age

Lumbar Epidural Blockade

Indications (see also box on the next page for advantages and disadvantages)

1. To reduce anesthetic requirements for thoracic or abdominal procedures
2. To provide postoperative analgesia for thoracic, lumbar, and sacral dermatomes
3. As part of the management of chronic pain syndromes, including reflex sympathetic dystrophy of the lower extremities and neoplasias of the thorax, abdomen, and lower extremities

ADVANTAGES AND DISADVANTAGES OF EPIDURAL BLOCKADE IN CHILDREN

Advantages

- Provides analgesia for thoracic, lumbar, and sacral dermatomes
- Easily reinforced through an indwelling catheter
- Early ambulation
- Shorter recovery time
- Diminished narcotic requirement
- Fewer pulmonary complications than with systemic analgesics
- Improved postoperative pulmonary function
- Can provide muscle relaxation if necessary
- Prevents hemodynamic instability by avoiding the variations in analgesia seen with intermittent IM injections

Disadvantages

- Technically difficult to perform in children because of the shallow epidural space
- Necessity for concurrent general anesthesia or sedation
- Increased risk of intrathecal block
- Risk of air embolism with LOR technique
- Risk of spinal cord trauma
- Complications of technique (headache, intravascular injection, catheter migration, epidural abscess or hematoma)
- Complications of neuraxis agents (motor blockade, paresthesias, urinary retention, pruritus, respiratory depression)

4. To provide analgesia and immobilization of the lower extremities (as for orthopedic procedures)

Contraindications

1. Treatment of lesions above T_2 to T_4
2. Local or systemic infection
3. Coagulopathy
4. Hemodynamic instability
5. Presence of a neurologic disease that may be exacerbated by conduction blocks (e.g., multiple sclerosis)

Technique

1. General anesthesia is induced except with highly cooperative, older children or adolescents.
2. Sterile preparation and draping are performed with the patient in the lateral decubitus position.
3. 18- or 19-gauge Tuohy needles with 20- or 21-gauge catheters are commonly used; 20- or 22-gauge needles with 23- or 27-gauge catheters are available for use in smaller children.
4. The catheter is placed by a loss of resistance (LOR) technique using air or saline. Although it may dilute the small volume of anesthetic, saline minimizes the risk of air emboli.
5. Either the L_3 to L_4 or the L_4 to L_5 interspace is selected because they are below the termination of the spinal cord.

Dosages and Solutions

- Bupivacaine 0.5% with epinephrine 1:200,000 is commonly selected to provide prolonged analgesia. The use of 0.25% bupivacaine will decrease total dosage and decrease incidence of motor block.
- Initial loading dose: 0.5 ml/kg; supplementary doses: 0.25 ml/kg.
- Bolus dose for postoperative pain relief: bupivacaine 0.25% plus epinephrine 1:200,000, 0.5 ml/kg q6-8h as needed.
- Continuous infusion: bupivacaine 0.125% plus epinephrine 1:200,000 at 0.04 to 0.06 ml/kg/hr (may cause urinary retention or motor blockade).

Complications

- Intrathecal injection
- Intravascular injection
- Headache from continued CSF leak
- Migration of catheter
- Epidural abscess or hematoma
- Paresthesia
- Urinary retention
- Retained catheter

Caudal Blockade

Indications (See also box below for advantages and disadvantages)

1. Intraoperative analgesia
   - Caudal blockade can markedly decrease (or eliminate) general anesthesia requirements for procedures of the sacral dermatomes (urologic procedures).

ADVANTAGES AND DISADVANTAGES OF CAUDAL BLOCKADE IN CHILDREN

Advantages

- Provides excellent analgesia for sacral and lower lumbar dermatomes
- Abdominal and thoracic levels of analgesia may be achieved with larger volumes of the drug
- Indwelling catheter can be placed for continuous use
- Technically easy to perform in children
- Improved recovery time
- Early ambulation
- Long history of safe and efficacious use

Disadvantages

- Children usually require general anesthesia for placement
- Requires a large volume of drug to provide thoracic analgesia
- Complications of technique:
  -Injection into adjacent structures: intravascular, intrathecal, intraosseous, intracolonic, intravesicular
  -Infection
  -Hematoma
- Complications of neuraxis agents:
  -Motor blockade
  -Urinary retention
  -Paresthesias

2. Postoperative analgesia
   - A single-dose caudal block using local anesthetics placed intraoperatively can provide postoperative analgesia. The duration of analgesia may be prolonged by the use of morphine in combination with low-dose local anesthetics.
   - Caudal catheters for continuous infusion have been described but carry a significant risk of infection because of proximity to the anus.

Contraindications

- Local or systemic infection
- Coagulopathy
- Immunocompromise

Technique

1. General anesthesia is induced.
2. The block may be placed with the patient placed in either the prone, lateral decubitus, or knee-chest position.
3. The sacral area is sterilely prepared and draped.
4. The sacral cornua and sacral hiatus are identified by palpation.
5. A "no-touch" technique can be used, whereby an alcohol wipe is placed under the examiner's thumb at the sacral hiatus.
6. The needle is advanced through the hiatus in the midline between the cornua at a 45 degree angle, bevel down (Fig. 22-1, *A*).
7. After "popping through" the sacrococcygeal ligament, the needle-to-skin angle is reduced so that the needle is advanced 2 to 3 mm into the caudal canal parallel to the spinal axis (Fig. 22-1, *B*).
8. A test dose of 0.1 ml/kg is injected before the remaining volume.
9. The palpating thumb remains over the sacrum during injection (after aspirating for blood and spinal fluid). In this manner, subcutaneous in-

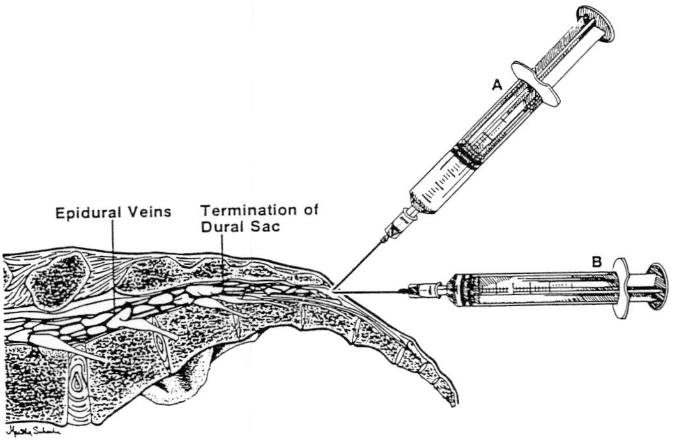

Fig. 22-1. Technique of caudal block insertion (see text). (With permission. Broadman LM: ASA Refresher Courses, vol 14, pp 43-60, 1986.)

jection can be immediately recognized because a bleb is raised under the thumb.

Dosages and Solutions

1. Bupivacaine 0.25% with or without epinephrine 1:200,000 in dosages of 0.05 ml/kg/segment.
2. Alternatively:
   - 0.35 ml/kg for a T_{12} to L_1 level
   - 0.5 to 0.75 ml/kg for a T_{10} level
   - 0.75 to 1.25 ml/kg for a T_4 to T_5 level
   - For children over 20 kg in weight and 100 cm in height: 1 ml/10 cm of height. (Use of the lumbar epidural route for larger children reduces the necessary quantity of local anesthetic.)
   - Infants less than 2 to 2.5 kg: a more dilute solution is used (0.125%), and volume can be increased to 1.5 ml/kg.

Neuraxis Opioids

See Tables 22-8 and 22-9 for doses and complications.

- Fentanyl, morphine, and sufentanil have been administered intrathecally or by either caudal or epidural techniques. They can be given in single bolus doses or by continuous infusion.
- Depending on the characteristics of the drug, pain relief can be obtained for varying periods of time without motor or sympathetic blockade.
- Children over 1 year of age receiving single-dose narcotics through spinal or epidural routes require apnea monitoring (preferably with oximetry) because of the risk of respiratory depression.
- Infants and children receiving continuous narcotic infusions into the neuraxis, and patients with preexisting medical problems should be monitored in the intensive care unit. Infants less than 1 year of age receiving a single-dose neuraxis narcotic may also be considered for ICU monitoring.

Peripheral Nerve Blockade (See Table 22-10 for techniques)

Basic principles of peripheral nerve blockade include the following:

- Epinephrine usually increases duration of blockade but should never be used with terminal circulation (e.g., penis).
- Volume and dose of anesthetic should never exceed toxic doses (e.g., bupivacaine, 2.5 mg/kg, lidocaine with epinephrine, 7 mg/kg).

NONPHARMACOLOGIC APPROACHES

Psychologic Intervention

Hypnotherapy

- Self-hypnosis or relaxation imagery is a technique by which the child induces different mental images in order to achieve an alternate state of awareness during periods of pain.
- Biofeedback systems provide the child with instant reports of his or her progress while learning to use relaxation imagery.
- These techniques are particularly useful for children who must undergo repeated procedures involving minor discomfort or who are in chronic pain.

TABLE 22-8. Neuraxis opioids for analgesia in children

Mode of delivery/drug	Dosage	Volume	Comments
Intrathecal morphine	0.01-0.025 mg/kg	As small as possible; less than 1 ml in children under 12 yrs	• High incidence of complications (about 50%) • Not indicated for infants and small children
Caudal morphine	0.03-0.05 mg/kg with bupivacaine 0.25% and epinephrine 1:200,000	Sacral levels: 0.5 ml/kg *or* 0.05 ml/kg/segment	• Respiratory depression reported with doses of 0.1 mg/kg
Epidural morphine (administered via lumbar space)	**Single dose** • Abdominal or lower extremities: 50 μg/kg • Thoracotomy: 120-150 μg/kg	0.05-0.056 ml/kg/segment	• Duration: 8-24 hr
	Infusion Bupivacaine 0.1% + morphine 0.1 mg/ml	0.1 ml/kg/hr	• Continuous levels of analgesia achieved
Epidural fentanyl	0.5-1 μg/kg single dose	0.05 ml/kg/segment	• Duration: 3-4 hr • Lipid solubility may necessitate higher volume of injectate to achieve levels similar to morphine
Epidural sufentanil	0.75 μg/kg single dose	0.05 ml/kg/segment	• Duration: 2 hr • High lipid solubility suggests continuous infusion will be more effective for long-term analgesia

Data from Broadman (1987); Krane, Tyler, and Jacobson (1989); Attia (1986); Benlabed (1987).

TABLE 22-9. Complications of neuraxis opioids

Complication	Treatment
Respiratory depression	• Maintain airway, ventilation with 100% oxygen • Naloxone 0.5-1 μg/kg IV bolus, repeated as needed • Then, naloxone infusion 3-5 μg/kg/hr IV
Nausea, vomiting	• Droperidol 10-30 μg/kg IV/IM *or* • Naloxone infusion 0.5-1 μg/kg/hr IV (low-dose)
Pruritus	• Diphenhydramine 1.25 mg/kg/dose • Naloxone infusion 0.5-1 μg/kg/hr IV (low-dose)
Urinary retention	• Naloxone infusion 0.5-1 μg/kg/hr IV • Bethanacol 0.05 mg/kg/dose SC • If still unable to void, straight catheterization is indicated for single-dose opioids • Indwelling urinary catheter may be necessary for patients on continuous epidural narcotic infusions

Behavior Therapy

- Desensitization exposes the child gradually to a painful procedure through a series of progressive steps designed to ready the child for the procedure. Sufficient time must be available before the procedure for adequate preparation.
- The term *positive reinforcement* implies the promise of a reward for the child who is cooperative during a painful procedure.

Acupuncture

Although acupuncture has gained respect for use in adult pain syndromes, its reported use in pediatrics is anecdotal.

Transcutaneous Electrical Nerve Stimulation (TENS)

General Principles

- Analgesia provided by the transmission of pulsed electricity to nerves, through electrodes attached to the skin, is gaining limited use in pediatrics, particularly with older children and adolescents.
- TENS units are available with three adjustable variables: rate, pulse width, and amplitude.
- There are five basic modes of transmission: conventional; high width, low rate; high rate, high width and amplitude; burst; and modulation.
- An effect is seen in approximately 15 to 20 minutes.

Indications

- After thoracotomies, repair of pectus excavatum or carinatum, and in chronic pain syndromes
- May significantly diminish postoperative narcotic requirement

TABLE 22-10. Peripheral nerve blocks for pediatric patients

Location	Indications	Drug	Dose	Technique	Comments
Ilioinguinal (L_1) or iliohypogastric (T_{12}, L_1)	• Urogenital surgery • Inguinal herniorrhaphy	Bupivacaine 0.25%	0.4 ml/kg	1. A 22-gauge needle is placed 1 cm medial and 1 cm caudal to the anterior superior iliac spine, above the inguinal ligament, deep to the internal and external oblique muscles. 2. Anesthetic is injected in a fanlike pattern as the needle is withdrawn.	• Useful for infants; not suitable in older children because the incision is above the level of these nerves. • Decreases requirements for general anesthesia intraoperatively. • Provides postoperative analgesia.
Femoral-obturator-lateral femoral cutaneous block (paravascular 3-in-1 block)	• Surgery on the anterior aspect of thigh above the knee • Useful for muscle biopsy in MH-susceptible patients • Femur fractures	Bupivacaine 0.5%	0.4 ml/kg	1. A 22-gauge needle is placed below the inguinal ligament lateral to the pulsation of the femoral artery in a 30- to 45-degree cephalad direction. 2. After negative aspiration, digital pressure is applied distal to needle placement during injection to direct anesthetic in a cephalad direction. 3. Use of a nerve stimulator is helpful for needle placement.	• Potential complications include intravascular injection, hematoma, and nerve injury.

Continued.

TABLE 22-10. Peripheral nerve blocks for pediatric patients—cont'd

Location	Indications	Drug	Dose	Technique	Comments
Sciatic nerve block	• Foot and ankle surgery	Bupivacaine 0.5%	0.15-0.2 ml/kg	Posterior approach (Sim's position): 1. A line is drawn between the greater trochanter and posterior superior iliac spine (A). 2. A second line (B) is drawn perpendicular to (A) at its midpoint. 3. A third line (C) is drawn from the greater trochanter to the sacral hiatus or tip of the coccyx. 4. A 25-gauge (3.5-inch) spinal needle is inserted at the point where line B crosses line C until a paresthesia radiating to the foot is obtained, or the foot moves if a nerve stimulator is being used.	• Complications include intravascular injection and nerve injury.

Axillary block of the brachial plexus	• Forearm and hand surgery	Bupivacaine 0.25% *or* lidocaine 0.5% + tetracaine 0.2% with epinephrine	0.3-0.5 ml/kg	1. The arm is abducted and externally rotated. 2. A 22-gauge needle is inserted at the site of axillary artery pulsation until a paresthesia is elicited or movement noted by use of the nerve stimulator.	• Complications include intravascular injection, hematoma, and nerve injury.
Penile ring block	• Circumcision • Hypospadias repair	Bupivacaine 0.25% (plain)	Volume limited to the amount that results in a circumferential skin wheal	Subcutaneous circumferential infiltration at base of penis	• Minimizes complications of dorsal nerve block, including intravascular injection and hematoma formation deep to the fascia, with arterial compression causing distal ischemia. • Compression and ischemia may still result from a large volume of drug injected subcutaneously.

Continued.

TABLE 22-10. Peripheral nerve blocks for pediatric patients—cont'd

Location	Indications	Drug	Dose	Technique	Comments
Intercostal block	• Thoracotomy • Rib fractures	Bupivacaine 0.25-0.5% with epinephrine 1:200,000	2 ml per rib	*Posterior approach* (for thoracotomy incisions) 1. The needle is inserted lateral to the sacrospinous muscles with the patient in the lateral decubitus position. 2. The needle is inserted perpendicular to the rib and "walked off" the caudal edge. 3. A pop is usually felt after inserting the needle an additional 1 or 2 cm. 4. The anesthetic is injected after negative inspiration. 5. The rib above and below must also be blocked.	• Improves pulmonary function tests after thoracotomy. • Usually several levels must be blocked to provide analgesia for thoracotomy incision. • Complications include pneumothorax and local anesthetic toxicity because large volumes of drug are injected.

Data from Sethna and Berde (1989); Ecoffey (1990).

Technique

- Two electrodes are placed parallel to the incision, 1 to 6 cm apart, before being covered with sterile dressing.
- The TENS unit is disconnected, the mode set, and the amplitude adjusted until muscle twitches are seen, at which point it is decreased until the muscle movement ends.

Possible Mechanisms

Gate theory. Stimulation of α neurons inhibits impulses from unmyelinated C and A delta fibers.

Endogenous opiate theory. Electrical stimulation causes increased production of endogenous endorphins.

Frequency-dependent conduction block theory. A pain-transmitting neuron can be blocked by increasing the frequency of an external impulse more rapidly than the ionic channels can respond and produce an action potential. If no action potential is produced, no pain is felt.

BIBLIOGRAPHY

Abajian JC, Melish RWP, and Brown AF: Clinical reports: spinal anesthesia for surgery in the high-risk infant, Anesth Analg 63:359-62, 1984.

Anand KJS and Hickey PR: Pain and its effect in the human neonate and fetus, N Engl J Med 317:1321-29, 1987.

Attia J and others: Epidural morphine in children: pharmacokinetics and CO_2 sensitivity, Anesthesiology 65:590-94, 1986.

Benlabed M and others: Analgesia and ventilatory response to CO_2 following epidural sufentanil in children, Anesthesiology 67:948-51, 1987.

Berde CB: Pediatric postoperative pain management. In Schechter NL, editor: Acute pain in children, Pediatr Clin North Am 36:921-40, 1989.

Berde CB, Anand KS, and Sethna NF: Pediatric pain management. In Gregory GA, editor: Pediatric anesthesia, vol 2, ed 2, New York, 1989, Churchill Livingstone.

Beyer JE and Wells N: The assessment of pain in children. In Schechter NL, editor: Acute pain in children, Pediatr Clin North Am 36:837-54, 1989.

Broadman LM and Rice LJ: Pediatric regional anesthesia and perioperative analgesia, Problems in anesthesia, 2:386-407, 1988.

Broadman LM and others: Intraoperative subarachnoid morphine for postoperative pain control following Harrington rod instrumentation in children, Can J Anaesth 34:S96, 1987.

Ecoffey C: Regional anesthesia techniques in children. In Tyler DC and Krane EJ, editors: Advances in pain research and therapy, vol. 15, Pediatric pain, New York, 1990, Raven Press.

Gleason CA and others: Optimal position for a spinal tap in preterm infants, Pediatrics 71:31-35, 1983.

Glenski JA and others: Postoperative use of epidurally administered morphine in children and adolescents, Mayo Clin Proc 59:530-33, 1984.

Greene MG, editor: Harriet Lane handbook, ed 12, St Louis, 1991, Mosby–Year Book.

Hannallah RS and others: Comparison of caudal and ilioinguinal/iliohypogastric blocks for control of post-orchiopexy pain in pediatric ambulatory surgery, Anesthesiology 66:832, 1987.

Hinkle AJ and Koka BU: Transcutaneous electrical stimulation after thoracic surgery in children, Reg Anaesth 8:163-65, 1983.

Koehntop DE and others: Pharmacokinetics of fentanyl in neonates, Anesth Analg 65:227-31, 1986.

Koren G and Maurice L: Pediatric uses of opioids, Pediatr Clin North Am 36:1141-56, 1989.

Koren G and others: Postoperative morphine infusion in newborn infants: assessment of disposition characteristics and safety, J Pediatr 107:963-67, 1985.

Krane EJ: Delayed respiratory depression in a child after caudal epidural morphine, Anesth Analg 67:79-82, 1988.

Krane EJ, Tyler DC, and Jacobson LE: The dose response of caudal morphine in children, Anesthesiology 71:48-52, 1989.

Mahe V and Ecoffey C: Clinical reports: spinal anesthesia with isobaric marcaine in infants, Anesthesiology 68:601-3, 1988.

Miser AW and Miser J: The treatment of cancer pain in children, Pediatr Clin North Am 36(4):990, 1989.

Olness K: Hypnotherapy: a cyberphysiologic strategy in pain management. In Schechter NL, editor: Pediatr Clin North Am 36:873-84, 1989.

Rodgers BM and others: Patient controlled analgesia in children, J Pediatr Surg 23:259-62, 1988.

Ronchi L and others: Femoral nerve blockade in children using bupivacaine, Anesthesiology 70:622-24, 1989.

Rothstein P and others: Bupivacaine for intercostal nerve blocks in children: blood concentration and pharmacokinetics, Anesth Analg 65:625-32, 1986.

Scott DB and Cousins MJ: Clinical pharmacology of local anesthetic agents. In Cousins MJ and Bridenbaugh CO, editors: Neural blockade in clinical anesthesia and management of pain, Philadelphia, 1980, JB Lippincott Co.

Sethna NF and Berde CB: Pediatric regional anesthesia. In Gregory GA, editor: Pediatric anesthesia, vol 1, ed 2, New York, 1989, Churchill Livingstone.

Shannon M and Berde CB: Pharmacologic management of pain in children and adolescents, Pediatr Clin North Am 36:855-72, 1989.

Stang HJ and others: Local anesthesia for neonatal circumcision: effects on distress and cortisol response, JAMA 259:1507-11, 1988.

Yaster M: The dose responses of fentanyl in neonatal anesthesia, Anesthesiology 66:433-35, 1987.

Zeltzer LK, Jay SM, and Fisher DM: The management of pain associated with pediatric procedures. In Schechter NL, editor: Pediatr Clin North Am 36:941-64, 1989.

23

MALIGNANT HYPERTHERMIA

Jonathan D. Halevy

The next day Michael's temperature was normal.
He really didn't seem sick.
BUT THE DAY AFTER THAT
the thermometer shot way past 98 point six.
MARGUERITE RUSH LERNER, M.D.
MICHAEL GETS THE MEASLES

DESCRIPTION

Malignant hyperthermia (MH) is a rare and serious clinical syndrome of great relevance to anesthesiologists. It is the only clinical entity specifically related to and caused by anesthetic agents. The disorder is an acute hypermetabolic state of skeletal muscle (skeletal muscle is approximately 40% of body weight), resulting in increased oxygen consumption, lactate accumulation, and heat production. The exact cellular mechanism or defect is unknown.

MH is of particular concern to the pediatric anesthesiologist because of its increased incidence in children and because of the association between MH and many of the musculoskeletal disorders that are more prevalent in children.

Incidence

Children	=	1:15,000
Adults	=	1:50,000

The increased incidence in children may be a reflection of the age at which surgery is first performed; or because many of the associated neuromuscular disorders are more prevalent in children. Also, anesthesia in children is more often induced with halothane and succinylcholine than in adults, a combination that is particularly effective at triggering malignant hyperthermia.

Etiology

MH is an inherited disorder, originally described as having autosomal dominant inheritance. It is now known that MH shows both variable penetrance and expression and that two to three genes are responsible for transmitting the disease.

Associated Disorders (See the box below)

The only syndrome uniformly associated with MH is the King-Denborough syndrome (short stature, growth retardation, and musculoskeletal abnormalities). Other disorders involving the musculoskeletal system have had an inconstant association with MH, with Duchenne's muscular dystrophy being described most commonly and consistently.

DISORDERS ASSOCIATED WITH MH

King-Denborough syndrome
Muscular dystrophy (MD)
Duchenne's MD
Myotonia congenita
Central core disease
Schwartz-Jampel syndrome
Sudden infant death syndrome (SIDS)
Neurolept malignant syndrome
Heat stroke
Caffeine sensitivity (in adults)
Ptosis
Kyphosis
Scoliosis
Pes excavatum
Club foot
Recurrent hip dislocation
Osteogenesis imperfecta
Arthrogryposis
Strabismus
Congenital hernias (inguinal, umbilical, diaphragmatic)

Triggering Agents

Agents which elicit the clinical manifestations of MH are called triggering agents (see Table 23-1 for triggering agents and the box on the next page for agents whose use is controversial). To date the halogenated agents and succinylcholine are the anesthetic drugs that are known to trigger MH. The exact mechanism for this remains unclear. Nonpharmacologic factors that trigger MH include anxiety, stress, and fatigue. Reports of the full syndrome in humans without anesthetic triggers are rare.

PATHOPHYSIOLOGY

1. The biochemical changes that occur with MH are present only in the skeletal muscle and hematopoietic system. However, the effects of this biochemical error may be seen in multiple organ systems.

ANESTHETIC TRIGGERS FOR MH

Triggering agents	Nontriggering agents
Halothane	Anticholinesterases
Enflurane	Barbiturates
Isoflurane	Narcotics
Succinylcholine	Nitrous oxide
Decamethonium	Benzodiazepines
	Pancuronium
	Vecuronium
	Atracurium
	Althesin
	Etomidate
	Ester local anesthetics

TABLE 23-1. Controversial agents for use in MH patients

Ketamine, phenothiazines	Do not trigger MH, but affect temperature regulation and sympathetic tone and may confuse the clinical diagnosis
Droperidol	May precipitate neurolept malignant syndrome, clinically similar to MH; Also may prevent a positive test result in muscle biopsy
Anticholinergics	Cause hyperpyrexia (by preventing sweating) and tachycardia that confuses the clinical diagnosis
Lidocaine	Originally thought to increase intracellular calcium, it is now considered safe in MH patients by most experts

2. The precipitating cellular event is a marked increase in intracellular ionized calcium—up to eight times normal resting levels—and blockage of calcium reuptake (see Table 23-2 for effects of elevated calcium in MH).
   a. The rise in ionized calcium may be caused by a defect in the sarcoplasmic reticulum, mitochondria, sarcolemma, or transverse tubule.
   b. Neuromuscular transmission is unaffected.
   c. Skeletal muscle cells also may have a decreased contracture threshold response.
3. Increased intracellular calcium combines with troponin, forming the actin-myosin cross-bridges that initiate MH muscle "contracture" (nonpropagated and prolonged, unlike normal contraction). Rigidity may result.
4. Continuous muscle contracture requires constant energy infusion supplied by means of ATP.
   a. Activation of glycogenolysis and phosphorylase kinase produce ATP and heat.
   b. The muscle enters into a hypermetabolic state that exhausts aerobic metabolism.

TABLE 23-2. Effects of elevated calcium in MH

Mechanism		Effect
Ionized intracellular Ca^{++} combines with troponin	→	Contractures of skeletal muscle
Glycogenolysis and phosphorylase kinase systems are activated to increase ATP production	→	Exhaustion of aerobic metabolism and conversion to anaerobic metabolism
Hypermetabolic state	→	Increased: • O_2 consumption • CO_2 production • Heat production
Altered muscle membrane permeability and rhabdomyolysis	→	Cellular efflux of: • Potassium • Calcium • Myoglobin • Sodium • CPK

c. Anaerobic metabolism begins with lactate accumulation and hyperpyrexia.
d. Accelerated metabolism results in the following:
- Increased oxygen consumption
- Increased CO_2 production
- Increased heat production

e. Massive muscle edema results in increased membrane permeability and rhabdomyolysis, causing the following problems:
- Hyperkalemia
- Hypercalcemia
- Myoglobinuria
- Elevated CPK
- Hypernatremia

CLINICAL SYNDROME

MH may be seen as an acute fulminant episode or it may develop slowly in the postoperative period. The multiple organ involvement that defines the clinical syndrome is secondary to the skeletal muscle hypermetabolism and injury.

Signs and Symptoms (See the box on the next page)

Cardiovascular

Tachycardia. Tachycardia is often one of the earliest signs of MH. Other more common causes of tachycardia should be excluded before the diagnosis of MH is considered, such as: light anesthesia, hypercarbia, hypoxemia, hypovolemia, and use of anticholinergic or sympathomimetic agents.
Arrhythmias. Arrhythmias associated with MH are caused by sympathetic stimulation and increased $PaCO_2$. Premature ventricular contractions (PVCs)

CLINICAL FEATURES OF MH

Tachycardia
Tachypnea
Arrhythmias
Hypercarbia
Hemodynamic instability
Hyperpyrexia
Cyanosis
Masseter spasm
Dark blood in surgical field
Muscle rigidity
Rash
Renal failure

and ventricular tachycardia (VT) are common. As hyperkalemia develops the ECG may show peaked T waves and widening QRS.

Hemodynamic instability. Initially there is a rise in blood pressure from excess sympathetic stimulation. However, as MH progresses hypotension may develop secondary to cardiac depression from severe acidosis, conduction abnormalities, and hyperkalemia.

Respiratory

Hypercarbia. Marked elevations in CO_2 production occur with skeletal muscle hypermetabolism. As a result, tachypnea is one of the earliest signs of MH in spontaneously breathing patients. Patients ventilated mechanically will exhibit a rapid rise in end-tidal CO_2, despite attempts to increase minute ventilation. In a semi-closed circle system, the CO_2 absorber becomes very hot due to accelerated exothermic reaction, and the color indicator will change quickly as the canister becomes exhausted. If hypercarbia is not present the diagnosis of MH is questionable.

Pulmonary edema. Pulmonary edema is a late event caused by cardiac decompensation and shifts in intravascular fluids.

Cyanosis. Cyanosis may occur from inability to keep up with oxygen requirements or from cardiorespiratory failure and circulatory collapse.

Cutaneous

Rash. A rash (reddish to mottled purple) frequently is observed about the head, neck, and upper thorax.

Diaphoresis. As the patient's temperature climbs, normal modes of heat loss, such as diaphoresis, take place.

Body Temperature

Body temperature usually rises in response to the increased metabolic state and not because of a defect in central thermoregulation. Heat production may not be apparent as hyperpyrexia if it does not exceed heat-loss mechanisms (cold room, large exposed surgical field, diaphoresis, or use of cardiopulmonary bypass).

Central Nervous System

CNS involvement including cerebral edema, permanent coma, or paralysis have been reported as late events with MH, usually caused by cerebral hypoxia and ischemia.

Renal

Renal failure is usually a consequence of tubular inspissation of myoglobin with inadequate renal perfusion. The osmotic diuresis caused by the mannitol present in dantrolene sodium (150 mg of mannitol/mg of dantrolene) will help prevent this sequela.

Hematologic

MH patients have direct involvement of the hematopoietic system both by increased red blood cell fragility and by a change in platelet infrastructure. Disseminated intravascular coagulation is often a late complication of profound rhabdomyolysis or hemolysis, or can be caused by release of tissue thromboplastin during shock and periods of stasis.

Neuromuscular

Muscle rigidity. Rigidity frequently is observed with MH and simply reflects contractures of the muscles. This finding should not be confused with normal muscle contraction caused by end-plate stimulation with acetylcholine. Neuromuscular blocking agents will not relieve these contractures.

Masseter spasm (trismus)

1. Definition: sustained contracture of jaw muscles after induction of anesthesia that prevents opening the mouth for laryngoscopy, although extremity relaxation is adequate.
2. Etiologies:
   a. Myotonia
   b. Malignant hyperthermia
   c. Normal response to succinylcholine given with halothane
   d. Unknown etiology
3. Incidence may be as high as 1% in patients when a halothane induction is followed by intravenous succinylcholine use. The coincidence of MH and trismus is about 50%.
4. Recommended treatment of masseter spasm:
   a. Stop the anesthetic and cancel surgery if the procedure is elective.
   b. Maintain mask ventilation with 100% oxygen.
   c. Do not repeat the dose of succinylcholine.
   d. Monitor temperature, CPK (q 4 to 6 hr), myoglobin and potassium for 12 to 24 hours.
   e. Maintain adequate hydration and urine output.
   f. Dantrolene sodium therapy need not be given if masseter rigidity resolves promptly without other clinical signs and symptoms (hypercarbia, acidosis, arrhythmias, etc.)
   g. Emergency surgery can proceed by discontinuation of all MH triggers, using a nontriggering technique, and careful monitoring (including

end-tidal capnography and intraarterial catheter). Prophylactic dantrolene sodium administration should be considered.

h. The patient and family should be counseled (see the section on Counseling and Follow-up).

TREATMENT OF THE ACUTE EPISODE OF MALIGNANT HYPERTHERMIA (Table 23-3)

Recognition

Early recognition and aggressive treatment are the two most important factors for a successful outcome in cases of malignant hyperthermia. After the diagnosis has been made, help should be immediately summoned. At least five people are suggested.

1. An anesthesiologist to direct the resuscitation
2. A second person to manage the airway and ventilation
3. A third person to establish additional IV access and place an arterial catheter
4. A fourth person to draw up drugs and keep a record of events
5. A fifth person to run laboratory specimens (see Table 23-4 for common laboratory findings)

MANAGEMENT OF THE MH SUSCEPTIBLE PATIENT

Population

MH Susceptible Child

1. Previous MH episode
2. First-degree relative of individual with a history of MH episode or positive muscle biopsy
3. Previous masseter spasm

High Index of Suspicion

1. Presence of associated stigmata; history of heat stroke, muscle cramps of large bulky muscles (especially calves), caffeine sensitivity, etc.
2. Presence of associated disorders; strabismus, ptosis, scoliosis, muscular dystrophy, etc.

Anesthetic Management of MH Susceptibility

Preoperative visit

The MH susceptible child will need a preoperative consultation with the anesthesiologist. Appropriate laboratory data can be ordered at that time (including CBC, CPK, electrolytes, urinalysis, and ECG). A thorough discussion of the relative risks and proposed anesthetic techniques should be undertaken with the parents.

Premedication

Premedication is advised to reduce stress in the child (see Chapter 4). Benzodiazepines and barbiturates are good choices for premedication. Oral, intranasal, or rectal routes of administration are preferred over intramuscular injections.

TABLE 23-3. Treatment protocol for an acute episode of MH

Protocol	Comments
1. Summon help	Persons are needed for: resuscitation, line placement, airway management, record keeping, lab delivery.
2. Discontinue all halogenated volatile agents	Ideally, an O_2 tank or clean machine and circuit without previous exposure to volatile agents should be brought into the room.
3. Hyperventilate with 100% O_2 at high gas flows to maintain normocarbia	Mask ventilation is not usually difficult even in the presence of trismus or rigidity, when intubation may be problematic. Intubation should be performed when clinically feasible to secure the airway.
4. Inform the surgeon	The surgical procedure should be terminated as quickly as possible.
5. Administer dantrolene sodium IV by mixing each 20-mg bottle with 50-60 ml sterile water	Initial dose: 2.5 mg/kg IV; • If *ALL* symptoms are not resolved within 45 minutes a repeat dose is administered either as: a. 2.5 mg/kg IV every 30 min until all symptoms dissipate, or b. single repeat bolus of 10 mg/kg IV is given
6. Establish additional IV access	Central venous catheter placement should be considered.
7. Place an intraarterial catheter	Invasive hemodynamic monitoring and frequent blood sampling will be required.
8. Send STAT arterial and venous blood gas, electrolytes and CPK	Bicarbonate is given intravenously as needed to correct acidosis (1-2 mEq/kg) if ventilation is adequate and PCO_2 is near normal. Supplemental potassium should be avoided (hyperkalemia may occur later). If dangerous hyperkalemia occurs: infuse 10 U regular insulin and 50 ml D_{50} slowly to effect.

9. Initiate cooling if necessary	Iced saline 10-15 ml/kg IV every 10 minutes × 3 Surface cooling with ice packs, hypothermia units (cooling blanket) Iced saline lavage of body cavities (stomach, bladder, rectum, peritoneal or thoracic cavities) Extracorporeal circulation with cooling if other methods are not successful
10. Maintain urine output (2 ml/kg/hr) and assess urine myoglobin	Place Foley catheter Mannitol 300 mg/kg IV (Note: The dantrolene vial contains 150 mg of mannitol/mg dantrolene) Furosemide 0.5-1.0 mg/kg IV Aggressive hydration with central venous pressure monitoring
11. Give procainamide if arrhythmias are still present after adequate dantrolene therapy	Presence of arrhythmias may indicate need for additional dantrolene sodium. Procainamide loading dose to avoid hypotension: a. 1.5 mg/kg IV over 1 min and repeat every 5 min until arrhythmia is controlled or a total dose of 15 mg/kg is given b. 15 mg/kg over 30 min Infusion: 0.02-0.08 mg/kg/min
12. Transfer to intensive care unit	Hemodynamic monitoring should be continued for 24-72 hr after initial episode; recrudescence can occur from 4-36 hr after the event. Laboratory data • ABG and electrolytes as dictated by clinical course • CPK q 4-6 hr × 24 hr • Urine myoglobin until clear Continue dantrolene administration 1-2.5 mg/kg IV q 6 hr × 24 hr. Multiorgan system involvement should be treated as dictated by clinical course.
13. Counsel patient and family	A discussion of pretreatment for future anesthetics, possible muscle biopsy for family members, and MHAUS referral should be completed prior to discharge.

TABLE 23-4. Common laboratory findings in MH

Arterial blood gas	Acidosis—both respiratory and metabolic Hypercarbia Hypoxemia Base deficit
Electrolytes	Hyperkalemia Hypermagnesemia Hypercalcemia (early) Profound hypocalcemia (late) Hypernatremia
Enzymes	Increased CPK—20,000 U/L is diagnostic Increased LDH Increased SGOT
CBC	Decreased hemoglobin Thrombocytopenia
Coagulation profile	Prolonged prothrombin and partial thromboplastin time Decreased fibrinogen Increased fibrin split products

Necessary Equipment and Monitors

1. Standard monitoring (ECG, blood pressure, temperature, oximetry, precordial stethoscope)
2. Particularly useful additions
   a. Capnography to see early rise in $ETCO_2$
   b. Arterial catheter and Foley catheter for repeat sampling during lengthy procedures
3. Clean anesthesia machine (never exposed to inhalation anesthetics), or
4. Previously used anesthesia machine
   a. Continuously flushed with oxygen at 10 L/min (recommendations vary from 4 to 18 hours)
   b. All vaporizers removed
   c. All plastic and rubber connections changed
   d. CO_2 absorbers changed
   e. New circuit and mask
5. Cooling blanket on operating room table

Pretreatment with Dantrolene Sodium (see Table 23-5 for pharmacology of dantrolene sodium)

1. Recent controversy exists over the need to pretreat patients. Administration of a nontriggering anesthetic rather than prophylactic dantrolene is believed to be more advantageous in the MH-susceptible patient.
   a. Crises are rare when nontriggering techniques are used.
   b. Carefully monitored patients can be treated quickly with IV dantrolene sodium if necessary.
   c. Complications of treatment including nausea, disequilibrium, fatigue, and weakness necessitating ventilatory assistance may outweigh the advantages.

TABLE 23-5. Pharmacology of dantrolene sodium

Pharmacokinetics	• Onset: 6-20 min • Duration (of adequate plasma concentration) is 5-6 hr • Metabolized by liver • Active metabolic is 5-hydroxydantrolene (half-life is 15 hr) • Elimination half-life: children 7-10 hr; adult 12 hr • Excretion: renal
Pharmacodynamics	**Muscular** • Inhibits excitation-contraction coupling • Increases contraction activation threshold voltage • Decreases intracellular calcium • Slows calcium release by the sarcoplasmic reticulum • No effect: Centrally On neuromuscular junction On actin-myosin binding Synergistically with nondepolarizing relaxants **Cardiovascular** • Primary antiarrhythmic (increases refractory periods) • Decreases cardiac contractility and cardiac index • Increases systemic vascular resistance • No effect on mean arterial pressure
Toxicity and side effects	• Hepatotoxic with prolonged oral use • Muscle weakness sufficient to warrant airway protection or prolonged ventilation • Decreases LD_{50} of bupivacaine • Side effects include drowsiness, dizziness, headache, and nausea • Synergistic toxicity if given with diltiazem or verapamil causing hyperkalemia and cardiac arrest

2. Dantrolene sodium 2.5 mg/kg IV administered 2 hours preoperatively will achieve adequate plasma levels for 5 hours.
3. It is not necessary to pretreat with dantrolene sodium or avoid triggering agents in children with associated disorders.

Frequently Used Anesthetic Techniques

1. Barbiturate induction with balanced technique (nitrous oxide/oxygen, narcotic, benzodiazepine and nondepolarizing muscle relaxant)
2. Regional anesthesia
3. Local anesthesia with sedation

Postoperative Monitoring

Postoperatively, the child is monitored in the postanesthesia recovery room for 2 to 4 hours. Intensive care unit admission may be necessary, particularly if prophylactic dantrolene sodium has resulted in residual muscle weakness.

NEUROLEPT MALIGNANT SYNDROME (NMS)

This syndrome was first described in 1968 in patients taking major tranquilizers. It is believed that NMS patients may also be MH susceptible, because the clinical features are similar and several NMS patients have had positive muscle biopsies. However, the specific association between the two disorders has not been established (see Table 23-6 for comparison of MH and NMS).

COUNSELING AND FOLLOW-UP

1. A patient who has experienced an acute MH crisis or episode of trismus and his or her family should be counseled at length on the disorder and implications for future anesthetics before discharge from the hospital.
   a. This information should be disseminated to first-degree relatives and all second-degree relatives with either a myopathy or elevated CPK activity.
   b. A formal letter describing the event, laboratory documentation, treatment, and future recommendations should be given to the family and mailed to the primary physician.
2. A medical alert bracelet is recommended for the patient and susceptible family members.
3. A muscle biopsy may be performed.
   a. The halothane-caffeine contracture test is the only widely accepted test for MH susceptibility.
   b. The test is not standardized; each laboratory uses different criteria for positive, negative, and indeterminate results.
   c. The patient must travel to a center where the test is performed, because fresh live muscle tissue is necessary. Dantrolene and droperidol are avoided because they can normalize a positive response.
   d. The recommendation for muscle biopsy is controversial, because all susceptible patients should be treated as positive whether or not a biopsy is obtained. Therefore it may be best to perform a muscle biopsy incidentally during other elective surgery. It may be useful for the following reasons:
      - To document an acute episode of MH
      - To identify modes of genetic transmission
      - To give peace of mind to family members
      - To resolve concerns about insurance coverage
4. All MH-susceptible families should be referred to the Malignant Hyperthermia Association of the United States (MHAUS) for advice and support.
   a. Address: PO Box 3231
Darien, CT 06820
   b. For nonemergency and patient referral calls: (203) 655-3007
   c. Names of on-call physicians available to consult in MH emergencies 24 hours a day: (203) 634-4917 ask for "Index Zero-Malignant Hyperthermia Consultant List."

TABLE 23-6. Comparison of neurolept malignant syndrome and MH

	NMS	MH
Clinical features	Hyperthermia Muscular rigidity and akinesia Altered consciousness Autonomic instability May lead to multiorgan system failure	Tachycardia Tachypnea Hyperthermia Skeletal muscle contracture Autonomic instability May lead to multiorgan system failure
Triggering agents	Phenothiazines, butyrophenones, thioxanthenes, miscellaneous antipsychotic agents Abrupt withdrawal of levodopa	Volatile halogenated anesthetics Succinylcholine
Incidence	0.5-1% of all patients exposed to neuroleptics	1:50,000 adults 1:15,000 children
Population	Predominately young men	Inherited disorder Males and females equally affected
Etiology	Central defect, possibly in dopamine-receptor blockage	Peripheral defect of calcium release and reuptake in skeletal muscle
Onset	Over days to weeks (unrelated to duration of triggering agent exposure)	Within minutes to hours after exposure to anesthetic agent
Laboratory abnormalities	Increased creatinine phosphokinase (CPK) Leukocytosis Increased liver function tests Myoglobinuria	Marked acidosis Increased CPK Hyperkalemia Myoglobinuria
Treatment	Cessation of neuroleptic drug Dantrolene sodium Dopamine agonists: • Bromocriptine • Amantadine • Levodopa with carbidopa Supportive therapy	Cessation of anesthetic Dantrolene sodium Supportive therapy
Mortality	20%-30%	Less than 10% with prompt recognition and use of dantrolene sodium

BIBLIOGRAPHY

Brandom BW, Carroll JB, and Rosenberg H: Malignant hyperthermia. In Motoyama EK and Davis PJ, editors: Smith's anesthesia for infants and children, ed 2, St Louis, 1990, The CV Mosby Co.

Fletcher JE and Rosenberg H: In vitro interaction between halothane and succinylcholine in human skeletal muscle: implications for malignant hyperthermia and masseter muscle rigidity, Anesthesiology, 63:190-94, 1985.

Flewellen EH: Malignant hyperthermia and associated conditions: dilemma, controversy, unanswered questions, Review Course Lectures, International Anesthesia Research Society, 1985.

Gronert EA: Malignant hyperthermia, Anesthesiology 53:395-423, 1980.

Guzé BH and Baxter LR: Neuroleptic malignant syndrome, N Engl J Med 313:163-66, 1985.

Larach MG and others: Prediction of malignant hyperthermia susceptibility by clinical signs, Anesthesiology, 66:547-50, 1987.

Lerman J, McLeod ME, and Strong HA: Pharmacokinetics of intravenous dantrolene in children, Anesthesiology, 70:625-29, 1989.

Ording H: Incidence of malignant hyperthermia in Denmark, Anesth Analg, 64:700-704, 1985.

Rosenberg H and Fletcher JE: Masseter muscle rigidity and malignant hyperthermia susceptibility, Anesth Analg, 65:161-64, 1986.

Ryan JF: Malignant hyperthermia. In Ryan JF and others: A practice of anesthesia for infants and children, Orlando, Fla, 1986, Grune & Stratton.

Schwartz L, Rockoff MA, and Koka BV: Masseter spasm with anesthesia: incidence and implications, Anesthesiology, 61:772-75, 1984.

Sessler DI: Malignant hyperthermia. In Gregory GA, editor: Pediatric anesthesia, ed 2, New York, 1989, Churchill Livingstone.

Van Der Spek AFL and others: The effects of succinylcholine on mouth opening, Anesthesiology, 67:459-65, 1987.

APPENDIXES

CONTENTS

ANTIBIOTIC CEPHALOSPORINS—FIRST GENERATION

ANTIBIOTIC CEPHALOSPORINS—SECOND GENERATION

ANTIBIOTIC CEPHALOSPORINS—THIRD GENERATION

ANTICHOLINERGICS

ANTICOAGULANT

ANTICONVULSANTS

ANTIDYSRHYTHMIC/INOTROPE

ANTIEMETIC

ANTIHISTAMINES

ANTIHYPERTENSIVES

ANTITHYROID PREPARATIONS

BARBITURATES

BENZODIAZEPINES

BETA BLOCKERS

BRONCHODILATORS

CALCIUM CHANNEL BLOCKERS

CHOLINESTERASE INHIBITORS

CORTICOSTEROIDS

DIURETICS

GASTRIC MOTILITY STIMULANT

PITUITARY HORMONES

HEPARIN ANTAGONIST

H_2 RECEPTOR ANTAGONISTS

INOTROPES

INSULINS

LOCAL ANESTHETICS

Amides

Esters

MUSCLE RELAXANTS

NARCOTICS

NARCOTIC ANTAGONIST

NONBARBITURATE INDUCTION AGENTS

PHENOTHIAZINES

PROSTAGLANDIN E_1

SEDATIVE/HYPNOTIC

THYROID PREPARATION

VASODILATORS

LIST OF ABBREVIATIONS

α	Alpha
β	Beta
BBB	Blood brain barrier
CBC	Complete blood count
CHF	Congestive heart failure
E	Elimination route (unchanged drug or metabolites)
ED	Effective dose
ETT	Endotracheal tube
g	Gram
GI	Gastrointestinal
GU	Genitourinary
hr	Hour
HSV	Herpes simplex virus
IM	Intramuscular
IN	Intranasal
IV	Intravenous
K^+	Potassium
kg	Kilogram
M	Metabolism
MAO	Monoamine oxidase
μg	Microgram
mEq	Milliequivalent
mg	Milligram
min	Minute
msec	Millisecond
Na^+	Sodium
NSS	Normal saline solution
PO	Per os (orally)
PR	Per rectum
PRN	As needed
Q	Every
SC	Subcutaneous
SL	Sublingual
SVR	Systemic vascular resistance
SVT	Supraventricular tachycardia
$T_{1/2}\beta$	Elimination half-life
VF	Ventricular fibrillation
VT	Ventricular tachycardia
yrs	Years
$>$	Greater than
$<$	Less than

A

DRUG LISTS

Drug	Class	Dose	Pharmacokinetics	Comments
Acetaminophen (Tylenol, Panadol)	Analgesic	0-3 mo: 40 mg/dose PO 4-11 mo: 80 mg/dose PO 12-24 mo: 120 mg/dose PO 2-3 yr: 160 mg/dose PO 4-5 yr: 240 mg/dose PO 6-8 yr: 320 mg/dose PO 9-10 yr: 400 mg/dose PO 11-12 yr: 480 mg/dose PO or 5-10 mg/kg Q 6 hr PO	Onset: 30-60 min Duration: 3-4 hr M = liver E = kidney $t_{1/2}\beta$ = 1-3 hr	• A metabolite of phenacetin but low risk of methemoglobinemia or hemolytic anemia • Hepatotoxicity occurs at doses >140 mg/kg. Treatment with N-Acetylcysteine is most effective if begun within 10 hr of ingestion
Acetazolamide (Diamox)	Diuretic	*Diuretic:* PO/IV: 5 mg/kg QD or QOD *Glaucoma:* IV: 20-40 mg/kg/day divided Q 6 hr IM: 20-40 mg/kg/day divided Q 6 hr PO: 8-30 mg/kg/day divided Q 6-8 hr	E = kidney IV onset: 2 min Duration: 4-5 hr PO onset: 1-1.5 hr Duration: 8-12 hr	• Carbonic anhydrase inhibitor • Side effects: hypokalemia, acidosis, alkaline urine, paresthesias, vomiting, and diarrhea
Acyclovir	Antiviral	*Herpes simplex virus:* Neonate: IV: 30 mg/kg/day divided Q 8 hr Child: <12 yr IV: 750 mg/meter²/day divided Q 8 hr	E = kidney $t_{1/2}\beta$ = 2.5 hr	• Can cause renal dysfunction (if rapidly infused), thrombophlebitis, headache, rash • Encephalopathy can occur with IV use • Widely distributed to all tissue and body fluids (including CSF)

Albuterol (Proventil, Ventolin)	Bronchodilator	*Enteral:* 2-5 yrs: 0.1 mg/kg/day divided Q 8 hr PO May increase to 12 mg/day 6-11 yrs: 2 mg PO TID May increase to 24 mg/day >12 yrs: 2-4 mg PO TID or QID *Inhaler:* 1-2 puffs Q 4-6 hr *Nebulizer:* 0.01-0.03 ml/kg in 2 ml NSS TID-QID (Concentration = 5 mg/ml with 1 ml maximum dose)	Peak Effect: 30-60 min after inhalation Duration: 4-6 hr	• Selective β_2 agonist • Tachyphylaxis with long-term use • Side effects: tachycardia, nausea, vomiting, nervousness, and hypokalemia
Alprostadil (Prostin VR)	Prostaglandin E_1	IV = 0.05 μg/kg/min continuous infusion Increase incrementally up to 0.4 μg/kg/min *Maintenance:* Increase until acceptable PO_2, then immediately decrease to lowest effective dose	M = lungs (70%) E = kidney	• Aids in maintaining a patent ductus arteriosus in ductus-dependent cyanotic heart defects • Side effects include apnea, seizures, bradycardia, hypotension, hyperpyrexia, and bronchoconstriction
Alfentanil (Alfenta)	Narcotic	*Load:* 30-50 μg/kg IV *Maintenance:* 10-15 μg/kg IV single boluses or infusion of 0.5-1.5 μg/kg/min	Onset: 1-2 min M = liver E = kidney	• Slow elimination in patients with liver disease • Hypotension potential when used with diazepam • May cause truncal rigidity

Continued.

Drug	Class	Dose	Pharmacokinetics	Comments
Amantadine (Symmetrel)	Antiviral	*Child:* 1-9 yr: PO: 4-8 mg/kg/day divided Q 8-12 hr 9-12 yr: PO: 200 mg/kg divided Q 12 hr	E = kidney $t_{1/2}\beta$ = 15-20 hr (prolonged with renal dysfunction)	• Side effects include depression, nausea, seizures, CHF and orthostatic hypotension • Give for 90 days after influenza exposure for prophylaxis if vaccine contraindicated • Adjust dose in renal failure
Amikacin (Amikin)	Antibiotic	*Neonate:* <7 days and <1000 gm IV/IM: 7.5 mg/kg Q 24 hr <7 days and 1000-2000 gm IV/IM: 7.5 mg/kg Q 12 hr <7 days and >2000 gm IV/IM: 10 mg/kg Q 12 hr >7 days IV/IM: 7.5-10 mg/kg Q 8 hr *Child:* IV/IM: 15 mg/kg/day divided Q 8 hr	E = kidney $t_{1/2}\beta$ = 2-3 hr (prolonged with renal dysfunction, neonates)	• Excellent gram negative coverage especially *Pseudomonas* • Side effects include ototoxicity, nephrotoxicity and potentiation of neuromuscular blockade • Infuse slowly IV • Therapeutic levels: Peak = 25-30 mg/l Trough = 5-8 mg/l

Aminophylline	Bronchodilator	*Load:* 6 mg/kg IV over 20-30 min *Maintenance:* IV infusion: Neonate 0.2 mg/kg/hr <1 yr 0.2-0.9 mg/kg/hr 1-9 yr 1 mg/kg/hr	Onset: IV rapid M = liver E = kidney $t_{1/2}\beta$ = 3-10 hr (children); 15-58 hr (neonates)	• Indicated for relief of bronchospasm and treatment of neonatal apnea • Side effects include tachycardia, dysrhythmias, nervousness, nausea, and vomiting • Metabolism slowed with CHF, cimetidine administration and β-blockers • Therapeutic levels Asthma: 10-20 mg/l Apnea: 6-13 mg/l
Amoxicillin (Amoxil)	Penicillin	PO: 20-40 mg/kg/day divided Q 8 hr	E = kidney	• Achieves serum levels twice those of ampicillin • Less GI effects than ampicillin
Amphotericin B (Fungizone)	Antifungal	*Test Dose:* IV: 0.1 mg/kg infants, up to 0.5 mg in children *Initial Dose:* IV: 0.25 mg/kg/day, increase daily by 0.125-0.25 mg/kg increments to a maximum total dose of 1.5 mg/kg/day	E = kidney $t_{1/2}\beta$ = 15 days	• Does not penetrate CNS • Premedicate with diphenhydramine and acetaminophen • Side effects include renal dysfunction, shaking chills, anemia, thrombocytopenia, allergic reactions, hypokalemia, hypomagnesemia, and seizures

Continued.

Drug	Class	Dose	Pharmacokinetics	Comments
Ampicillin (Omnipen, Polycillin)	Antibiotic	*Neonate:* IV or IM* 0-7 days: 50-100 mg/kg Q 12 hr >7 days: 75-100 mg/kg Q 8 hr *Child:* Mild-moderate infection: IV/IM/PO: 50-100 mg/kg/day divided Q 6 hr Maximum dose = 2-4 gm/day Severe infection: IV/IM: 200-400 mg/kg/day divided Q 4-6 hr Maximum dose = 12 gm/day	M = liver (about 50%) E = kidney, liver $t_{1/2}\beta$ = 2-4 hr (age dependent)	• Has gram negative activity, including enterococcus • Higher doses are for treatment of *H. flu* meningitis in conjunction with chloramphenicol After 5-10 days: • Delayed skin rash is common and may not indicate hypersensitivity • May cause interstitial nephritis
Amrinone (Inocor)	Inotrope	*Load:* IV: 0.75 mg/kg over 2-3 min may repeat in 30 min if needed *Infusion:* IV: 5-10 μg/kg/min	Onset: 2-5 min Duration: 0.5-2 hr (depending on dose) M = liver E = kidney $t_{1/2}\beta$ = 3.6 hr (adults)	• Inotropic agent that acts via inhibition of phosphodiesterase • May act as a negative inotrope in infants • Has direct relaxant effect on vascular smooth muscle to decrease preload and afterload • Do *not* dilute with dextrose solutions or mix with furosemide • Side effects include thrombocytopenia, hepatotoxicity, hypotension, and arrhythmias • Avoid in patients sensitive to bisulfites

*Doses increase for meningitis.

Atracurium (Tracrium)	Nondepolarizing muscle relaxant	*Intubation:* IV: 0.3-0.5 mg/kg *Maintenance:* IV: 0.25 mg/kg Infusion: 6 μg/kg/hr	Onset: 1-2 min Duration: 20-30 min M = Hoffman elimination Ester hydrolysis	• Lacks cumulative effects • Laudanosine metabolite can cause CNS stimulation • Significant histamine release only occurs at 3 × ED_{95}
Atropine	Anticholinergic	IV: 10-20 μg/kg IM: 20 μg/kg Maximum dose for resuscitation = 1 mg IV	Onset: IV = rapid; IM = 2-5 min Duration: 4 hr M = liver E = kidney $t_{1/2}\beta$ = 2 hr	• Indicated to prevent reflex bradycardia with suction, intubation, etc. and to treat symptomatic bradydysrhythmias • Side effects include hyperpyrexia, urinary retention, dry mouth, confusion, and rash
Bretylium (Bretylol)	Antiarrhythmic	*Initial:* IV: 5-10 mg/kg over 10-30 min may repeat in 20-30 min × 1 *Maintenance:* IV bolus: 5-10 mg/kg Q 6 hr over 10 min IV infusion: 1-2 mg/min	Onset: 2 min-2 hr Duration: 6-24 hr M = minimal E = kidney $t_{1/2}\beta$ = 5-10 hr	• Indicated for management of recurrent life-threatening ventricular dysrhythmias • Causes initial catecholamine release followed by sympathectomy-like state manifested by orthostatic hypotension
Bupivacaine (Marcaine)	Local amide anesthetic	Maximal safe dose: 2.5 mg/kg With epinephrine: 3 mg/kg	Duration: 240-480 min M = liver E = kidney $t_{1/2}\beta$ = 2-6 hr	• Slow onset and long duration agent with high in vivo toxic potential • Severe cardiotoxicity has limited use of 0.75% solution • Toxic levels = 1.5 μg/ml

Continued.

Drug	Class	Dose	Pharmacokinetics	Comments
Calcium Chloride	Inotrope	IV bolus: 10 mg/kg, may repeat	Onset: rapid	• Should be given centrally to avoid phlebitis • Do not mix with bicarbonate • Once injected, calcium is bound to protein and incorporated into muscle, bone, and other tissues
Calcium Gluconate*	Inotrope	IV bolus: 100 mg/kg may repeat IV infusion: 200-500 mg/kg/day	Onset: rapid	• May produce arrhythmias in digitalized patients • Do not mix with bicarbonate • Formulation of choice for peripheral IV administration • Can cause tissue necrosis if extravasation occurs • Protein binding and incorporation into tissue occurs as with calcium chloride

*See page 606 for infusion preparation.

Captopril (Capoten)	Antihypertensive	*Neonate:* PO: 0.1-0.4 mg/kg Q 6-24 hr *Infant:* PO: 0.5-0.6 mg/kg/day divided Q 6-12 hr *Child:* PO: 25 mg/day divided Q 12 hr	Onset: 30 min-2 hr M = liver E = kidney	• Indicated in renovascular hypertension and in the management of congestive heart failure • Competitively inhibits angiotensin converting enzyme • Side effects include hyperkalemia, elevated creatinine, neutropenia, proteinuria, cough, and acute hypotension after first dose
Carbamazepine (Tegretol)	Anticonvulsant	*<6 years:* PO: 10 mg/kg/day divided Q 12-24 hr initially Maximum dose = 20 mg/kg/day *6-12 years:* PO: 10 mg/kg/day divided QD or BID initially Maintenance = 20-30 mg/kg/day divided Q 6-8 hr Maximum dose = 1000 mg/day *Adolescent:* PO: 200 mg BID initially Maintenance: 600-1200 mg/day divided Q 6-8 hr Maximum dose = 1000 mg/day	Onset: 2-6 hr Duration: 6-8 hr M = 98% liver $t_{1/2}\beta$ = 13-17 hr	• Indicated for trigeminal/glossopharyngeal neuralgias, and psychomotor epilepsy • Obtain pretreatment CBC • Side effects include: sedation, diplopia, vertigo, nausea, vomiting, and ataxia • *Life Threatening:* aplastic anemia, thrombocytopenia, oliguria, hypertension, acute heart failure and hepatic dysfunction • Therapeutic drug levels 4-12 mg/l

Continued.

Drug	Class	Dose	Pharmacokinetics	Comments
Carbenicillin (Geopen)	Antibiotic	*Neonate:* IV or IM 0-7 days: 50-75 mg/kg Q 6 hr *Children:* IV or IM UTI: 50-200 mg/kg/day divided Q 4-6 hr Severe infection: 400-500 mg/kg/day divided Q 4-6 hr Maximum dose = 40 gm/day	M = liver E = kidney $t_{1/2}\beta$ = 1-4 hr, age dependent	• Indicated for *Pseudomonas* and *Proteus* resistant to ampicillin • Interferes with normal platelet aggregation such that bleeding time is prolonged • 1 gram contains 4-7 mEq Na^+ • May lead to urinary K^+ loss and cardiac failure
Cefazolin (Ancef/Kefzol)	Antibiotic cephalosporin—first generation	*Infant/child:* IV or IM 25-100 mg/kg/day divided Q 6-8 hr	M = minimal E = kidney $t_{1/2}\beta$ = 2 hr	• Reduce dose in renal failure • Use caution in penicillin-allergic patients • Active against *Staphylococcus, E. coli* and *Klebsiella*
Cefamandole (Mandol)	Antibiotic cephalosporin—second generation	*Child:* IV/IM: 50-150 mg/kg/day divided Q 4-8 hr	M = minimal E = kidney $t_{1/2}\beta$ = 30-60 min	• 1 gm = 3.3 mEq Na^+ • Not recommended in children <1 mo • Can produce hypoprothrombinemia • Greater gram negative and less gram positive coverage than 1st generation drugs

Cefoperazone (Cefobid)	Antibiotic cephalosporin—third generation	*Infant/child:* IV/IM: 25-100 mg/kg/day divided Q 12 hr	M = minimal E = bile $t_{1/2}\beta$ = 2 hr (neonate 6-12 hr)	• Penetrates into CNS when meninges are inflamed • Dose reduction not necessary in renal insufficiency • Can produce hypoprothrombinemia • Less gram positive coverage than 1st generation drugs but has excellent pseudomonas coverage
Cefotaxime (Claforan)	Antibiotic cephalosporin—third generation	*Neonate:* IV/IM <7 days: 50-100 mg/kg/day divided Q 12 hr 7-30 days: 75-150 mg/kg/day divided Q 8 hr *Infant/child:* (<50 kg) IV/IM: 50-180 mg/kg/day divided Q 4-6 hr	M = liver (50%) E = kidney $t_{1/2}\beta$ = 1-1.5 hr	• Broad gram negative coverage, especially against *Serratia* • Little dose adjustment in renal insufficiency • Good CNS penetration
Cefotetan (Cefotan)	Antibiotic cephalosporin—second generation	IV: 40-60 mg/kg divided Q 12h	M = minimal E = kidney, bile $t_{1/2}\beta$ = 3-5 hr	• Special role in clinical use is against *B. fragilis*
Cefoxitin (Mefoxin)	Antibiotic cephalosporin—second generation	*Infant/child:* IV/IM: 80-160 mg/kg/day divided Q 4-6 hr	M = minimal E = kidney $t_{1/2}\beta$ = 45-60 min	• Special role in clinical use is against *B. fragilis*

Continued.

Drug	Class	Dose	Pharmacokinetics	Comments
Ceftazidime (Fortaz)	Antibiotic cephalosporin—third generation	*Neonate:* IV: 60 mg/kg/day divided Q 12 hr *Infant/child:* IV: 75-150 mg/kg/day divided Q 8 hr	M = none E = kidney $t_{1/2}\beta$ = 2-4 hr	• Active against gram positive, gram negative and anaerobes, but not *B. fragilis* • Not active against most enterococci
Ceftizoxime (Cefizox)	Antibiotic cephalosporin—third generation	*Infant/child:* IV/IM: 150-200 mg/kg/day divided Q 6-8 hr	M = none E = kidney $t_{1/2}\beta$ = 1.3-1.6 hr	• Active against gram positive, gram negative and anaerobic organisms, including *B. fragilis* • Inactive against most enterococci
Ceftriaxone (Rocephin)	Antibiotic cephalosporin—third generation	*Infant/child:* IV/IM: 50 mg/kg/day Q D *Meningitis:* IV: 75 mg/kg × 1 dose then 100 mg/kg/day divided Q 12 hr	M = none E = kidney $t_{1/2}\beta$ = 4-8 hr	• Good CNS penetration • Active against gram positive, gram negative and anaerobes • Inactive against most enterococci
Cefuroxime (Zinacef)	Antibiotic cephalosporin—second generation	*Neonates:* IV/IM: 10 mg/kg/day divided Q 12 hr *Infant/child:* IV/IM: 50-100 mg/kg/day divided Q 6-8 hr *Meningitis:* IV: 200-240 mg/kg/day divided Q 6-8 hr	M = none E = kidney $t_{1/2}\beta$ = 1-4 hr, age dependent	• Broad gram positive coverage, except enterococci • Good gram negative coverage except *Pseudomonas*, most strains of *Serratia* and *Proteus vulgaris*

Cephalothin (Keflin)	Antibiotic cephalosporin—first generation	*Neonate:* IV or IM 0-7 days: 40 mg/kg/day divided Q 12 hr >7 days: 60 mg/kg/day divided Q 8 hr *Child:* 80-160 mg/kg/day divided Q 4-6 hr	M = liver (50%) E = kidney $t_{1/2}\beta$ = 0.5-1 hr	• See cefazolin • For treatment of *Staphycoccal* infections
Cephapirin (Cefadyl)	Antibiotic cephalosporin—first generation	40-80 mg/kg/day divided Q 6 hr IV, IM	M = liver (50%) E = kidney $t_{1/2}\beta$ = 0.5-1 hr	• Similar to Cephalothin
Cephradine (Velosef)	Antibiotic cephalosporin—first generation	*Children:* IV: 50-100 mg/kg/day divided Q 6 hr IM: 50-100 mg/kg/day divided Q 6 hr PO: 25-100 mg/kg/day divided Q 6-12 hr	M = minimal E = kidney $t_{1/2}\beta$ = 0.7-2 hr	• For treatment of gram positive infections as well as *E. coli*, *Proteus mirabilis*, and *Klebsiella*

Continued.

Drug	Class	Dose	Pharmacokinetics	Comments
Chloral Hydrate (Noctec)	Sedative/hypnotic	PO: 20-40 mg/kg Q 8 hr Up to 500 mg for sedation Up to 1.0 g for hypnotic PR: 20-40 mg/kg Q 8 hr	Onset: PO/PR: 13-60 min Duration: PO/PR: 4-8 hr M = liver and RBC to active trichloroethanol E = kidney (some liver)	• Useful for preoperative sedation • Excellent PO/PR absorption, but has a bitter taste • Side effects include gastric irritation, myocardial depression (in cardiac diseases), and potentiation of oral anticoagulants • Contraindicated in marked hepatic or renal dysfunction
Chloramphenicol (Chloromycetin)	Antibiotic	Loading dose (all ages) IV/PO: 20 mg/kg *Neonates:* IV <7 days: 10 mg/kg/day divided Q 12-24 hr, initiate 24 hr after load 7-21 days: 20 mg/kg/day divided Q 8-12 hr >21 days: 30 mg/kg/day divided Q 6-12 hr *Children:* IV/PO: 50-100 mg/kg/day divided Q 6-8 hr	M = liver E = kidney $t_{1/2}\beta$ = 1.5-3.5 hr	• Few indications for use exist but indicated for typhoid fever and ampicillin-resistant *H. flu* meningitis • Must monitor drug levels (15-20 mg/l) • May cause aplastic anemia • Inhibits hepatic microsomal enzymes

Chlorpromazine (Thorazine)	Phenothiazine	PO: 0.5 mg/kg Q 4-6 hr IV/IM: 2 mg/kg/day divided Q 6-8 hr *Maximum Daily Doses:* <5 yrs: 40 mg 5-12 yrs: 75 mg	Onset: IV: rapid IM: 30 min PO: 30-60 min Duration: IM: 3-4 hr PO: 4-6 hr M = liver E = liver, kidney $t_{1/2}\beta$ = 10-20 hr	• A neuroleptic • Also useful as an antiemetic, major tranquilizer • Side effects include sedation, orthostatic hypotension (α-blockade), extrapyramidal reactions, cholestatic jaundice and leukopenia • Not recommended in children <6 mo or in those with suspected Reyes syndrome
Cimetidine (Tagamet)	H_2 receptor antagonist	*Neonate:* PO/IV: 10-20 mg/kg/day divided Q 4-6 hr *Child:* PO/IV: 20-40 mg/kg/day divided Q 6 hr	Onset: 45-90 min PO Duration: IV/IM/PO: 4-5 hr M = liver E = kidney $t_{1/2}\beta$ = 2 hr	• Side effects include drowsiness, dizziness, gynecomastia, and neutropenia • May cause increased levels of active propranolol, benzodiazepines, phenytoin, theophylline by inhibiting hepatic microsomal enzymes
Clindamycin (Cleocin)	Antibiotic	IV/IM: 15-40 mg/kg/day divided Q 6-8 hr PO: 8-25 mg/kg/day divided Q 6-8 hr	E = kidney $t_{1/2}\beta$ = 2-4 hr	• Use with caution in neonates, infants and in hepatic and renal insufficiency • Gram positive and anaerobic activity • Associated with pseudomembranous colitis

Continued.

Drug	Class	Dose	Pharmacokinetics	Comments
Clonazepam (Klonopin)	Benzodiazepine	Children up to 10 yrs, 30 kg: PO: 0.01-0.03 mg/kg/day divided Q 8 hr May be increased to maximum 0.1-0.2 mg/kg/day divided Q 8 hr	M = liver E = kidney $t_{1/2}\beta$ = 24-48 hr	• Side effects include depression, drowsiness, ataxia, behavioral changes and increased bronchial secretions • May cause GI, CV, GU, renal and hematopoietic toxicity
Cloxacillin (Cloxapen)	Antibiotic	<20 kg: 50-100 mg/kg/day divided Q 6 hr PO >20 kg: 1-2 gm/day divided Q 6 hr PO Maximum dose = 4 gm/day	M = liver (50%) E = kidney and liver $t_{1/2}\beta$ = 6 hr	• Rapid, but incomplete PO absorption • Better PO absorption achieved with Dicloxacillin • Antistaphylococcal activity
Cocaine	Ester local anesthetic	*Topical:* 4% solution (1 drop = 2 mg) Maximum safe dose = 3 mg/kg (1.5 mg/kg if used with a volatile anesthetic)	M = liver, plasma esterases E = kidney $t_{1/2}\beta$ = 1 hr	• Sympathomimetic which blocks reuptake of norepinephrine • May cause tremors, seizures, tachycardia, and hyperpyrexia
Codeine	Narcotic	*Analgesic:* IV: 0.5-1.0 mg/kg Q 4-6 hr PO: 0.5-1.0 mg/kg Q 4-6 hr *Antitussive:* PO: 0.25-0.5 mg/kg Q 4 hr Maximum dose = 30 mg/day	M = liver E = kidney $t_{1/2}\beta$ = 3-3.5 hr	• Semisynthetic opioid • Best used in combination with acetaminophen for analgesia • Side effects include sedation, nausea, and vomiting

Corticotropin (ACTH)	Hormone	*Aqueous:* IV/IM/SC: 1.6 unit/kg/day divided Q 6-8 hr *Gel:* IV/IM/SC: 0.8 unit/kg/day divided Q 12-24 hr	Onset: rapid by any route Duration: 2 hr	• Used diagnostically to evaluate suspected primary adrenal insufficiency • Side effects include sodium retention and hypokalemic metabolic alkalosis • Contraindicated in Cushing's disease, peptic ulcer disease, psychosis, TB, fungal disease and pork sensitivity
Co-trimoxazole (Bactrim, Septra)	Sulfonamide	*Moderate infections:* PO: 8 mg/kg/day trimethoprim *plus* 40 mg/kg/day sulfamethoxazole divided Q 12 hr *Severe infections or pneumocystis:* PO/IV: 20 mg/kg/day trimethoprim *plus* 100 mg/kg/day sulfamethoxazole divided Q 6 hr *Prophylaxis* in immunocompromised patients: PO: 5 mg/kg/day trimethoprim *plus* 25 mg sulfamethoxazole divided Q 12 hr	M = liver E = kidney $t_{1/2}\beta$ = 10 hr	• Side effects include rash, glossitis, stomatitis • May cause jaundice or worsen renal dysfunction • In folate-deficient patients, anemia, leukopenia and thrombocytopenia can occur

Continued.

Drug	Class	Dose	Pharmacokinetics	Comments
D-tubocurarine	Nondepolarizing muscle relaxant	*Intubation:* Premature = 0.125 mg/kg IV 0-2 mo = 0.25 mg/kg IV >2 mo = 0.3-0.6 mg/kg IV Supplemental doses ½ initial dose	Onset: 3-5 min Duration: 30 min M = liver (minimal) E = kidney $t_{1/2}\beta$ = 1-3 hr	• Neonates and infants are more sensitive to drug effects • Causes significant histamine release resulting in hypotension in the usual dose range
Desmopressin Acetate (DDAVP)	Posterior pituitary hormone	IN: (solution = 100 μg/ml) 3 mo-12 yr = 5-30 μg/kg/day divided Q 12-24 hr (endocrine replacement) IV: 0.3 μg/kg over 30 minutes (hematologic dose)	Duration: 6-20 hr	• Drug of choice for central diabetes insipidus, *not* useful for nephrogenic diabetes insipidus • Side effects include nausea, hypertension, water retention, and hypotension (especially with rapid administration) • Will stimulate release of von Willebrand's factor (VIII_A)
Dexamethasone (Decadron)	Corticosteroid	*Increased Intracranial Pressure:* Initial: 0.5-1.5 mg/kg IV/IM Maintenance: 0.2-0.5 mg/kg/day divided Q 6 hr IV/IM *Croup/Airway Edema:* IV: 0.25-0.5 mg/kg Q 6 hr PRN (begin 24 hr prior to planned extubation then repeat × 4-6 doses)	Duration: 36-54 hr M = liver E = kidney $t_{1/2}\beta$ = 2-4 hr	• Glucocorticoid activity 40 times hydrocortisone • Little mineralocorticoid activity

Diazepam (Valium)	Anticonvulsant, anxiolytic	*Premedicant:* IM: 0.3-0.4 mg/kg PO: 0.1-0.2 mg/kg *Status Epilepticus:* 1 mo-5 yr: 0.2-0.5 mg/kg IV Q 10-30 min to effect, then repeat Q 2-4 hr Maximum Dose = 5 mg >5 yr: 1 mg IV Q 15-30 min to effect then repeat Q 2-4 hr Maximum dose = 10 mg	Onset: IV: rapid IM: 15-30 min M = liver (Active metabolites-oxazepam + desmethyl diazepam) E = kidney $t_{1/2}\beta$ = 7-20 hr (Metabolites 5-20 hr)	• Indicated for sedation, treatment of status epilepticus, and induction anesthesia • Avoid in children <1 yr due to prolonged drug action • IM route may cause pain on injection, poor absorption, and aseptic necrosis
Diazoxide (Hyperstat)	Antihypertensive	*Hypertensive Crisis:* IV: 1-3 mg/kg slow bolus, may repeat Q 15-30 min then Q 6-8 hr PRN *Refractory Hypoglycemia:* (insulin producing tumors) Newborn/infant: 8-15 mg/kg/day divided Q 8-12 hr PO/IV Child: 3-8 mg/kg/day divided Q 8-12 hr PO/IV	Onset: 1-2 min IV Duration: 2-12 hr M = liver E = kidney	• Primary site of action is arteriolar resistance vessels • Chemically related to thiazide diuretics • Side effects include sodium and water retention, hyperglycemia, hypotension, and reflex tachycardia

Continued.

Drug	Class	Dose	Pharmacokinetics	Comments
Digoxin (Doses given are for treatment of CHF)	Antidysrhythmic, inotrope	*Total Digitalizing Dose (TDD):* Premature: 20 μg/kg IM or IV Full Term: 30 μg/kg IM or IV <2 yrs: 30-50 μg/kg IM or IV 35-60 μg/kg PO 2-10 yrs: 15-30 μg/kg, IM or IV, 20-40 μg/kg PO >10 yrs: 10-15 μg/kg IV or PO *Maintenance:* PO Premature: 5 μg/kg Full Term: 8-10 μg/kg <2 yrs: 10-12 μg/kg 2-10 yrs: 8-10 μg/kg >10 yrs: 2-5 μg/kg	Onset: IV: 5-30 min IM: 30 min PO: 1-2 hr M = Minimal E = kidney $t_{1/2}\beta$ = 42 hr	• TDD given as ½ dose stat then ¼ TDD Q 6h × 2 followed by maintenance • Maintenance dose divided bid in children <10 yrs • IV/IM doses are 75% of PO dose except IV = PO in children >10 yrs • Side effects of toxicity include anorexia, nausea, vomiting, disorientation, and AV block • Toxicity potentiated by hypokalemia, hypomagnesemia, and hypercalcemia • Therapeutic level = 0.8-2.0 μg/l
Diphenhydramine (Benadryl)	Antihistamine	*Sedation:* IV/IM/PO = 5 mg/kg/day divided Q 6 hr *Anaphylaxis/Phenothiazine Overdose:* IV: 1-2 mg/kg slowly	Onset: IV: rapid IM/PO: 15-30 min M = liver E = kidney $t_{1/2}\beta$ = 3-7 hr	• Indicated for sedation, treatment of allergic/anaphylactic reactions/extrapyramidal reactions or as an antiemetic • Side effects include dry mouth, tachycardia, hypotension, and respiratory depression

Dobutamine* (Dobutrex)	Inotrope	IV: 1-10 μg/kg/min continuous infusion Maximum recommended dose = 40 μg/kg/min	Onset: 2 min IV Duration: 10 min IV M = liver E = kidney, liver $t_{1/2}\beta$ = 2 min	• Synthetic catecholamine with primarily β_1 stimulation properties • Increases cardiac output with minimal effect on heart rate or peripheral resistance
Dopamine* (Intropin)	Inotrope	IV: 1-20 μg/kg/min continuous infusion	Onset: 5 min IV Duration: 10 min IV M = kidney, liver, nerve endings E = kidney $t_{1/2}\beta$ = 2 min	• Natural catecholamine with effects on dopaminergic, β-, and α-adrenergic receptors • Indicated in low output states associated with hypotension • Side effects include tachycardia, tachydysrhythmias, hyperglycemia and intense vasoconstriction with skin sloughing if accidental extravasation occurs
Droperidol (Inapsine)	Antiemetic	IM/IV: 30-70 μg/kg PRN	Onset: 5-8 min IV/IM Duration: 3-6 hr M = liver E = kidney $t_{1/2}\beta$ = 100 min	• Inhibits dopamine receptors in chemoreceptor trigger zone of medulla to decrease nausea and vomiting • Side effects include extrapyramidal reactions and hypotension (α blockade) • May cause dysphoria

Continued.

*See page 606 for infusion preparation.

Drug	Class	Dose	Pharmacokinetics	Comments
Edrophonium (Tensilon)	Cholinesterase inhibitor	IV: 0.5-1 mg/kg	Onset: 1-5 min Duration: 60 min M = liver (30%) E = kidney (70%) $t_{1/2}\beta$ = 1.8 hr	• Less muscarinic side effects than longer acting cholinesterase inhibitors • Duration of action similar to neostigmine but less than pyridostigmine
Epinephrine (Adrenalin)*	Inotrope	IV: 0.1-1 μg/kg/min continuous infusion or 10 μg/kg IV bolus PRN *Cardiac Arrest:* 50 μg/kg IV of 1:10,000 solution (100 μg/ml)	Onset: rapid IV Duration: 10 min IV M = liver, nerve terminals E = kidney, liver	• Natural catecholamine with α_1, β_1, and β_2 adrenergic activity • Side effects include dysrhythmias, hypertension, tachycardia, nausea, vomiting, and necrosis at site of repeated injection • May be given via endotracheal tube • Pediatric infusion dose is ten times usual adult infusion

* See page 606 for infusion preparation.

Erythromycin (numerous)	Antibiotic	*Children:* IV: 10-20 mg/kg/day divided Q 6 hr (slow infusion) PO: 30-50 mg/kg/day divided Q 6-8 hr *Rheumatic Fever Prophylaxis:* PO: 500 mg/day divided Q 12 hr	M = liver E = kidney $t_{1/2}\beta$ = 1.4 hrs	• Effective against *Legionella*, *Mycoplasma*, *Streptococci* and *Neisseria gonorrhea* • GI side effects common • Avoid IM (pain/necrosis) • Use with caution in liver disease (cholestatic hepatitis) • May increase digoxin, theophylline, and carbamazepine levels • Indicated for penicillin allergic patients
Esmolol (Brevibloc)	Beta blocker	*Load* (Extrapolated from adult doses): IV: 500 μg/kg over 1 minute may repeat after infusion started if response inadequate *Infusion:* IV: 50-200 μg/kg/min	Onset: rapid IV M = blood esterases E = kidney $t_{1/2}\beta$ = 9 min	• β_1 selective β-blocker • Drug must be diluted to a concentration of <10 mg/ml to avoid venous irritation • Side effects include bradycardia, hypotension and *rarely* sedation, confusion and bronchospasm
Etidocaine (Duranest)	Local amide anesthetic	Infiltration: 4 mg/kg	Onset: slow Duration: 2-4 hr (infiltration) M = liver E = kidney $t_{1/2}\beta$ = 6 hr	• Resembles lidocaine but is 50× more lipid soluble and lasts 2-3× longer • Toxic levels = 2 μg/ml • Indicated for local infiltration, peripheral nerve block and epidural anesthesia

Continued.

Drug	Class	Dose	Pharmacokinetics	Comments
Etomidate (Amidate)	Nonbarbiturate induction agent	*Induction of Anesthesia* IV: 0.3 mg/kg (Children >10 yrs)	Onset: 30 sec Duration: 3-12 min M = liver E = kidney $t_{1/2}\beta$ = 2.5 hr	• Awakening more rapid than with thiopental • Causes less hemodynamic depression than barbiturates • Side effects include pain on injection, myoclonus, and adrenocortical suppression
Fentanyl (Sublimaze)	Narcotic	*Analgesia:* IV: 1-2 μg/kg initial dose *As the sole agent for cardiovascular surgery:* IV: 50-75 μg/kg	Onset: 1-2 min Peak: 10 min Duration: 20-30 min M = hepatic (85%) E = kidney $t_{1/2}\beta$ = 2-4 hr	• Synthetic opioid that is 75-125 times more potent than morphine • Side effects include bradycardia, respiratory depression and truncal rigidity
Furosemide (Lasix)	Diuretic	PO: 2 mg/kg Q 6-8 hr IV: 1 mg/kg Q 12 hr IM: 1 mg/kg Q 12 hr May increase dose by 1 mg/kg with maximum single dose 6 mg/kg	Onset: IV: 2-10 min IM: 5-30 min PO: 30-60 min Duration: IV: 2 hr PO: 6-8 hr M = minimal E = kidney $t_{1/2}\beta$ = 1 hr	• Side effects include ototoxicity, hypokalemia, alkalosis, increased urinary calcium excretion, and volume depletion

Gentamycin	Antibiotic	*Neonate:* under 2000 gm <30 wks: 2.5 mg/kg/day divided Q 24 hr IV/IM 30-34 wks: 2.5 mg/kg/day divided Q 18 hr IV/IM >34 wks: 2.5 mg/kg/day divided Q 12 hr IV/IM over 2000 gm <7 days: 2.5 mg/kg/day divided Q 12 hr IV/IM >7 days: 2.5 mg/kg/day divided Q 8 hr IV/IM *Children:* IV/IM: 5-7 mg/kg/day divided Q 8 hr	M = liver (40%) E = kidney $t_{1/2}\beta$ = 2-3 hr (nonneonates)	• See amikacin • Therapeutic levels peak = 6-10 mg/l trough = <2 mg/l • Adjust dose with renal dysfunction • Give intrathecally for CNS infections
Glycopyrrolate (Robinul)	Anticholinergic	IV: 5-10 μg/kg IM: 10 μg/kg	Onset: Rapid IV M = minimal E = probably kidney	• Primarily indicated as an antisialagogue and in conjunction with neostigmine and pyridostigimine for reversal of neuromuscular blockade • Poorly lipid-soluble and doesn't cross BBB well

Continued.

Drug	Class	Dose	Pharmacokinetics	Comments
Heparin Sodium	Anticoagulant	IV: 50 units/kg bolus for cardiac bypass: 400 units/kg (4 mg/kg) *Maintenance:* IV: 10-25 units/kg/hr as continuous infusion or 100 units/kg Q 4 hr	Onset: immediate Duration: 2-6 hr M = liver E = kidney $t_{1/2}\beta$ = 1-2 hr	• Potency of commercial preparations range from 140-190 units/mg • Acts by accelerating AT-III neutralization of activated clotting factors • Follow drug effect with PTT and/or ACT • Contraindicated in patients with known bleeding tendencies or who are to undergo intraocular or intracranial procedures • Side effects include hemorrhage, thrombocytopenia, allergic reactions, and altered protein binding (displacement of basic drugs)
Hydralazine (Apresoline)	Antihypertensive	*Hypertensive Crisis:* IV/IM: 0.1-0.5 mg/kg Q 4-6h *Chronic Hypertension:* PO = 0.75-3 mg/kg/day divided Q 6-12 hr	Onset: IV: 2.5-20 min IM: 10-30 min PO: 20-30 min M = liver E = kidney $t_{1/2}\beta$ = 2-4 hr	• Acts by direct smooth muscle dilatation (arterioles > venules) • May cause SLE and arthritis-like syndrome • May cause enhanced deflurination of enflurane • Reflex tachycardia is common

Hydrochlorothiazide (Hydrodiuril)	Diuretic	PO: 2-3 mg/kg/day divided Q 12 hr	E = kidney	• Side effects include hyperbilirubinemia, hypokalemia, alkalosis, hyperuricemia, hyperglycemia, and hyponatremia
Hydrocortisone (Solu-cortef)	Corticosteroid	*Physiologic Replacement:* 10-14 mg/meter^2/day IM/IV *Stress Dose:* 4-8 mg/kg/day in 3 divided doses or 2-4 × physiologic replacement IV *Acute Adrenal Insufficiency* 1-2 mg/kg/dose bolus, then 25-200 mg/day in divided doses IV *Status asthmaticus:* Load: 4-8 mg/kg IV Maintenance: 8 mg/kg/day divided Q 6 hr IV	Duration: 4-6 hr M = liver E = kidney $t_{1/2}\beta$ = 1-2 hr	• Side effects include psychosis, GI ulceration, impaired wound healing, adrenal suppression, hyperglycemia, water retention, hypernatremia, hypokalemia, and myopathy • Appropriate for sole replacement in adrenocortical insufficiency
Hydroxyzine (Atarax/Vistaril)	Antihistamine	IM: 0.5-1 mg/kg Q 4-6 hr PO: 2 mg/kg/day divided Q 6 hr	Onset: 15-20 min PO Duration: 4-6 hr PO M = liver E = kidney, liver $t_{1/2}\beta$ = 3 hr	• Same indications as for diphenhydramine • Minimal cardiorespiratory depression • IV injection can cause thrombosis, hemolysis; arterial injection can cause necrosis

Continued.

Drug	Class	Dose	Pharmacokinetics	Comments
Insulin—Regular	Insulin	Diabetic ketoacidosis: Load: 0.1 unit/kg IV bolus to saturate insulin receptors Infusion: 0.1 unit/kg/hr	Onset: 30-60 min Peak: 2-5 hr Duration: 5-8 hr	• Rapid onset and short duration
Insulin—Semi-lente	Insulin	As indicated SC, never IV	Onset: 30-90 min Peak: 5-10 hr Duration: 12-16 hr	• Rapid onset and short duration
Insulin—Lente	Insulin	As indicated SC, never IV	Onset: 1-2.5 hr Peak: 7-15 hr Duration: 24 hr	• 30% semi-lente + 70% ultra-lente • Intermediate onset and duration
Insulin—NPH	Insulin	As indicated SC, never IV	Onset: 1-2 hr Peak: 6-12 hr Duration: 18-24 hr	• Intermediate onset and intermediate duration • Human NPH may be more potent and shorter acting than pork-derived NPH
Insulin—Protamine Zinc (PZI)	Insulin	As indicated SC, never IV	Onset: 4-8 hr Peak: 14-24 hr Duration: 36 hr	• Delayed onset, long duration
Insulin—Ultra-lente	Insulin	As indicated SC, never IV	Onset: 4-8 hr Peak: 10-30 hr Duration: 36+ hr	• Delayed onset and long duration

Isoetharine (Bronkosol)	Bronchodilator	*Inhaler:* 1-2 puffs Q 3-4 hr *Nebulizer:* 0.25-0.5 ml 1% solution diluted to 2 ml with NSS Q 4 hr	Peak Effect: 15-60 min Duration: 2-4 hr	• See albuterol
Isoproterenol (Isuprel)*	Bronchodilator/inotrope	*Inhaler:* 1-2 puffs Q 3-4 hr *Nebulizer:* 0.01 ml/kg diluted to 2 ml with NSS Q 4 hr Maximum dose = 0.05 ml/dose *Inotrope/Chronotrope/Severe Bronchospasm:* IV: 0.1-1 μg/kg/min continuous infusion	Onset: rapid IV: rapid Inhaled: 2-5 min Duration: IV: 1-2 min Inhaled: 1-3 hr M = liver, nerve endings E = kidney, liver	• Synthetic catecholamine that is the most potent activator of β_1 and β_2 adrenergic receptors • Indicated as an inhaler to produce bronchodilation, to increase the heart rate in complete heart block, and to decrease pulmonary resistance • IV infusion for severe refractory bronchospasm or circulatory support • Side effects include dysrhythmias and hypertension (especially with epinephrine) • Tachyphylaxis is common

Continued.

*See page 606 for infusion preparation.

Drug	Class	Dose	Pharmacokinetics	Comments
Kanamycin (Kantrex)	Antibiotic	*Neonate:* under 2000 gm <7 days: 15 mg/kg/day divided Q 12 hr IV/IM >7 days: 20 mg/kg/day divided Q 12 hr IV/IM over 2000 gm <7 days: 20 mg/kg/day divided Q 12 hr IV/IM >7 days: 30 mg/kg/day divided Q 8 hr IV/IM *Infant/child:* IV/IM: 15-30 mg/kg/day divided Q 8-12 hr *Suppression of Bacterial Flora* PO = 50-100 mg/kg/day divided Q 6 hr	E = kidney $t_{1/2}\beta$ = 2-3 hr	• See amikacin • Used to suppress intestinal flora prior to GI surgery • Therapeutic levels: peak = 15-30 mg/L trough = 5-10 mg/L

Ketamine (Ketalar)	Nonbarbiturate induction agent	*Induction:* IV: 1-3 mg/kg IM: 5-10 mg/kg PO: 6 mg/kg *Analgesia:* IV: 0.2-0.5 mg/kg	Onset: IV: 30-60 sec IM: 3-5 min PO: 30 min Duration: IV: 5-10 min IM: 10-20 min M = liver E = kidneys, liver $t_{1/2}\beta$ = 2.5 hr	• Produces a "dissociative" state as well as profound analgesia, bronchodilation • Side effects include tachycardia, hypertension, salivation, elevated intracranial pressure, prolongation of non-depolarizing muscle relaxants, and emergence delirium • Emergence delirium is diminished by prior administration of barbiturates and benzodiazepines, not by recovery in a quiet room
Levothyroxine (Synthroid)	Thyroid preparation	*Neonates:* PO: 25-50 μg/day IV: 20-40 μg/day *<1 Year:* PO: 50-75 μg/day IV: 40 μg/day *Children:* PO: 3-5 μg/kg/day IV: 75% PO dose	M = liver	• Levothyroxine 100 mg = thyroid 65 mg • Titrate dose to serum free T_4 and thyroid stimulating hormone levels • Increases catabolism of vitamin K-dependent factors

Continued.

Drug	Class	Dose	Pharmacokinetics	Comments
Lidocaine (Xylocaine)*	Amide local anesthetic	*Local Anesthesia:* Maximal safe dose: 5 mg/kg With epinephrine: 7 mg/kg	M = liver E = kidney Duration: 60-120 min	• Extensive metabolism results in plasma clearance being proportional to hepatic blood flow • Monoethylglycinexylide metabolite has 80% of parent drug's activity against arrhythmias
	Antiarrhythmic	*Ventricular Dysrrhythmias:* Bolus = 1 mg/kg IV, may repeat Q 5-10 min to maximum dose of 3-5 mg/kg Infusion = 30-50 μg/kg/min	Onset: immediate M = liver E = kidney (10% unchanged) $t_{1/2}\beta$ = 1.5 hr	• Indicated for ventricular dysrhythmias • Contraindicated in WPW syndrome, amide-type drug hypersensitivity, and severe SA, AV, or intraventricular block in the absence of a pacemaker • Therapeutic levels 1-5 μg/ml • Toxicity occurs at levels >7 μg/ml
Lorazepam (Ativan)	Benzodiazepine	*Sedation:* IV = 0.03-0.05 mg/kg Q 6 hr PRN PO = .05 mg/kg > age 6	Onset: IV: 5-20 min Duration: IV: 10 hr M = liver E = kidney $t_{1/2}\beta$ = 10-20 hr	• Long $t_{1/2}\beta$ makes it less attractive than other benzodiazepines for preop sedation • May cause mild respiratory depression and paradoxical excitation • Has some antiemetic properties • Hallucinations reported in children <6 yr

*See page 606 for infusion preparation.

Meperidine (Demerol)	Narcotic	*Premedication:* IM: 1-2 mg/kg *Analgesia:* IV/IM/PO/SC: 1-1.5 mg/kg Q 3-4 hr	Onset: IV: 5 min IM/SC: 10 min PO: 15 min Duration: 2-4 hr M = liver 95% E = kidney $t_{1/2}\beta$ = 1.5-4 hr	• Synthetic opioid with 1/10 the activity of morphine • Major metabolite normeperidine is active and has an elimination half-life of 15-40 hr (CNS stimulant) • Side effects include orthostatic hypotension, negative inotropy, seizures, and respiratory depression • Tachycardia and mydriasis reflect atropine-like activity
Mepivacaine (Carbocaine)	Amide local anesthetic	Maximal dose: 5-6 mg/kg	M = liver E = kidney $t_{1/2}\beta$ = 2 hr Duration: 90-180 min	• Similar to lidocaine but lacks vasodilator activity and is a better choice when addition of epinephrine is undesirable • Toxic levels = >5 mg/ml
Metaproterenol (Alupent)	Bronchodilator	*Inhaler:* 1-2 puffs Q 3-4 hr *Nebulizer:* 0.2-0.3 ml of 5% solution in 2-5 ml NSS Q 4-6 hr	Peak Effect: 30-60 min Duration: 3-4 hr	• See albuterol • May repeat Q 1 hr for severe bronchospasm with careful monitoring

Continued.

Drug	Class	Dose	Pharmacokinetics	Comments
Methicillin (Staphcillin)	Antimicrobial	*Neonate:* 0-7 days 50-100 mg/kg/day divided Q 12 hr IV/IM >7 days 100-200 mg/kg/day divided Q 6-8 hr IV/IM *Child:* IV/IM = 100-400 mg/kg/day divided Q 4-6 hr	E = kidney	• Contains 2.5 mEq Na^+/gram • Very effective against *S. aureus* • Poor PO absorption
Methimazole (Tapazole)	Antithyroid preparation	*Child:* Initial dose: 0.4-0.7 mg/kg/day divided Q 8 hr *Maintenance:* 50% initial daily dose divided Q 8 hr once euthyroid	Onset: days to weeks Duration: 8-12 hr E = kidney $t_{1/2}\beta$ = 6-13 hr	• Inhibits iodine incorporation into thyroglobin • Only available as PO form • Improvement usually seen in 1-2 days • Side effects include urticarial rash, pruritis, and granulocytopenia
Methohexital (Brevital)	Barbiturate	*Induction:* PR: 20-30 mg/kg of 10% solution IM: 10 mg/kg of 5% solution IV: 1-2 mg/kg of 1% solution	Onset: IV: Rapid PR: 5-10 min M = liver E = kidney $t_{1/2}\beta$ = 1-2 hr	• Psychomotor recovery is more rapid than thiopental after repeated doses due to greater hepatic clearance • Side effects include involuntary muscle movements, hiccoughs, mild cardiovascular depression • Intraarterial injection can cause necrosis • Avoid in porphyria

Methyldopa (Aldomet)	Antihypertensive	PO = 10 mg/kg/day divided Q 6-12 hr Maximum dose = the lesser of 65 mg/kg or 3 mg/day *Hypertensive Crisis:* IV: 20-40 mg/kg/day divided Q 6 hr	Onset: IV: 1-2 hr PO: 4-6 hr M = liver E = kidney $t_{1/2}\beta$ = 2 hr	• Converted to α methylnorepinephrine which inhibits central α-adrenergic receptors • Side effects include sedation, liver dysfunction, positive direct Coomb's test, and rebound hypertension
Methylprednisolone (Solumedrol)	Corticosteroid	*Immunosuppression:* PO = 0.4-1.6 mg/kg/day divided Q 6-12 hr *Status Asthmaticus:* Load: 1-2 mg/kg IV *Maintenance:* 1.6 mg/kg/day divided Q 6 hr IV	Duration: 12-36 hr $t_{1/2}\beta$ = 2-4 hr	• Preferred over prednisone in liver disease or methylation may be impaired • Glucocorticoid activity 5 × hydrocortisone but little mineralocorticoid activity
Metoclopramide (Reglan)	Gastric motility stimulant	*Gastric Dysmotility:* 1-6 yr: 0.1 mg/kg Q 6 hr PO/IV 6-12 yr: 3-9 mg Q 6 hr PO/IV *Antiemetic:* IV: 1-2 mg/kg Q 2-6 hr	Onset: peak PO levels in 40-120 min M = liver E = kidney $t_{1/2}\beta$ = 2-4 hr	• Dopamine antagonist; increases esophageal sphincter tone, stimulates small bowel motility, acts as an anti-emetic • Contraindicated in pheochromocytoma, GI obstruction, and in patients with extrapyramidal symptoms or those receiving phenothiazines, butyrophenones, MAO inhibitors or tricyclic antidepressants • Side effects include sedation, dry mouth, dysphoria, and extrapyramidal reactions • Decrease dose in renal failure

Continued.

Drug	Class	Dose	Pharmacokinetics	Comments
Mezlocillin (Mezlin)	Penicillin	Moderate infection: IV, IM: 50-100 mg/kg/day divided Q 6 hr Severe infection: IV, IM: 200-300 mg/kg/day divided Q 6 hr	E = kidney $t_{1/2}\beta$ = 1.5 hr	• Contains approximately 2 mEq Na per gram • Active against *Klebsiella* and *Pseudomonas*
Metronidazole (Flagyl)	Antibiotic	*Initial Dose*: Neonate = 15 mg/kg IV Child = 15 mg/kg IV *Maintenance:* Neonate = <7 days = 7.5 mg/kg divided Q 12 hr IV >7 days = 7.5 mg/kg divided Q 8 hr IV Children = 7.5 mg/kg divided Q 6 hr IV	M = liver E = kidney	• Effective against anaerobic organisms • Potentiates anticoagulants and causes disulfuram-type reaction with alcohol • Side effects include nausea, diarrhea, leukopenia and vertigo • Infuse over 1 hour • Good CNS penetration
Midazolam (Versed)	Benzodiazepine	*Sedation:* IM = 0.07-0.08 mg/kg IV = 0.03 mg/kg PRN IN = 0.2 mg/kg *Induction of Anesthesia:* IV = 0.2-0.3 mg/kg	Onset: IV: 3-5 min IM: 15-30 min IN: 5-10 min Duration: IV: <2 hr IM: 2 hr M = liver E = kidney $t_{1/2}\beta$ = 1-4 hr	• Water soluble so less pain on IM injection • 2-3 times more potent than diazepam

Morphine Sulfate	Narcotic	*Premedication:* IM: 0.1-0.2 mg/kg *Analgesia:* IV/IM/SC: 0.1-0.2 mg/kg Q 2-4 hr	Onset: IV: 5-10 min IM: 30-60 min SC: 30-90 min Duration: 4-6 hr M = liver E = kidney $t_{1/2}\beta$ = 2-4 hr	• Side effects include orthostatic hypotension due to histamine release, bradycardia, respiratory depression, miosis, nausea, vomiting, and biliary spasm • Useful in treatment of cyanotic spells in Tetralogy of Fallot
Nafcillin (Unipen)	Antibiotic	*Neonate:* 0-7 days: 40 mg/kg/day divided Q 12 hr IV/IM >7 days: 60 mg/kg/day divided Q 6-8 hr IV/IM *Child:* IV: 100-200 mg/kg/day divided Q 4 hr IM: 100-200 mg/kg/day divided Q 12 hr PO: 50-100 mg/kg/day divided Q 6 hr	M = liver (90%) E = kidney	• See Methicillin • Poor PO absorption • Causes more vein irritation than oxacillin

Continued.

Drug	Class	Dose	Pharmacokinetics	Comments
Neomycin	Antibiotic	*Neonate:* PO: 50 mg/kg/day divided Q 6 hr *Infant/child:* PO: 50-100 mg/kg/day divided Q 6 hr *Hepatic Encephalopathy:* Acute: 2.5-7 gm/meter^2/day divided Q 6 hr × 5-7 days PO Chronic: 2.5 gm/meter^2/day divided Q 6 hr PO *Bowel prep:* PO: 90 mg/kg/day divided Q 4 hr × 3 days	E = GI tract (PO drug does not undergo systemic absorption)	• Indicated to decrease intestinal flora prior to intestinal surgery and to manage hepatic encephalopathy
Naloxone (Narcan)	Narcotic antagonist	IV/IM: 5-10 mcg/kg repeat Q 3-5 min PRN	Onset: IV: 1-2 min IM: 2-5 min Duration: IV: 60 min IM: 1-4 hr M = liver E = kidney $t_{1/2}\beta$ = 1-1.5 hr (adult); 3 hr (neonate)	• Side effects include nausea, vomiting, tachycardia, hypertension, and pulmonary edema • May need 100-200 μg/kg for large narcotic overdoses followed by a continuous infusion of 1-2 μg/kg/hr, especially if a long acting narcotic was given

Neostigmine (Prostigmine)	Cholinesterase inhibitor	IV: 0.05-0.07 mg/kg	Onset: 1-5 min Duration: 60 min M = liver (50%) E = kidney (50%) $t_{1/2}\beta$ = 1.3 hr	• Duration more similar to glycopyrrolate than atropine
Nifedipine (Procardia)	Calcium channel blocker	PO: 0.25-0.5 mg/kg Q 6-8 hr SL: 0.25-0.5 mg/kg Q 6-8 hr	Onset: 15-30 min PO M = liver E = liver/kidney $t_{1/2}\beta$ = 4-5 hr	• Side effects include hypotension, tachycardia, and syncope • Little effect on automaticity
Nitroglycerin	Vasodilator	IV: 0.5-20 μg/kg/min continuous infusion	Onset: 1-2 min IV Duration: 10 min IV M = smooth muscle, liver $t_{1/2}\beta$ = 2 min	• Acts primarily on venous capacitance vessels but at higher doses has effects on systemic resistance vessels • Side effects include headache, flushing, hypotension, reflex tachycardia and methemoglobinemia
Norepinephrine (Levophed)	Inotrope	IV: 0.1-1.0 μg/kg/min continuous infusion, increase as required	Onset: rapid IV Duration: 1-2 min IV M = liver, nerve terminals E = kidneys (minimal)	• Natural catecholamine with primarily α activity (some β_1) • Indicated for hypotension due to low SVR states (septic shock) • Side effects include hypertension, reflex bradycardia and skin sloughing after extravasation

Continued.

Drug	Class	Dose	Pharmacokinetics	Comments
Oxacillin (Prostaphlin)	Antibiotic	Neonate: IV or IM >7 days: 100-200 mg/kg/day divided Q 8 hr *Child:* PO PO: 50-100 mg/kg/day divided Q 6 hr	E = kidney, liver $t_{1/2}\beta$ = 1 hour	• Good staphlococcal coverage • Hepatitis can occur with high doses • Well-absorbed PO
Pancuronium (Pavulon)	Nondepolarizing muscle relaxant	*Intubation:* IV: 0.07-0.1 mg/kg *Maintenance:* IV: 0.05 mg/kg	Onset: 1-3 min Duration: 35-55 min M = liver (minimal) E = kidney 80% liver 20% $t_{1/2}\beta$ = 1-2 hr	• Neonates and infants are more sensitive to drug effects • Tachycardia occurs and is due to blockade of cardiac muscarinic receptors and vagolysis
Penicillin G	Antibiotic	*Neonate:* IV or IM 0-7 days: 50-100,000 unit/kg/day divided Q 12 hr >7 days: 100-250,000 unit/kg/day divided Q 8 hr *Child:* IV/IM: 25-500,000 unit/kg/day divided Q 4-6 hr PO: 40-80,000 unit/kg/day divided Q 6 hr (125 mg = 200,000 u for all PCN)	E = kidney $t_{1/2}\beta$ = 1 hr	• Na^+ salt: 1 million units contains 1.68 mEq Na^+ • K^+ salt: 1 million units contains 1.68 mEq K^+ • Side effects include skin rash, anaphylaxis, and serum sickness

Pentobarbital (Nembutal)	Barbiturate	*Premedication:* IM/PO: 3-5 mg/kg, maximum 100 mg	Onset: IM: 10-30 min PO: 30-60 min M = liver E = kidney $t_{1/2}\beta$ = 20-50 hr	• Paradoxical excitation may occur in presence of pain • IM injection painful • Avoid in porphyria
Phenobarbital (Luminal)	Barbiturate	*Sedation:* IM: 2-3 mg/kg divided Q 8 hr PO: 2-3 mg/kg divided Q 8 hr *Status Epilepticus:* IV: 15-25 mg/kg no faster than 30 mg/min *Maintenance:* PO: 4-6 mg/kg/day divided Q 12 hr	Onset: 2-3 hr PO M = liver microsomes E = kidney $t_{1/2}\beta$ = 96 hr	• Indicated for grand mal and focal epilepsy as well as for prophylaxis against the recurrence of febrile seizures • Paradoxical reaction may occur in children resulting in agitation and hyperactivity • Contraindicated in porphyria • Stimulates hepatic microsomes • Therapeutic levels 10-20 μg/ml
Phenylephrine (Neosynephrine)	Inotrope	IV = 0.1-1 μg/kg/min continuous infusion or 10 μg/kg IV bolus PRN	Onset: rapid IV Duration: IV: 5-20 min M = liver intestine	• Synthetic catecholamine that acts primarily on α_1 receptors to increase SVR • May cause carotid reflex-mediated bradycardia • Useful in treatment of cyanotic spells in Tetralogy of Fallot

Continued.

Drug	Class	Dose	Pharmacokinetics	Comments
Phenytoin (Dilantin)	Anticonvulsant	*Status Epilepticus:* IV: 15-25 mg/kg no faster than 50 mg/min *Maintenance:* 4-7 mg/kg/day divided Q 12-24 hr IV/PO *Antiarrhythmic:* IV: 2-4 mg/kg over 5 min PO: 2-5 mg/kg/day	Onset: IV: 3-5 min PO: slow M = 98% liver (metabolites inactive) E = kidney $t_{1/2}\beta$ = 7-42 hr	• Indicated for control of all types of seizure disorders (except petit mal) as well as ventricular and digitalis-induced dysrhythmias • Side effects include nystagmus, ataxia, diplopia, vertigo, allergic reactions, peripheral neuropathy, and gingival hyperplasia • Therapeutic drug levels 10-20 μg/ml • Above plasma levels of 10 μg/ml elimination follows zero-order kinetics • 90% protein bound; increased free level in patients with low albumin

Potassium Iodide	Antithyroid preparation	*Thyrotoxicosis:* Child: 200-300 mg/day PO divided Q 8-12 hr	E = kidney	• Indicated for preoperative preparation before thyroidectomy for hyperthyroidism as well as in treatment of thyrotoxicosis • Inhibits thyroid hormone formation and release • Effects can be seen in 24 hr • Side effects include angioedema, laryngeal edema, nausea, vomiting, rash, rhinitis • SSKI contains 1 gm of KI in 1 ml
Prednisone	Corticosteroid	*Physiologic Replacement:* PO = 4-5 mg/m^2/day divided Q 12 hr *Stress Dose:* 2-4 × physiologic replacement *Asthma:* Acute: 0.5-1.0 mg/kg/day PO up 20-40 mg/day × 3-5 days *Antiinflammatory:* 0.5-2 mg/kg/day PO divided Q 6-12 hr	Duration = 18-36 hr $t_{1/2}\beta$ = 1-1.5 hr	• Glucocorticoid activity 4 × hydrocortisone; slightly less mineralocorticoid activity than hydrocortisone • Appropriate for sole replacement in adrenal insufficiency

Continued.

Drug	Class	Dose	Pharmacokinetics	Comments
Procainamide (Pronestyl)	Antiarrhythmic	*Loading Dose:* IV: 2-5 mg/kg over 30 min *Maintenance:* IV: 20-80 μg/kg/min continuous infusion Maximum dose = 50-60 mg/kg/day	Onset: IV: <5 min M = liver, plasma E = kidney $t_{1/2}\beta$ = 2.5-5 hr (active metabolites 6 hr)	• Indicated for ventricular and atrial dysrhythmias • Contraindicated in myasthenia gravis and complete heart block • Hepatic acetylation yields NAPA, an active metabolite that is renally excreted • Side effects include hypotension, lupus-like syndrome, asystole and thrombocytopenia • Therapeutic levels 4-12 μg/ml and likelihood of toxicity increases at >8 μg/ml and is indicated by QRS >0.2 msec
Prochlorperazine (Compazine)	Phenothiazine	PO: 0.4 mg/kg/day divided Q 6-8 hr PR: 0.4 mg/kg/day divided Q 6-8 hr IM: 0.2 mg/kg/day divided Q 6-8 hr	Onset: PO: 30-40 min IM: 10-20 min PR: 60 min Duration: IM/PR: 3-4 hr M = liver E = kidney $t_{1/2}\beta$ = 10-20 hrs	• Indicated for postoperative nausea and vomiting • Side effects and cautions regarding use are similar to chlorpromazine • Do not use in children <10 kg or under 2 years

Promethazine (Phenergan)	Antihistamine	*Sedation:* IM: 0.5-1 mg/kg Q 6 hr PRN *Antiemetic:* IM/PO/PR: 0.25-0.5 mg/kg Q 4-6 PRN *Antihistamine:* PO = 0.1 mg/kg Q 6 hr	Onset: IV: 3-5 min IM/PO: 20 min M = liver E = kidney, liver $t_{1/2}\beta$ = 4.4-7 hr	• Same indications as for diphenhydramine • Low incidence of extrapyramidal reactions
Propranolol (Inderal)	Beta blocker	*Arrhythmias:* IV: 0.01-0.1 mg/kg slow IV push may repeat Q 5-10 min PRN *Maintenance:* PO: 0.5-4 mg/kg/day divided Q 6-8 hr Maximum daily dose 60 mg *Hypertension:* PO: 0.5-1.0 mg/kg/day divided Q 6-12 hr Maximum daily dose 2 mg/kg/day *Tetralogy Spells:* IV: 0.15-0.25 mg/kg slowly may repeat × 1 after 15 min PO: 1-2 mg/kg divided Q 6 hr	Onset: IV: 2 min PO: 20 min M = liver E = kidney $t_{1/2}\beta$ = 2-6 hr	• Non-selective β-blocker • Contraindicted in asthma and advanced heart block • Use cautiously in CHF, diabetes mellitus and with hepatic and renal disease • Extensive hepatic first pass effect • 4-OH propranolol metabolite is active

Continued.

Drug	Class	Dose	Pharmacokinetics	Comments
Propylthiouracil (PTU)	Antithyroid preparation	*Child:* 0-10 yrs: 50-150 mg/day PO divided Q 8 hr >10 yrs: 150-300 mg/day PO divided Q 8 hr Maintenance: 30-50% initial daily dose divided Q 8 hr	Onset: Days to weeks Duration: 2-3 hrs E = kidney $t_{1/2}\beta$ = 2 hr	• Blocks thyroid hormone synthesis as well as peripheral conversion of T4 to T3 • 100 mg PTU = 10 mg methimazole • *Not* available in parenteral form • Side effects rare and include rash and granulocytopenia
Protamine Sulfate	Heparin antagonist	IV = According to heparin dose-response curve or give 1-1.3 mg for every 100 units of heparin given in previous 2 hrs	Onset: 5 min Duration: 2 hr	• Binds with heparin to form an inactive complex • Can cause myocardial depression and peripheral vasodilation with resultant sudden hypotension or bradycardia • Allergic reactions are more common in patients with fish allergy and those on protamine zinc insulin (NPH)
Pyridostigmine (Regonal, Mestinon)	Cholinesterase inhibitor	IV: 0.25 mg/kg	Onset: 2-5 min Duration: 90 min M = liver (30%) E = kidney (70%) $t_{1/2}\beta$ = 1.9 hr	• See neostigmine

Ranitidine (Zantac)	H_2 receptor antagonist	PO: 2-4 mg/kg/day divided Q 12 hr IV: 1-2 mg/kg/day divided Q 6-8 hr	Onset: PO: 30-60 min Duration: IV/PO: 8-12 hr M = liver E = kidney (50% unchanged) $t_{1/2}\beta$ = 2-3 hr	• Fewer androgenic effects than cimetidine
Ribavirin (Virazole)	Antiviral	*Aerosol:* Dilute 6 gm vial in 300 ml (20 mg/ml) Administer by aerosol 12-18 hrs/day × 3-7 days		• Treatment for severe lower respiratory RSV (respiratory syncytial virus) infection • Particles may obstruct ventilator
Scopolamine	Anticholinergic	IV: 5-10 μg/kg IM: 10 μg/kg	Onset: Rapid IV E = kidney	• Indicated for preoperative sedation and antisialagogue activity • Crosses BBB
Secobarbital (Seconal)	Barbiturate	*Premedication:* IM/PO: 3-5 mg/kg	Onset: IM: 7-10 min PO: 15-30 min M = liver E = kidney $t_{1/2}\beta$ = 20-28 hr	• See pentobarbital

Continued.

Drug	Class	Dose	Pharmacokinetics	Comments
Sodium Nitroprusside (Nipride)*	Vasodilator	IV: 0.5-10 μg/kg/min continuous infusion	Onset: rapid IV Duration: 1-10 min IV M = RBC and liver (thiocyanate) E = kidney	• Smooth muscle dilator affecting primarily resistance vessels • Absolutely contraindicated in Leber's hereditary optic atrophy and tobacco amblyopia, avoid with B_{12} deficiency and severe liver or renal disease • Side effects include hypotension, reflex tachycardia, and cyanide toxicity
Spironolactone (Aldactone)	Diuretic	PO: 1-3 mg/kg/day divided Q 6-12 hr	E = kidney	• Competitive aldosterone antagonist • May potentiate ganglionic blocking agents and other antihypertensives • Side effects include hyperkalemia, nausea and vomiting
Streptomycin	Antibiotic	*Neonate:* IM: 20-30 mg/kg/day divided Q 12 hr × up to 10 days *Child:* IM: 20-40 mg/kg/day divided Q 8 hr × up to 10 days *Tuberculosis:* IM: 20-50 mg/kg × 1 dose (use higher dose for Tb meningitis)	M = liver E = kidney $t_{1/2}\beta$ = 2-3 hr	• See amikacin • Need to follow with auditory tests • Commonly used with other antibiotics for synergistic action against bacterial endocarditis, tularemia, and plague • Rarely cause nephrotoxicity

*See page 606 for infusion preparation.

Succinylcholine (Anectine)	Depolarizing muscle relaxant	IV: 1-2 mg/kg IM: 4-5 mg/kg	Onset: IV: 30-60 sec IM: 2-3 min Duration: IV: 10-15 min IM: 10-30 min M = plasma pseudocholinesterase E = kidney	• Use upper dose limit in infants • Fasciculations rare in children less than 3 yrs old • Pretreat with atropine 0.01 mg/kg IV or 0.02 mg/kg IM to prevent vagally-mediated bradycardia • Prolonged action with severe liver disease, hypothermia, treatment with antibiotics (aminoglycosides), hypothermia, hyperkalemia, and pseudocholinesterase deficiency
Terbutaline (Brethine)	Bronchodilator	PO: $<$12 yrs: 0.05 mg/kg Q 8 hr up to 0.3 mg/kg/day $>$12 yrs: 2.5 mg Q 8 hr up to 5 mg Q 8 hr SC: $<$12 yrs: 0.005-0.01 mg/kg Q 15-20 min × 2 maximum dose of 0.25 mg $>$12 yrs: 0.25 mg Q 15-30 min do not exceed 0.5 mg/4 hr	Peak Effect: PO: 60 min SC: 15-30 min Duration: PO: 8 hr SC: 4-6 hr	• See albuterol • Less β_2 selectivity with SC administration

Continued.

Drug	Class	Dose	Pharmacokinetics	Comments
Tetracaine (Pontocaine)	Ester local anesthetic	Maximum safe dose: 1.5 mg/kg	M = plasma cholinesterase E = kidney Duration: 60-180 min	• PABA metabolite may be an antigen responsible for future allergic reactions
Tetracycline	Antibiotic	*Child:* PO: 25-50 mg/kg/day divided Q 6 hr IM: 15-25 mg/kg/day divided 8-12 hr (not to exceed 250 mg/dose)	M = liver E = biliary, kidney $t_{1/2}\beta$ = 6-9 hr	• IV administration scleroses veins • Broad spectrum of activity against gram positive and negative organisms • Not recommended in children <8 yrs due to tooth staining and impaired bone growth • May cause nausea and vomiting • May cause increased ICP in infants • Outdated drug has been associated with a form of Fanconi's anemia
Thiopental Sodium (Pentothal)	Barbiturate	*Induction:* IV: 3-5 mg/kg PR: 20-30 mg/kg	Onset: rapid IV M = liver E = kidney $t_{1/2}\beta$ = 5-10 hr	• Intraarterial injection can cause necrosis • Avoid in porphyria • Side effects include anaphylactic/anaphylactoid reactions and histamine release

Ticarcillin (Ticar)	Penicillin	Moderate infection: IV/IM 50-100 mg/kg/day divided Q 6 hr Severe infection: IV/IM: 200-300 mg/kg/day divided Q 6 hr	E = kidney $t_{1/2}\beta$ = 1.5 hr	• Contains >5 mEq Na^+ per gram • Effective against *Pseudomonas*
Tobramycin (Nebcin)	Antibiotic	*Neonate:* See gentamycin *Children:* IV/IM: 7.5 mg/kg/day divided Q 8 hr	M = liver (40%) E = kidney $t_{1/2}\beta$ = 2-3 hr	• See amikacin
Valproic acid (Depakene, Depakote)	Anticonvulsant	PO = 10-15 mg/kg/day divided Q 12 hr Increase by 5-10 mg/kg/day Q week Maximum dose = 60 mg/kg/day	Onset: peak PO levels in 1-4 hr M = 70% liver (inactive metabolites) $t_{1/2}\beta$ = 12 hr	• Indicated in petit mal epilepsy • Side effects include impairment of platelet aggregation, false-positive urine ketone test, hepatotoxicity, nausea and vomiting • Results in increased plasma levels of phenytoin, diazepam, and phenobarbital • Therapeutic levels 50-100 mg/l

Continued.

Drug	Class	Dose	Pharmacokinetics	Comments
Vancomycin (Vancocin)	Antibiotic	*Neonate:* Under 1000 gm: <7 days: 10 mg/kg Q 24 hr IV >7 days: 10 mg/kg Q 18 hr IV 1000-2000 gm <7 days: 10 mg/kg Q 18 hr IV >7 days: 10 mg/kg Q 12 hr IV Greater than 2000 gm: <7 days: 10 mg/kg Q 12 hr IV >7 days: 10 mg/kg Q 8 hr IV *Infant/child:* IV: 30 mg/kg/day Q 8 hr (45 mg/kg for CNS infections)	E = kidney (90%) $t_{1/2}\beta$ = 6 hours	• Side effects include ototoxicity and nephrotoxicity • Therapeutic levels: 10-25 mg/l • Drug induced rashes and hypotension caused by histamine release; must be given slowly over 1 hour • Must adjust dose in renal insufficiency
Vasopressin (Pitressin)	Posterior pituitary hormone	*Aqueous:* 0.5-3 ml/day divided Q 8 hr SC (ampule contains 20 u/ml) *Tannate in Oil:* 0.25 ml Q 1-3 day IM/SC PRN (ampule contains 5 u/ml) *Nose Drops:* 1-2 drops in each nostril, Q 4-6 hr PRN	Duration: Tannate: 48-96 hrs SC/IM Aqueous: 2-8 hrs SC/IM M = liver/kidney E = kidney $t_{1/2}\beta$ = 10-20 min	• Indicated for treatment of central diabetes insipidus • Side effects include nausea, vomiting, abdominal pain, tremor, sweating, urticaria, and anaphylaxis • Physiologic half-life does not correlate with $t_{1/2}\beta$

Vecuronium (Norcuron)	Nondepolarizing muscle relaxant	*Intubation:* IV: 0.05-0.1 mg/kg	Onset: Infant—1.5 min Child—2.4 min Duration: Infant—73 min Child—35 min M = liver (80%) E = kidney (20%)	• $t_{1/2}\beta$ is prolonged by liver failure when dose exceeds 0.2 mg/kg • Devoid of circulatory effects except when given with high-dose narcotics, when bradycardia is sometimes seen • Less renal excretion than pancuronium
Verapamil (Isoptin/Calan)	Calcium channel blocker	IV: 0.1-0.3 mg/kg not to exceed 5 mg	Onset: IV: 1-10 min PO: 15-30 min Duration: 6 hr M = liver E = liver/kidney $t_{1/2}\beta$ = 5-7 hr	• Indicated for treatment of SVT • Contraindicated in 2nd or 3rd degree heart block, CHF, hypotension, and right-to-left shunt • Use in infants <1 yr can result in apnea, bradycardia, and hypotension
Vidarabine (Ara-A)	Antiviral	*HSV encephalitis/neonatal HSV infection:* IV: 15 mg/kg/day over 12 hr × 10 days	E = kidney	• Poorly soluble in water so must be diluted in large volumes

B

PEDIATRIC RESUSCITATION DRUG DOSAGES

Drug	Dose (mg/kg)	Stock solution	Preparation
*†Atropine	0.01-0.02	Many, commonly: 0.4 mg/ml, 0.5 mg/ml	*Undiluted:* **0.4 mg/ml stock solution:** 0.025 ml/kg = 0.01 mg/kg 0.05 ml/kg = 0.02 mg/kg **0.5 mg/ml stock solution:** .02 ml/kg = 0.01 mg/kg .04 ml/kg = 0.01 mg/kg Minimum dose = 0.1 mg Maximum dose = 1.0 mg
†Calcium Chloride	10-30	10% solution (100 mg/ml)	*Undiluted:* 0.1 ml/kg = 10 mg/kg
Calcium Gluconate	100	10% solution (100 mg/ml)	*Undiluted:* 1 ml/kg = 100 mg/kg
*†Epinephrine	0.01 (0.05 for cardiac arrest)	1:1000 (1 mg/ml)	*Diluted* 1:10 gives: 1:10,000 solution = 0.1 mg/ml 0.1 ml/kg = 0.01 mg/kg

Drug	Dose (mg/kg)	Stock solution	Preparation
*†Lidocaine	1	4% solution (40 mg/ml)	*Diluted:* 2 ml of 4% lidocaine + 6 ml diluent = 1% solution (10 mg/ml) 0.1 ml/kg = 1 mg/kg
*Naloxone	0.01-0.02	0.4 mg/ml Neonatal = 0.02 mg/ml	*Undiluted* (neonatal): 0.5-1.0 ml/kg = 0.01-0.02 mg/kg 0.4 mg/ml DILUTED 1:4 gives 0.1 mg/ml, then .01 ml/mg = .01 mg/kg
†Phenylephrine	0.01	1% solution (10 mg/ml)	*Diluted* 1:10 twice to a 0.01% solution (0.1 mg/ml) 0.1 ml/kg = 0.01 mg/kg
Sodium Bicarbonate	1 mEq/kg	1 mEq/ml	*Undiluted:* 1 ml/kg = 1 mEq/kg Dilute: 1:1 OR 1:2 for infants and neonates
Tolazoline (Priscoline)	1 followed by infusion	25 mg/ml	*Diluted:* 1:10 gives: 2.5 mg/ml 0.4 ml/kg = 1 mg/kg

*Drugs can be given via endotracheal tube.
†Because of small volumes these drugs should be administered with a Tb syringe in infants <10kg.

C

DRUG INFUSIONS FOR PEDIATRIC RESUSCITATION

Drug	Dose (μg/kg/min)	Undiluted concentration (mg/ml)	Preparation (mg in diluent to equal 100 ml total volume)	Infusion rate
Calcium Gluconate	200-500 mg/kg/day	100 mg/ml	—	Dilute total dose in desired volume and infuse over 24 hr
Dopamine	1-15	40	A/ (wt in kg) × 6 or B/ 30 mg or C/ Alternative: 150 mg (3.75 ml) in 250 ml	A/ 1 ml/hr = 1 μg/kg/min B/ 1 ml/kg/hr = 5 μg/kg/min or wt in kg = ml/hr = 5 μg/kg/min C/ 1 ml/kg/hr = 10 μg/kg/min or wt in kg = ml/hr = 10 μg/kg/min

Drug	Dose (μg/kg/min)	Undiluted concentration (mg/ml)	Preparation (mg in diluent to equal 100 ml total volume)	Infusion rate
Dobutamine	1-15	50	Same as dopamine A	Same as dopamine A
Sodium nitroprusside	1-10	25	Same as dopamine A	Same as dopamine A (do not mix with saline)
Epinephrine	0.1-1	1	(wt in kg) × 0.6	1 ml/hr = 0.1 μg/kg/min
Isoproterenol	0.1-1	0.2	Same as epinephrine	Same as epinephrine
Lidocaine	20 (10-50)	40	120 (3 ml)	1 ml/kg/hr = 20 μg/kg/min
Tolazine	1	25	100 (4 ml)	1 ml/kg/hr = 1 mg/kg/hr (begin after 1 mg/kg IV loading dose)
Trimethaphan (Arfonad)	10-200	50	60 mg	1 ml/kg/hr = 10 μg/kg/min
PGE-1	0.01-1	0.5	0.06 (0.12 ml)	1 ml/kg/hr = 0.01 μg/kg/min

D

ANTIBIOTIC PROPHYLAXIS AGAINST BACTERIAL ENDOCARDITIS

CARDIAC CONDITIONS FOR WHICH PROPHYLAXIS IS RECOMMENDED:

Prosthetic heart valves (including bioprosthetics)
Previous history of endocarditis
Most congenital heart disease
Idiopathic hypertrophic subaortic stenosis
Surgically constructed systemic-pulmonary shunts
Mitral valve prolapse with mitral insuficiency
Permanent endocardial pacemaker electrode
Rheumatic and other valvular dysfunction

CARDIAC CONDITIONS FOR WHICH PROPHYLAXIS IS NOT RECOMMENDED:

Isolated secundum atrial septal defect (ASD)
Secundum ASD repaired WITHOUT a patch more than six months earlier
Patent ductus arteriosus ligated and divided more than six months earlier
Permanent epicardial pacemaker electrode

PROCEDURES FOR WHICH PROPHYLAXIS IS INDICATED:

All dental procedures likely to induce gingival bleeding
Tonsillectomy and/or adenoidectomy
Surgical procedure involving respiratory mucosa
Bronchoscopy
Incision and drainage of infected tissue
Most GI and GU procedures especially in high risk, except

- Percutaneous liver biopsy
- Upper GI endoscopy *without* biopsy
- Proctosigmoidoscopy *without* biopsy
- Straight catheterization of bladder

In high risk patients or if infection is suspected, give prophalactic antibiotics even in these lower risk procedures

DRUG REGIMENS FOR CARDIAC PROPHYLAXIS:

Dental/respiratory tract procedures:

1. Standard regimen
   Penicillin V, 1.0 g PO 1 hour before procedure, then 500 mg (double doses if >27 kg) 6 hours after initial dose
2. Unable to take oral medication
   Aqueous Penicillin G 50,000 units/kg (maximum 2 million units) IM/IV 30-60 min before procedure, and 25,000 units/kg (maximum 1 million units) 6 hours after initial dose
3. Penicillin allergic
   Erythromycin 20 mg/kg (maximum 1.0 g) PO 1 hour before procedure, then 10 mg/kg (maximum 500 mg) 6 hours after initial dose
   OR
   Vancomycin 20 mg/kg (maximum 1.0 g) IV slowly over 1 hour before procedure (only 1 dose necessary)
4. Maximum protection (prosthetic valves)
   Ampicillin 50 mg/kg (maximum 2.0 g) IM/IV *plus*
   Gentamycin 2 mg/kg IM/IV 30 minutes before procedure
   THEN
   Penicillin V 500 mg PO 6 hours after initial dose (1.0 g if >27 kg) or repeat the parenteral regimen 8 hours after the initial dose

Gastrointestinal or genitourinary procedures:

1. Standard regimen
   Amoxicillin 50 mg/kg (maximum 2.0 g) IV/IM *plus*
   Gentamycin 2 mg/kg IV/IM 30-60 minutes before procedure; may repeat entire regimen 8 hours after initial dose
2. Minor or repetitive procedures in low risk patients
   Amoxicillin 50 mg/kg (maximum 3.0 g) PO 1 hour before procedure and 25 mg/kg (maximum 1.5 g) PO 6 hours after initial dose
3. Penicillin allergic
   Vancomycin 20 mg/kg IV slowly over 1 hour *plus*
   Gentamycin 2 mg/kg IM/IV 1 hour before procedure
   May repeat entire regimen once 8-12 hours after initial dose

APPENDIX
BIBLIOGRAPHY

American Hospital Formulary Service: American Hospital Formulary, Bethesda, Md, 1989, American Society of Hopsital Pharmacists.

Behrman RE and Vaughan VC III: Nelson textbook of pediatrics, ed 13, Boston, 1987, Little Brown.

Benitz WE and Tatro DS: The pediatric drug handbook, ed 2, Chicago, 1988, Year Book Medical Publishers, Inc.

Committee on Rheumatic Fever and Infective Endocarditis, American Heart Association: Circulation 70:1123a-1127a, 1984.

Drug facts and comparisons, St Louis, 1988, JB Lippincott Co.

Gilman A et al: The pharmacological basis of therapeutics, ed 8, New York, 1990, Pergamon Press.

Greene MG, editor: The Harriet Lane handbook, ed 12, Chicago, 1990, Mosby–Year Book.

Physicians' desk reference, ed 44, Oradell, NJ, 1990, Medical Economics Co.

Stoelting RK: Pharmacology and physiology in anesthetic practice, Philadelphia, 1987, JB Lippincott.

Ziai M: Pediatrics, ed 3, Boston, 1984, Little Brown.

CREDITS

The following poems were excerpted from Daniel M, editor: A child's treasury of poems, New York, 1986, Dial Books for Young Readers: MacDonald, G: "Where did you come from baby dear?"; Anon: "The owl"; Rosetti, CG: "The swallow"; Stevenson, RL: "Good and bad children"; and Anon: "Star light, star bright".

Dear Little Mumps Child by Marguerite Rush Lerner, M.D., copyright 1960 by Lerner Publications Company, 241 First Avenue North, Minneapolis, MN 55401. Used by permission of the publisher.

Hunches in Bunches by Dr. Seuss. Copyright © 1982 by Theodor S. Geisel and Audrey S. Geisel. Reprinted by permission of Random House, Inc.

Now We Are Six, by A.A. Milne. Used by permission of the Canadian Publishers, McClelland & Stewart, Toronto.

Michael Gets the Measles by Marguerite Rush Lerner, M.D., copyright 1960 by Lerner Publications Company, 241 First Avenue North, Minneapolis, MN 55401. Used by permission of the publisher.

White Rabbit, Lyrics and music by Grace Slick. Copyright 1967, Irving Music, Inc. All rights reserved. International Copyright Secured.

INDEX